the
kind
diet

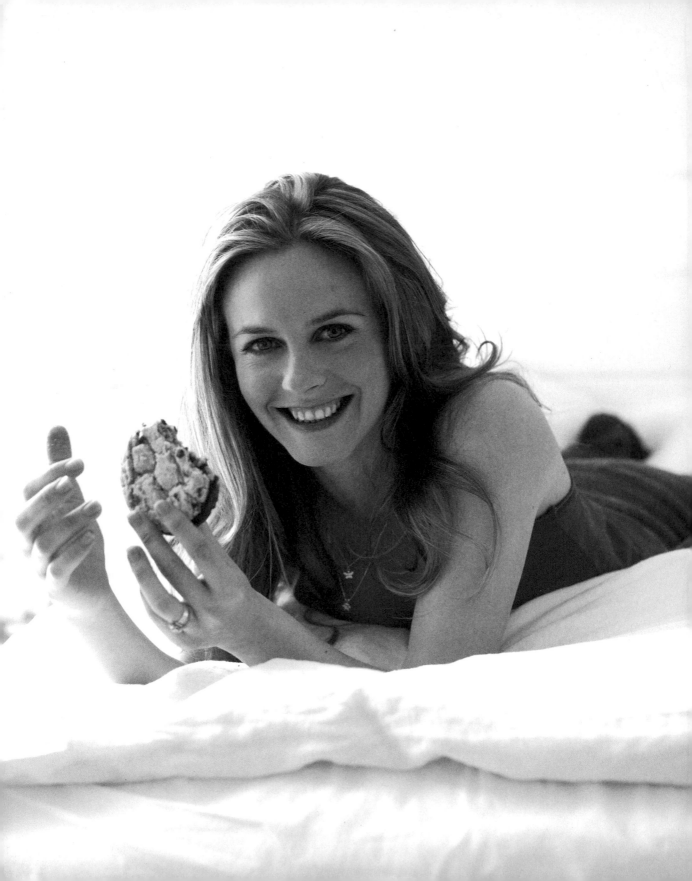

the
kind
diet

A Simple Guide to Feeling Great,
Losing Weight, and Saving the Planet

alicia silverstone

photographs by victoria pearson

RODALE

© 2009 by Alicia Silverstone
First published in hardcover by Rodale Inc. in 2009
This paperback edition published in 2011

Photographs copyright © 2009 by Victoria Pearson
Additional photo credits: Page 9, bottom, Jeremy and Claire Weiss; page 19, Connie Pugh © Farm Sanctuary, Inc.; page 29, Natalie Bowman © Farm Sanctuary, Inc.; page 30, Natalie Bowman © Farm Sanctuary, Inc.; page 32, © Randall Perez Photography; page 35, © Animal Acres; page 67, © Shawn Laksmi; page 77, Jeremy and Claire Weiss; page 88, bottom, 2nd from left, © Lisa Siskind; page 124, © Michael Tran/Filmmagic.com; page 129, © Farm Sanctuary, Inc.
"Arame Turnovers," "Hiziki-Tofu Croquettes," "Rice Pilaf with Caramelized Onions" from *Christina Cooks* by Christina Pirello, © 2004 by Christina Pirello. Used by permission of Berkley Publishing Group, a division of Penguin Group (USA) Inc.
"Black-Eyed Pea Croquettes" from *The Hip Chick's Guide to Macrobiotics* by Jessica Porter, © 2004 by Jessica Porter. Used by permission of Avery Publishing, an imprint of Penguin Group (USA) Inc.
"Pecan-Crusted Seitan," "Seitan Piccata with White Wine and Capers" from *The Candle Cafe Cookbook* by Joy Pierson and Bart Potenza with Barbara Scott-Goodman, © 2003 by Joy Pierson and Bart Potenza. Used by permission of Three Rivers Press, a division of Random House, Inc.

Preface © 2009 by Paul McCartney
Foreword © 2009 by Neal Barnard, MD

Rodale books may be purchased for business or promotional use or for special sales. For information, please write to: Special Markets Department, Rodale Inc., 733 Third Avenue, New York, NY 10017

Printed in the United States of America
Printed with inks containing soy and/or vegetable oils.
Printed on 100% Recycled Post Consumer Waste paper.
Book design by Wayne Wolf/Blue Cup Creative

Library of Congress Cataloging-in-Publication Data is on file with the publisher.

ISBN-10 1–60961–135–7
ISBN-13 978–1–60961–135–4

Distributed to the trade by Macmillan

2   4   6   8   10   9   7   5   3   1   paperback

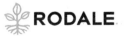

RODALE

We inspire and enable people to improve their lives and the world around them.
www.rodalebooks.com

For Sampson,
for all animals who suffer needlessly,
and
for those who do their best to tread lightly on the earth

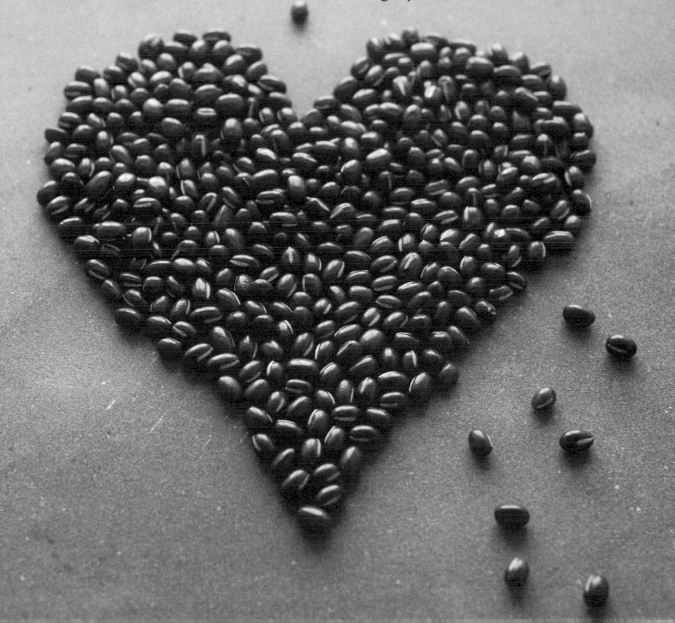

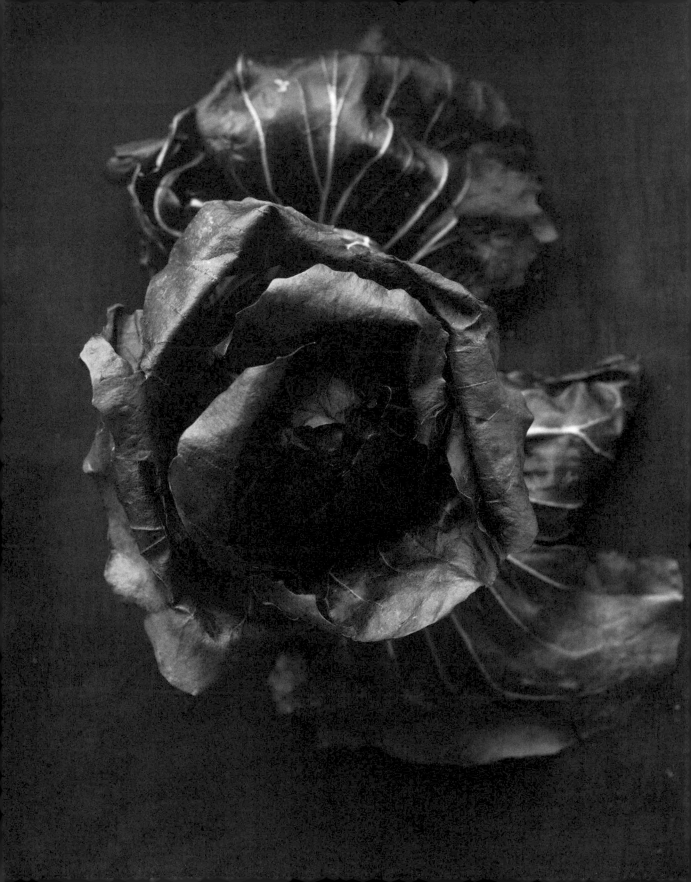

Preface

Having been vegetarian now for many years, I am always pleased when someone spreads the good word. Originally, I became a vegetarian when my wife, Linda, and myself were eating leg of lamb and, at the same time, watching a group of very cute baby lambs gamboling in the field. We made the connection, and so our original reason was that of compassion. Through the years, we have learned of the health benefits of a veggie diet and most recently have become aware of the extreme danger the livestock industry poses to the environment. When the United Nations (not a vegetarian group!) issued its report in 2006 saying that the livestock industry was responsible for more damage to the environment than all of the transport industry put together, I was glad to see a further reason for going veggie being made public. I believe that more and more people are looking at ways to change their diet and lifestyles, and I believe Alicia's book will be very helpful to them and all of us.

Paul McCartney

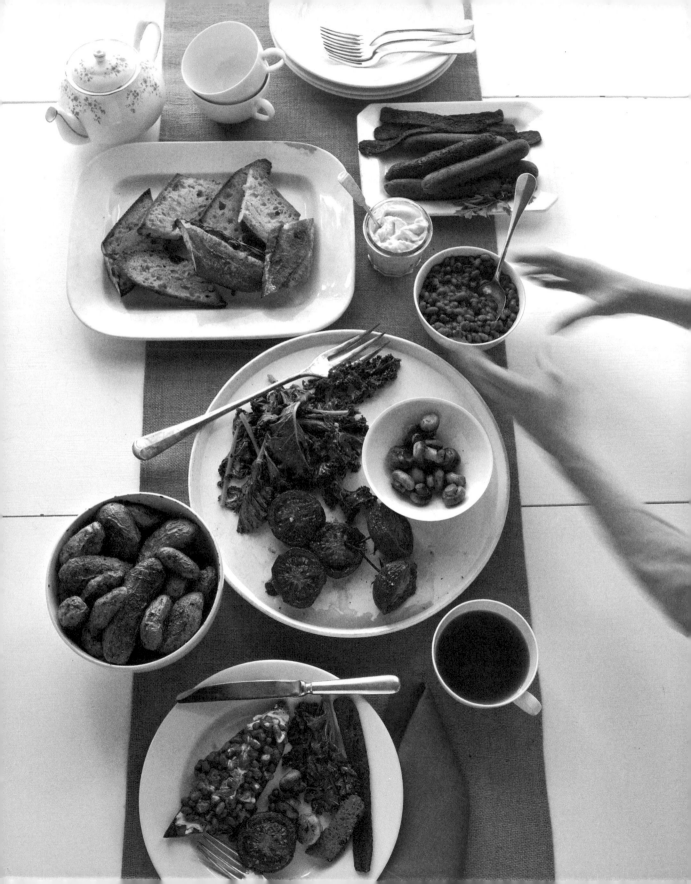

Contents

Foreword
by Neal Barnard, MD

Can this book really change the way you look, feel, and think about the world around you? Can it give you the tools to make serious changes—changes that will impact not only your own health, but that of the planet and every being that lives on it? Strong claims for something as simple as a diet plan, but it's true. If you follow the path that Alicia Silverstone has laid out in this thoughtful, empowering book, you will discover a new way of thinking about your body and the foods that nourish it. If you're aiming to trim away weight, regain your energy, and feel like yourself again, you'll find the answers here. If you are dealing with more serious health concerns, this guide will revolutionize your health.

In our modern culture, there is a strange disconnect between how we eat and how we feel. In my practice, I've always maintained the belief that food can and should be the first line of defense against disease and have seen my patients respond powerfully to a change in their diet, whether reducing the incidence of diseases like diabetes or reversing weight gain, which can be a contributing factor to so many health concerns. Of course, I am not alone in these beliefs; researchers have been putting foods to the test for many years, and their findings show that the results of an improved diet can be dramatic, even life-changing. Dr. Dean Ornish showed that simple changes in diet and lifestyle can reverse heart disease.

If weight loss is your goal, you no longer need to torture yourself with skimpy portions and a load of guilt if you happen to stray. As my own research team has proven, not only are certain foods naturally modest in calories, they also increase your metabolism—your calorie-burning speed—after every meal, allowing you to liberate some of their calories as body heat rather than storing them as body fat. The result is gentle, continuing weight loss.

After weighing the pros and cons of many diets, from low fat to high protein and everything in between, I have come to believe a plant-based diet like the one described in this book helps my patients achieve their health goals most effectively. Funded by the U.S. government's National

Institutes of Health, our research team showed that a low-fat vegan diet helps people with diabetes lower their blood sugars and reduce or even eliminate their need for medications. We found that a similar menu adjustment helps young women eliminate painful cramps and PMS. The secret is that these healthful foods gently rebalance the hormones that contribute to menstrual symptoms.

A change in diet will make you look healthier, too. Harvard researchers found that a plant-based menu is very kind to your skin, while dairy-laden, sugary diets have the opposite effect. You will also feel healthier, as headaches and joint pains melt away.

How can changing what you eat solve so many problems? Think of it like changing the fuel you put in your car. If your car is not accelerating well, it stalls a lot, the ride is rough, and the exhaust looks terrible, you might take a look through your owner's manual. And suddenly, you discover that your car actually does not take the diesel fuel you've been using; it takes unleaded. You switch to the right fuel, and suddenly, everything starts to get better. The acceleration improves, the ride evens out, and the exhaust clears up. Your body is the same way. The wrong foods slow you down. They interfere with your digestion, your blood circulation, your energy, and every other aspect of your body. With the right fuel, your whole body works better.

But how do you start? Some people like to dive right into a new way of eating. Others prefer to wade in gradually, and still others want to stick their toe into the pool and test the waters for a while. This book allows you to fit the menu to your personality and needs. Whether you would like to jump straight into a healthy menu, flirt with healthful foods for a bit, or go for the maximal benefit from a superhero approach, they are all here for you. Whichever way you choose, you'll find the process truly eye-opening.

One other thing: This is more than a way of eating; it is also a way of living. Our food choices affect the earth in ways that many of us tend not to think about. And needless to say, we also affect animals if we are putting them on the stove. So if you have ever wanted to learn about a way of eating that is kind to the earth and to animals, you've found it.

Alicia Silverstone knows about all these things as one who has not only studied for many years how foods affect the body, but as one who has lived it. In her uplifting, friendly, and honest way, Alicia explains how she did it and shows exactly how you can do the same. These wise words and delicious recipes will forever change the way you think about food.

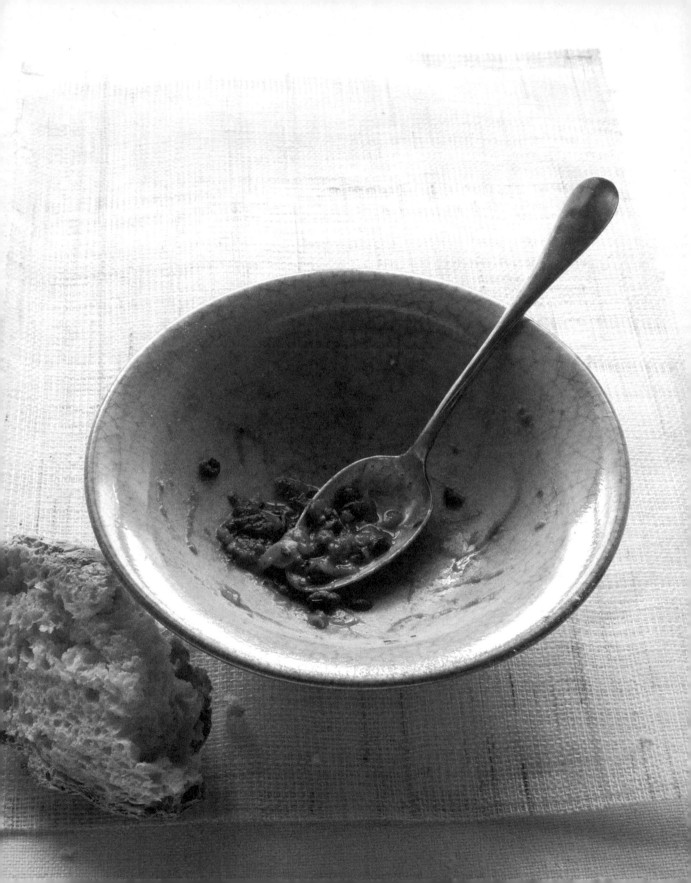

The Journey Starts Here

These days, it seems like there are a million and one problems in the world; global warming, droughts, rising food costs, toxic waterways, cancer, heart disease, diabetes, starvation . . . it's enough to make anyone want to crawl into a hole with a big bowl of ice cream!

Of course you know ice cream's not the solution. But what if I told you that the ice cream you're craving is actually one of the *causes* of every single one of those problems? What if I said that by choosing nondairy ice cream instead, you'd be taking a huge step toward solving them all?

And what about your health? Do you feel like your body is some mystery that only your doctor understands? Do you feel like getting older is just another way of saying "falling apart"? What if I told you that, by eating a varied, plant-based diet, you will strengthen your immune system, beautify your skin, increase your energy, and reduce your risk (significantly) of cancer, heart disease, diabetes, arthritis, osteoporosis, allergies, asthma, and almost every other disease? What if I said that I feel myself getting younger, more powerful, and more beautiful as I age simply because of *what I eat*? Of course the food we choose is not the only factor in our health and well-being, but it's definitely one of the most important—and, luckily, it's one we have control over. How does that nondairy ice cream sound now?

If you want to lose weight, you've come to the right place. But, unlike other diet books, I won't ask you to freak out about calories, carbs, or the glycemic index. With the Kind Diet, your relationship to your body, food, and the concept of dieting itself will transform. By staying away from nasty foods and making friends with grains and vegetables, a whole new, beautiful body will emerge.

And finally, do you feel like you're at peace with yourself? Comfortable in your own body? In your life? Or are you constantly battling yourself (or others), never feeling whole or balanced? Do you feel like you're in touch with your heart—your authentic self? I know it might sound crazy to say that your diet is behind that, too, but it is. When you begin to eat whole grains and abstain from crazy-making foods like white sugar, you will see how amazing and joyous and peaceful life really is.

By following the Kind Diet, you will lose weight easily, your skin will absolutely glow, you will have tons of energy, and you will become more sensitive to all the important things in life—like love, nature, and your deepest, truest self. By eating this way, you will become stronger. Your immune system will work more efficiently as your body releases excess fats and toxins. Released from the grip of certain foods, your body will begin to heal itself.

So here's your end of the bargain: Prioritize food. I know, I know, you're thinking, "I already prioritize food—I'm always on a diet! I think about food all the time!" But that's not what I mean. It's time to really reacquaint yourself with actual *food*, the stuff that comes out of the ground, the stuff that's designed to go in our bodies, supporting not only our physical functions but our hearts and even our souls.

Here's another promise that perhaps your tongue needs to hear: You will *not* feel deprived! If you make that single decision to prioritize food, try out some recipes, and explore some great healthy restaurants, you will be amazed at how delicious this food is. I didn't grow up vegetarian—as a kid my favorite food was pork chops—so I've made the transition that I'm asking you to consider. Not only was it possible, it was the best thing I've ever done. Period.

By the way, this isn't a lifestyle designed for celebrities and rich people. I'm not selling you some glamorous program that requires ridiculous equipment, fancy private sessions, or expensive creams. This radiant health is available to every single one of us because it's nature's way. I *love* that! And these days, the food is even cheap; trade in steak for grains and beans, and your grocery bill goes down. Find a local farmers' market for great prices on organic vegetables. Or even grow your own! You may find, over time, that you see your doctor less often. That you walk more and drive less. That you don't need that frappuccino, antacid, or sleeping pill.

But that's not all. One of the things I love best about the Kind Diet is that you will actually become part of the solution to our global problems. Following a plant-based diet dials down our insane consumption of resources like fresh water, oil, coal, and the precious rain forest. It helps to heal the environment by denying support to toxic food industries. It is a significant move toward ending world hunger and distributing food more equitably.

I believe that at the core of every human is love, and it seeks to spread itself—that's what love's all about. Your heart will open more than ever and that love will start to spread, affecting all the people in your life. And because the Kind Diet is sustainable, you are—by making simple, delicious choices—loving the whole planet with every single bite. I mean, come on . . . How cool is *that*?

Finally, deciding to follow a plant-based diet has introduced me to the most amazing individuals—so many of them kind, interesting, and awake. Wonderful people like Woody Harrelson. So I'll end this introduction with a story: About 10 years ago, right after becoming vegan, I was feeling sort of alone and disconnected. I had bumped into Woody at a number of events, but we'd never really talked, so one day I called him. "Woody," I said, "I'm so frustrated. I keep learning about food, and the planet, and I feel like I'm going crazy!"

After a moment he said, in his Woody way, "I'm taking a trip to Peru, down the Amazon. Wanna come? We're trying to save the rain forest."

"Uhh . . ."

"I'm bringing my wife, Laura, maybe the kids. Bring your boyfriend . . . it'll be fun."

Two months later, I met Woody Harrelson officially, for the first time, in the Lima airport. Three days later, he and Christopher were racing canoes down the Amazon, stark naked and paddling furiously, with me and Laura behind them, laughing. Vegan friends are the best.

Since then, I've been inspired by the joy Woody and Laura take in living life while simultaneously caring for themselves, their kids, and the earth. Their consciousness magically and mysteriously raises mine. Through this book, I hope I can do the same for you. As you get into this stuff, you will meet people full of hope and light, with a real love for this planet. They will make your life richer and more meaningful than you ever thought possible. And that is the greatest gift of all.

Peace out,

Alicia

P.S.: I've created an amazing Web site, thekindlife.com, which includes videos, photos, and blogs posted by me and many of the doctors and other people I've highlighted in this book. It's an interactive online community where we can share inspiration and continue to support each other in living the kind life. There will be fashion, beauty products, recipes, and all kinds of fun stuff. You can send me questions, too.

Throughout the book, I have indicated people or topics you can explore further on the Web site with bold green type. Look for this symbol 🌱 at the bottom of the page. So go to thekindlife.com right now and sign up for a profile.

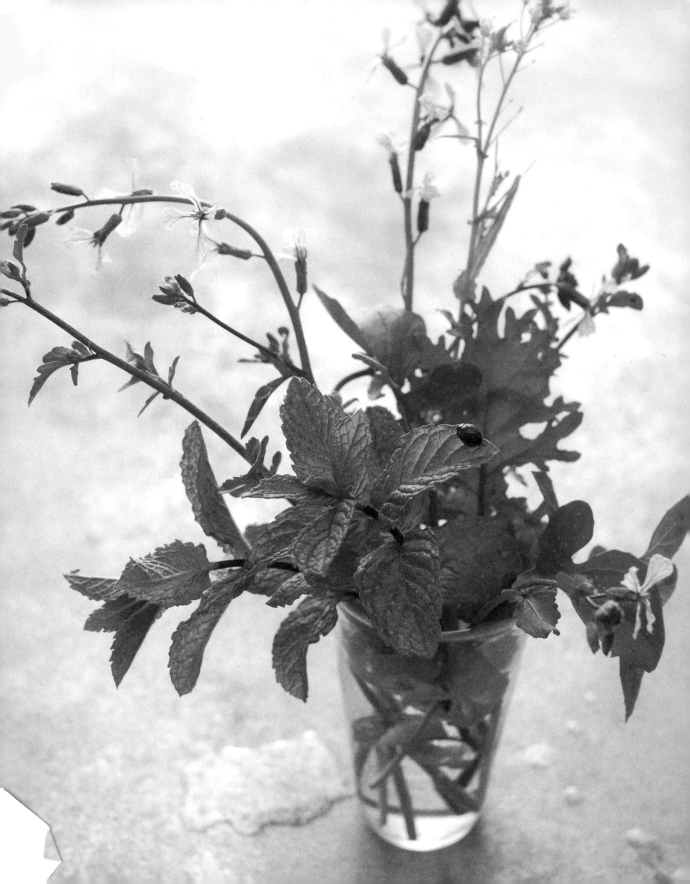

PART I

kind versus nasty

I

What's So Kind about Dieting?

diet: (noun) a way of living, or thinking, a day's journey

This was the definition of *diet* when it entered the English language in the mid-1600s. So simple! So sane! How did this cute little word become synonymous with deprivation, suffering, and—let's be honest—total hell?

With the Kind Diet, we are returning the word to its original definitions, for this journey is about changing how you think and live, one day at a time. And by allowing your mind and your choices to change, you will see amazing—even magical—results. It won't happen overnight, but it will happen, I promise, because it happened to me: By eating satisfying, delicious, plant-based foods, I was released from the prison of dieting.

Oh, the freedom of that! How amazing it is never to have to start another diet! To be able to think about my life, and the world, instead of spazzing out about calories and constantly asking myself, "Can I eat that?" It's like I got my brain back! These days, I get to eat as much as I want of foods that I *love,* and I never have to fear them. I feel truly and deeply nourished by food. I'm so grateful for that.

But what do I mean by "kind"? Well, let's start with you. This is about being really, really good to yourself. The Kind Diet will give you tons of energy, mental clarity, gorgeous skin, and a zest for life you won't want to miss. Plus, it's powerful; doctors like Dean Ornish and John MacDougall have discovered that plant-based diets have the power to reverse heart disease, diabetes, even cancer. So this is about treating yourself like a total goddess and putting yourself first.

And you deserve that kindness, my friend. I used to equate having self-worth with being selfish, but now I understand that taking care of myself is the most beautiful thing I can do. And quite frankly, I can't be a good actor, I can't be a good wife, friend, or mother (to my dogs) . . . I can't be a good *anything* until I've taken care of myself first. So this kindness to yourself is paramount.

And it doesn't stop there. This kindness extends to the earth itself; because it requires less fuel, water, and other precious resources, a plant-based diet is much lighter on the planet. And because it is clean, this diet helps our soil, water, and atmosphere get healthy as well. You will see that the Kind Diet reduces planetary suffering on all levels; following a plant-based diet is just about the greenest thing you can do.

But let's not get ahead of ourselves; this is a process. My own journey, which started quite a while ago and continues to this day, has had its own back-and-forths and big opportunities for learning, growth, and letting go. None of it happened overnight; it took some time, as most transformations do.

We'll start with my story. It began innocently enough—just a young girl wanting to save some dogs. Little did I know that I was actually stepping into the Magical-Life-Altering-Save-the-World-Soul-Expansion Machine!

You see, I've always been an animal-lover. Since I was a little, little girl. And my mom was the same way; if we saw a dog running in the street that looked in need, she'd slam on the brakes, and I'd hop out of the car to run after it—even on the freeway. We were a little dynamic duo. I'm still rescuing dogs to this day.

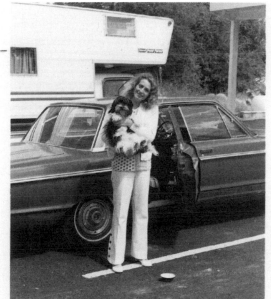

Every little kid is born with an innate love of animals. Animals are complete and individual creatures, each with a distinct personality, and children connect with that.

But the second you get old enough, people say that relating to animals is juvenile and they try to talk you out of it. I know a lot of people who grew up on farms and were given a piglet or a calf to raise. They loved it and cared for it, like any kid would. And then one day the parent has the animal slaughtered and says, "Toughen up. This is what it is to be a grown-up."

My love of animals came crashing down on my love of meat at the ripe old age of 8. My brother and I were on an airplane, and when my dinner came, it was a lamb chop. Just as I stuck my fork in, my brother started making sheep sounds and bleating *baa baa* like a baby lamb. (He was 13 at this point and knew exactly how to torment me.) Suddenly it all came together in my head and I freaked. I might as well have killed the lamb with my own hands. I decided right there on that flight that I was now a vegetarian.

But what did I know about nutrition or dietary concerns at 8? For the next month I ate nothing but ice cream and eggs. And then my resolve slipped. I stopped and started a lot or "forgot" I had sworn off meat. Truth be told, I think I conveniently forgot because I sure loved pork chops, bacon, steak, and everything else. . . .

At 12, I went to my first acting class. I loved it. I loved being with all the older kids. I loved feeling like I could touch a different world, one that provided so much excitement and possibility. In acting class, I discovered my passion and began to consider the meaning of commitment.

My commitment to not eating animals, however, was faltering. I'd wake up and declare, "I'm a vegetarian today!" but it was sort of hard to keep the resolution. I'd sit with a friend and she'd order a steak and I'd say, "Umm . . . are you going to finish that?" and take a bite. "But I thought you were a *vegetarian*!" she would remind me, and I'd counter with, "But you can't eat all that. I don't want it to go to waste!" I'd use any excuse.

I was 18 when *Clueless* came out. Going through adolescence is strange enough, but becoming famous at the same time is *really* weird. It felt good to be recognized as an actor, but after *Clueless*, it was like I was sucked up into a hurricane. You might assume that fame brings you more friends, but I actually became very isolated. I was no longer simply a girl with the freedom to make mistakes and have fun. There was enormous pressure, which put me in full survival mode. And being in survival mode made it hard to stay in touch with my truth; I just couldn't hear it anymore.

Well, almost. One of the really *good* things about being a public person was that animal rights groups were hearing about my passion for their cause and began soliciting my help. I worked on all sorts of campaigns: antidissection, antifur, spay and neuter, as well as animal rescue. All of that stuff made perfect sense to me; in an otherwise chaotic life, these gestures were simple and straightforward and good. But, at that point, nobody had talked to me seriously about vegetarianism, and I was still doing my little dance back and forth.

After a heart-wrenching day at an animal shelter, from which I took home a grand total of *11* dogs who were scheduled for execution, I found myself thinking, "Now what?" I was doing what I needed to do for my heart, but deep down I realized it wasn't a practical solution; the next day the shelter would just put down another batch of dogs . . . and then another . . . and then another. I was committing my heart, soul, time, and pocketbook to these poor creatures, and that's when it hit me: How could I spend so much energy saving one group of animals, then turn around and eat other ones? There was a fundamental hypocrisy in my thinking. Weren't they all living beings? Why did we buy some of them cute little doggy beds while slaughtering others? I had to ask myself—in all seriousness— why don't I just eat my *dog*?

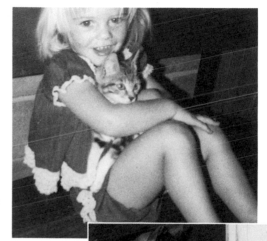

That realization helped me make up my mind once and for all. I realized that, until I stopped using my dollars to purchase meat or other products that are created through violence or cruelty, the suffering would never end. It wouldn't stop because I wanted it to. It wouldn't stop because I *wished* it would. If I really wanted to end cruelty to animals, I had to boycott it completely.

When I got home, I declared to my boyfriend (now husband), Christopher, "I'm going vegan. Forever. You don't have to," and I blathered on about wanting to save the pigs and the cows, and the logistics of living with the newly vegan me. I was getting all worked up planning everything

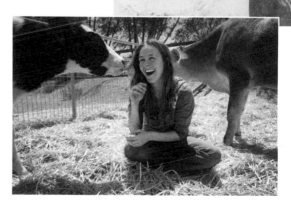

out, and he looked at me and said in the sweetest way, "Baby, I don't want to hurt the pigs either!" Which confirms that I am the luckiest girl on Earth, because he was totally on board with me from day one.

That night we grilled the final steak in our freezer and sat down to our last nonvegan supper. It was quite solemn. I remember crossing myself like a Catholic even though I'm Jewish, because this was a total act of faith; I had never tried to cook without meat. I wasn't sure I would ever eat a yummy meal again.

But after only 2 weeks of being vegan, people were beginning to ask, "What is going on with you? You look amazing!" I was still eating lots of white pasta, french fries, and all sorts of sludgy things (in fact, I still do sometimes). All I'd given up was meat and dairy, and yet I began to look better in just 2 weeks!

Something really wild was happening *inside* of me, too. I noticed that my whole body felt lighter. I was more vibrant and spunky. I felt like my heart had sort of opened a bit and my shoulders could relax, as if an overall softening had taken place. I no longer carried heavy animal protein in my body, which takes tons of energy to digest. Plus, I didn't have the heaviness of the suffering in me; frightened animals produce lots of cortisol and adrenaline right before slaughter, and we can become stressed from eating their meat.

Something seemed to be happening on a deeper level as well. The decision to be vegan was one I made purely for me, an expression of my truest self and deepest beliefs. It was the first time I'd stood up and said a definitive "NO!" My real self began to emerge. It was powerful.

One afternoon, a few years later, Christopher came home and announced that he wanted to try a macrobiotic diet. He'd read interviews with people who claimed that this diet made them feel balanced and happy and he was intrigued. I'd heard (incorrectly, as it turns out) that macrobiotics was only for sick people and that fish was a requisite part of the diet. No way was that for me! He looked at me with that sweet face of his and said, "Alright, baby. I'm going to do macrobiotics, but you don't have to."

Ironically, I was exploring another diet dimension myself at the time—raw foods. I was eating tons of fruit, nuts, and other cool, uncooked delicacies. Although I felt fine in sunny California, when I went to snowy, cold Manhattan to appear opposite Kathleen Turner and Jason Biggs in *The Graduate* on Broadway, it was another story. After a few days of work, my body felt cold and my energy was low, but I was determined to stick to my raw regimen. Between rehearsals, I would go out into the winter weather to hunt down wheatgrass juice, pineapples, and mangoes. I found them—it was New York, after all—but I wasn't feeling all that good. My brain didn't want to know, but my body was giving me signals that I was out of balance.

At work, I was teased by the other members of the cast for my "extreme" diet. I swear Jason deliberately ordered veal and rabbit just to make me crazy. Whenever I yawned or seemed tired, the director announced, "It's because you're not eating any meat!"

It's funny how the puzzle pieces of your life drop into place; during that same stint in New York, I went to Candle Café (one of my favorite restaurants), and I noticed Temple, a waitress who I hadn't seen in years. She was absolutely on fire. Her hair, her skin, and her body just looked amazing. She told me she'd seen a macrobiotic counselor, and now she was the healthiest she'd ever been in her life. I decided I would give Christopher a consultation with her counselor for his birthday. If she looked so fantastic, there had to be something to this macro business, right?

By the time the appointment rolled around, though, my defenses had reemerged. When we got to the counselor's office, I sat with my arms crossed, thinking, "This is stupid." She politely ignored me and worked with Christopher to design a regimen for him. Just as we were getting ready to leave, she turned to me and said, "Maybe you should try this, too. You could have more energy, and I could help you clear up your acne." Damn. She had noticed. But of course everyone did. Since going off the pill a few years before, my skin had become a nightmare, with really cystic acne. I'd even had to reshoot a scene for a movie because my skin looked so bad.

But she wasn't done. "Do you know how much energy is consumed to transport some of the food you're eating?" she asked. "These coconuts and pineapples and mangoes are flown in from all over the world. That's a huge waste of fuel." I had never thought about it, but of course she was right.

Sensing that my resistance was faltering, she pressed on. "How can these foods be good for you, in the dead of winter, in New York? If you eat something from another climate, how is your body supposed to cope with it? Your body is here, in cold New York. And the mango is designed to cool people off in tropical climates." She definitely had my attention now. "You need to eat what's indigenous to the area to avoid stressing your body." This made perfect sense to me on a holistic level. Between the acne and the mangoes and the excessive energy consumption, she had won me over. I decided to give it a try, and within a week of following her recommendations, my acne—which had haunted me for such a long time—had improved significantly. It was like magic.

But that's the Superhero diet, and I don't expect anyone to go full Superhero overnight. The simplest elements of the counselor's recommendations were to add whole grains to my diet at every meal. I also had miso soup almost every day and totally cranked up the vegetables. I made sure that everything I was eating was local and seasonal, choosing apples over pineapples. In terms of letting go, I said good-bye to white sugar, substituting sweeteners like rice syrup and maple syrup. I also gave up white flour and processed foods and, of course, still no meat or dairy.

A few tweaks and everything changed.

Although I felt good as a vegan, I had even more energy when I adopted the macrobiotic suggestions. At the same time, I was very calm and at peace within myself. My mind focused easily and my thinking became really clear. Although I had lost weight by going vegan, the macrobiotic diet helped me shed the few extra pounds I was holding on to and brought me to my perfect body effortlessly.

Over time, I became more sensitive. I started to feel things more acutely and sense my intuition. People used to say, "Listen to your body," and I had no idea what they meant. "What is my body saying? I don't know . . . it's just *here*!" But soon I really understood; my body was trying to tell me things all the time, and once I stripped away all the layers of crap inside, I could hear it.

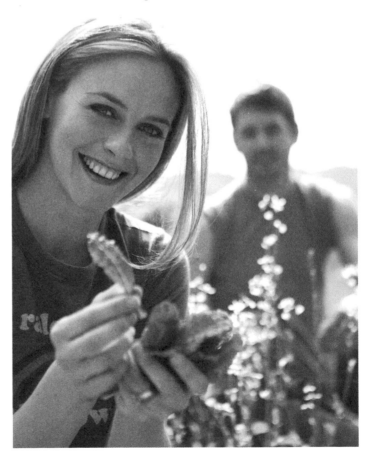

As I aligned more with nature and the seasons, I aligned more with myself. Instead of constantly relying on the people around me for direction, I felt I was on my own journey and I was beginning to sense—from inside of me—each next right step.

Which brings me to this book. I've known for quite a while that I wanted to help other people become their best selves. And, in fact, for the last few years, I've seen how my practice has influenced the people around me. The information I have to share is powerful because the food is powerful. Literally. Your deepest, truest self is released through food.

I encourage you to let this book gently lift your awareness, and you will begin to make the changes that work for you. There are plenty of little choices you can make—choices that will make huge impacts—without getting all uptight and thinking you have to be perfect.

Based on these stages I went through, I have designed three different approaches to the Kind Diet—each one for a different level of readiness—and you can choose according to what feels right to you. The first plan is called Flirting, and it's simply sticking your toe in the pool of the Kind Diet. The second plan is Vegan; it's for experienced Flirts and those of you who, after reading this book, want to commit to a plant-based diet. The third plan, Superhero, emphasizes whole grains, organic vegetables, and sea vegetables and will make you levitate. (Well, almost.)

So as you read, keep in mind that these different levels exist; that no matter where you're coming from, there's plenty of room for you on this path. Whether it takes you 2 weeks or 10 *years* to make my delicious rice crispy treats matters not a jot. It's your path, based on what you think and feel while reading this book. You will know what's right for you.

But before you choose your path, let's dine on some information. It's only by digesting and absorbing pertinent facts that you can make an informed choice. In the following chapters, we look closely at specific foods and the very real impact they have on our bodies and our world. *Bon appétit!*

A Weighty Issue

Although I wasn't an overweight kid, I do remember starting to develop self-consciousness around my body at a pretty early age. And it didn't help that I was in the movie industry, not exactly known for its relaxed attitudes toward an extra 10 or 15 pounds. By the time I was 14, I was fully hypnotized by calorie-counting, and my manager at the time took me to a Weight Watchers meeting. While preparing to play Batgirl in *Batman & Robin*, the press was so cruel about my teenage curves that I was chased through the L.A. airport by paparazzi yelling, "Fatgirl!" Of course, all the pressure made me rebel and eat even more. Although I was probably a normal weight, I was certainly moving in the wrong direction.

That feels like such a long time ago.

On the Kind Diet, you will experience freedom not only from excess pounds, but from the crazy, obsessive fixation on points, fats, calories, and all those horrible weight loss goals and deadlines. Over time, those things will simply slip away, I promise. Whole grains will give you a calm and peaceful mind. Vegetables—packed so densely with nutrients—will give you the most amazing, happy, and youthful vitality. And beans, full of fiber, will keep you feeling full and satisfied while everything moves through you like a dream. You're getting more than a new waistline, my friend. You're getting a new reality.

Dr. John MacDougall has been running a 10-day residential program in Santa Rosa, California, for 20 years now, is the author of several books, and has even developed a line of vegetarian foods for people on the go. By adopting a low-fat, plant-based diet, patients of Dr. MacDougall not only reach their optimal weight, they are often able to throw away their medications and reverse serious illness, such as heart disease and even cancer. Go Dr. MacDougall!

Dr. Joel Fuhrman encountered the same thing. Author of *Eat to Live: The Revolutionary Formula for Fast and Sustained Weight Loss,* Dr. Fuhrman devised a program that involves packing as much nutrition as possible into every calorie consumed. And what does he consider the best sources of nutrient-dense calories? Not meat. Not dairy. Plant-based foods. Like Dr. MacDougall, he has seen countless patients not only lose weight on their vegan food plans, but experience total transformations in health and emotional well-being as well, including reversals in heart disease, diabetes, rheumatoid arthritis, allergies, osteoporosis, lupus, and more. Amazing what happens when you eat *real food*!

For tips on quicker weight loss, go to page 138.

For more information visit us at: www.thekindlife.com

2

Nasty Food #1: Meat

Let food be thy medicine and thy medicine be thy food.

Hippocrates, the father of Western medicine, 460–377 BC

Things have changed a lot since Hippocrates uttered that beautiful statement. In fact, it's almost as if he never said it at all. These days, we tend to think of being healthy as just getting through the day, making a living, or not dropping dead. We consider health the absence of disease. When symptoms do arise, we throw chemicals at them, hoping they will go away rather than looking for the underlying cause. This is modern medicine.

Because we look at the body as a bunch of bits and pieces, we have all sorts of different doctors—the ear, nose, and throat guy; the skin guy; the heart guy—and when things go wrong, we have doctors who concentrate on the disease itself—like the oncologist, the cancer guy. Modern science is constantly focusing its microscope, seeing tinier and tinier bits and pieces, trying to figure out the puzzle of disease. Not health . . . disease.

Strangest of all, we've convinced ourselves that our health has nothing to do with what we eat. People who will spend that extra 20 cents on a gallon of premium gasoline because they realize their car performs better on it will drive straight to McDonald's for a Big Mac. We create a mental separation between food and illness in our culture, and our modern Western medical system—for the most part—supports this denial. When asked what causes an illness, we are told it's due to genetics or just bad luck. "Kids just get allergies" and "We don't have all the answers." These statements are usually swiftly followed by a prescription.

There are major forces trying to keep us all in this denial—megarich corporations and institutions that would not only prefer you stay in the dark, but are pouring billions of dollars into the effort to keep the lights off. But our mental disconnect between food and disease is not simply lining corporate pockets; it is literally destroying our health and that of the planet. This chapter and the next two shed some light on meat, dairy, sugar, and processed foods. I think you'll see why I call them "nasty."

MEAT: NASTY TO YOUR BODY

I grew up eating beef, pork, chicken, and eggs. And turkey and fish. Oh, and lamb, too. So it's no mystery to me why people love their flesh; the palate loves the taste and the belly feels full and warm with a greasy hunk of meat inside. I get it.

But that's just one side of the story.

Meat is bad for your ticker: Heart disease is the number one killer of women in the United States. Number one. Not breast cancer . . . not mascara poisoning. . . . Heart disease! And meat eating is a major contributor. You see, meat contains lots of saturated fat. Saturated fat elevates your blood cholesterol, and that causes plaque to clog your arteries. Clogged arteries lead to high blood pressure or—even worse—a stroke or a nice, juicy heart attack. But you knew that already. It's one of the few facts about meat eating that the meat industry has not been able to conceal.

According to the American Heart Association, high-cholesterol foods also raise blood cholesterol. Eggs contain 250 milligrams of cholesterol, and 64 percent of an egg's calories come from fat. Chicken contains as much cholesterol as beef, and trout is right behind that.[1]

No meat is a truly low-fat food. Because saturated fat is marbled throughout the muscle, and the cholesterol is found in the cell membranes of the meat itself, trimming the excess fat off your steak doesn't do much good. It seems that only a plant-based diet protects the heart. Dr. William Castelli, director of the Framingham Heart Study, says a low-fat plant-based diet would lower an individual's risk of heart attack by 85 percent. You heard me. Eighty-five percent.

Meat contributes to cancer: There are so many studies linking meat to cancer, it's hard to choose! Here are some of the stats on cancer and the possible reasons that meat is linked to it:

A 2007 study of more than 35,000 women published in the *British Journal of Cancer* found that women who ate the most meat were more likely to develop breast cancer than those who consumed the least.

Perhaps this is the reason: Researchers at the University of California at San Diego have isolated a sugar molecule (with the sexy name Neu5Gc) that shows up in many cancerous human tumors. But the human body doesn't produce Neu5Gc, so where could it be coming from? You guessed it: red meat. Not only does Neu5Gc seem to build tumors, our human bodies produce antibodies against Neu5Gc, which causes inflammation, helping the tumors to grow even more!

And maybe toxins play a role: Dioxin is the most toxic chemical known to science and is recognized as a human carcinogen. It is estimated that 93 percent[2] of our exposure to dioxin comes through eating animal products—beef, lamb, pork, chicken, dairy, eggs, and especially fish. Dioxin settles and accumulates in fat, so the more animal food we eat, the more dioxin we get. According to a study published in 1998,[3] the dioxin level in the blood of vegans was found to be much lower than that of the general population.

Finally, how we cook meat is a piece in the cancer puzzle as well: When either red or white meats hit a grill, they create cancer-causing compounds called heterocyclic amines. FYI: Grilled chicken has more than 17 times the number of these compounds than grilled steak.[4]

Meat contributes to osteoporosis: When you eat meat, your blood becomes acidic, and that's not cool; acidic blood can lead to all sorts of nasty problems, including . . . death. In order to balance all the acidity, your bones come to the rescue by releasing some of their minerals. This leaves your blood nice and balanced but your bones weak. It's a neat physiological trick to keep you healthy in the moment, but your poor bones pay the price over time. According to Dr. Neal Barnard, animal protein is the chief cause of osteoporosis (followed by sodium, caffeine, tobacco, and inactivity).[5]

In 1994, a report in the *American Journal of Clinical Nutrition* showed that when people went from a standard American diet to a vegetarian diet, they had over 50 percent less bone loss. Gnaw on that!

Meat is hard to digest: Fiber is the broom that sweeps out your intestines, moving food through your digestive tract and helping to eliminate waste. Meat contains absolutely no fiber. It gets stuck down there, creating a funky, stuck, acid environment. High meat consumption is a recognized factor in conditions such as colitis, diverticulitis, and even colon cancer.[6–8]

More health issues: Meat eating is also believed to exacerbate gout, contribute to rheumatoid arthritis, and to be a major factor in the formation of kidney stones.[9–11]

Meat is full of antibiotics: Because animals raised in confined, dirty, stressful environments

For more information visit us at: www.thekindlife.com

have a tendency to get sick, they are given antibiotics as a routine preventive measure. According to the Union of Concerned Scientists, 70 percent of the antibiotics sold in the United States go to livestock, including farm-raised fish. In fact, farmed salmon have more antibiotics administered by weight than any other form of livestock. These antibiotics are then passed on to you. Before yelling, "Yay! Free drugs!" you should know a thing or two: When you take unnecessary antibiotics by eating meat, (a) your own healthy intestinal bacteria get wiped out, making you less able to fight off disease, and (b) the bacteria that the drugs are designed to kill eventually morph into smarter and stronger versions of themselves. In true horror movie fashion, they are literally becoming superbugs against which none of us has natural resistance. Science has not yet caught up with these superbugs, so we have no efficient antibiotics to use against them. By dosing the cows and pigs with antibiotics, we are actually endangering ourselves.

Meat carries freaky pathogens: Have you ever seen the inside of a slaughterhouse? Suffice it to say they're not exactly the cleanest places on Earth. When animals are eviscerated, it's not unusual for their bowels to be punctured (workers kill up to 330 animals an hour), leaving all sorts of intestinal bacteria splatter on the meat and skin. In 1998, an amendment to an agriculture appropriations bill was proposed to give the USDA the power to fine meatpacking plants for unsanitary conditions. The House Appropriations Committee voted it down 25 to 19. Why would they do that? Turns out the 25 "nays" receive six times more money from the meat and poultry industries than the 19 "yays."

A USDA report published in 2000 estimated that a staggering 89 percent of U.S. beef ground into patties contained traces of deadly E. coli.[12]

Another bug called campylobacter is the leading cause of food-borne illness in the United States, and it usually arrives via chicken flesh. A dangerous little bacterium, campylobacter is

Superhero: Dr. William Castelli

In 1948, scientists at the National Heart, Lung, and Blood Institute began a huge research project called the Framingham Heart Study, which continues today. It is the longest-running study of its kind in medical history, covering three generations of roughly 5,000 participants per generation over the last 60 years. Dr. William Castelli served as director of the project from 1979 through 2008. After analyzing all the evidence, he concluded vegetarians have the lowest rates of coronary heart disease of any group in the country. He added that when individuals keep their cholesterol below 150, they are virtually guaranteed never to suffer a heart attack.

estimated to infect more than 2.4 million Americans each year.[13] It is also estimated that 70 percent of American chickens and 90 percent of our turkeys are contaminated with campylobacter, the result of the birds being housed in ridiculously crowded conditions and their regular dosing with antibiotics. In fact, factory-farmed chicken is so unclean that Gerald Kuester, former USDA microbiologist, says, "The final product is no different than if you stuck it in the toilet and ate it."[14]

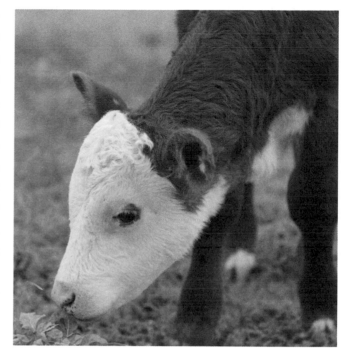

When the flesh we're putting in our mouths is full of disease, is it any surprise we get sick ourselves? It would be nice to think that Uncle Sam is there to protect us, but unfortunately, the Federal Humane Slaughter Act is so full of exceptions and loopholes that 90 percent of U.S. animals are exempted.

Another disturbing thing about meat is that it's secondhand food; in other words, because you are eating an animal, you are eating everything *stored* in that animal's tissues—including all the toxins he couldn't get rid of. And while we're on the topic of all things disgusting, consider what the animal you're eating has eaten; livestock feed is routinely beefed up with slaughterhouse wastes like blood, bone, and viscera as well as the remains of euthanized cats and dogs.[15] The drug used to kill these pets, sodium pentobarbital, survives the rendering process, so it gets passed into the feed as well. Ugh.[16]

Meat is full of hormones: Cattle, pigs, and chickens are routinely pumped full of hormones to promote muscle mass, and these hormones are passed directly on to you. Eggs are chockfull of hormonal goodies as well, as are farmed fish. That might sound good to the bodybuilders out there, but excess hormones have been linked to many cancers, including breast and prostate. We have our own hormones, and the body is constantly working to keep them in balance—simply put, we don't need more!

Plus, when an animal is led to slaughter, the adrenaline and stress hormones coursing through her veins get passed onto the dinner plate. Might this cause excess anxiety and aggression in us? Are we eating fear and anger? Although there's very little hard science on this, many people report becoming much calmer and more peaceful when they give up meat.

Fish has its own dangers: These days fish contain mercury and other industrial toxins. Coal-burning power plants release mercury into the air, which then falls into the ocean. Bacteria consume this mercury, which then is consumed by little fish and is concentrated up the fishy food chain. Smaller fish and seafood like salmon, cod, shrimp, and trout have lower levels of mercury, while swordfish, tile, mackerel, and tuna have the highest. But they ALL contain mercury, which has been shown to damage the brain, kidneys, and lungs and is particularly dangerous to pregnant women and their growing babies.

Does that mean farm-raised fish are better? Well, besides the fact that they are pumped full of antibiotics, farmed salmon were found to contain levels of industrial toxins called PCBs *16 times* higher[17] than their wild counterparts, so neither choice can be considered clean.

Why don't we know this stuff?

The meat industry has created entities like the National Cattlemen's Beef Association, the American Meat Institute, and the National Pork Producers Council, which spend millions and millions of dollars on print and television ads to cast their products in a positive light, despite evidence to the contrary.

Approximately 650,000 Americans die of heart disease each year. Half a million die of cancer.

Superhero: *Olympic Wrestler* Chris Campbell

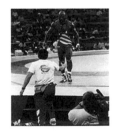

Chris became vegetarian after doing research on how to maximize his athletic potential for the 1980 Olympics, but because of the U.S. boycott, he was not allowed to compete that year. After an injury kept him out of the 1984 Olympic Games, he stopped competing and went on to earn a law degree. Still in world-class shape 8 years later, Chris qualified for the Barcelona Olympics and took home the bronze medal in 1992 at the ripe old age of 37, making him the oldest American wrestling medalist and one of the greatest comeback kids in wrestling history. He feels that his vegetarian diet allowed his body to use more energy for training because less was needed to process meat.

For more information visit us at: www.thekindlife.com

Those two diseases are slaying our population like modern plagues. And you know what? They're basically preventable—and often even reversible—through diet and lifestyle changes. Some people are trying to get the word out there: Groups like the American Heart Association, the World Health Organization, and the American Institute for Cancer Research. They all agree that a plant-based diet will help prevent these horrible illnesses that are killing our friends and families.

However, unlike the Cattlemen, these groups aren't in it for the money—they're simply trying to disseminate information as a public service. But it's hard to compete with big business: Did you know that the meat industries are subsidized by the U.S. government and continually lobby Congress to keep the subsidies alive? On its Web site, the National Chicken Council clucks with pride that it pays off politicians: "[We] collect funds through [our] Political Action Committee to distribute to congressional candidates who support the industry."

The doctor of the future will give no medication, but will interest his patients in the care of the human frame, diet, and in the cause and prevention of disease.

—Thomas A. Edison

MAYBE WE'RE JUST NOT BUILT FOR THIS

Many argue that we're not actually *designed* to consume much animal flesh. True carnivores, like cheetahs, have razor-sharp teeth and long claws and run as fast as a speeding car. You can't run that fast and your molars are flat, meant for grinding grains. Yes, we have four vestigial canine teeth, but good luck ripping flesh with them, much less your nails.

Our intestines tell a story, too. A carnivore's intestines are only about 6 feet long, because meat isn't meant to hang out in the gut forever. Our intestines are 20 feet long; when we eat meat, it takes a full 72 hours to pass through us. That's *3 days,* and your body, my friend, is 98.6 degrees inside! It's like having a steak sit out in the hot sun for 3 days straight. Eventually it will start to rot and putrefy. And that's what's happening inside of you. You may not feel that process now, but I challenge you to abstain from animal products for a month and then eat some meat. You will feel how heavy and dense it feels in your gut.

And maybe it's not in our nature to eat meat. If I were to put a child in a room with a live lamb and say, "That's your dinner . . . go for it!" what do you think she would do? Chances are

I'd come back an hour later to find them cuddling on the floor together. A young tiger would know what to do . . . but a human? I understand that some of our ancestors had to kill, but they did it for survival, used the whole animal, and expended enormous amounts of energy in the hunt. That's a world away from scarfing down a double cheeseburger for lunch at your desk.

The argument is often put forth that, in the Bible, man was given dominion over the animals, which is interpreted as, "Hey, let's go get a ham sandwich!" But it's hard to believe that God was encouraging us to torture and slaughter His living creatures for profit or fleeting sensual pleasure. Dominion means stewardship, implying a certain respect that just doesn't exist in our factory-farming world.

Finally, maybe we should ask ourselves if we really even *want* to be meat-eaters. The carnivores of the natural world have quick, precise energy, but then they're tuckered out and sleep for days. They are aggressive hunters with very little endurance. The herbivores, like horses or giraffes, not only have long-lasting energy and strength, but are generally a peaceful lot. Hmmm . . .

NASTY TO THE PLANET

Nothing will benefit human health and increase chances for survival of life on Earth as much as the evolution to a vegetarian diet.
—Albert Einstein

Our collective environmental consciousness has been raised enormously in the past few years, which is awesome. We've made great strides. But there's a big piece missing in our education. Despite all of our recycling, energy saving, and water conservation (all of which are great), most people still don't know that they can have the greatest impact on our precious Planet Earth by adopting a plant-based diet. With *20 billion* heads of livestock walking the earth—that's more than triple the number of humans—we are spending precious natural resources on *them* instead of us. They, in turn, wreak havoc on the environment. Crazy.

Here's the deal:

Meat contributes to global warming and climate change: One of our biggest environmental concerns is controlling the emission of gases into the atmosphere that get trapped and cause the greenhouse effect. You know how in a greenhouse the glass ceilings allow the sun's warmth to enter while trapping all the heat inside? Well, by burning fossil fuels and creating gas emissions at an unprecedented rate, we are raising global temperatures and changing climate

Pills versus Plants

Did you know that drug companies spend $19 billion annually to cultivate their relationships with physicians?[18] That's $52 million a day for free gifts, free drugs, and education about the drug companies' products. Obviously, the situation creates a conflict of interest for doctors, and it has been documented that all these freebies do influence physicians' prescribing habits.[19]

Unfortunately, your doctor is not tossing and turning at night, debating the benefits of pushing drugs or food. He doesn't have enough information to be conflicted; although medical schools are supposed to provide students with approximately 25 hours of nutritional education, it's believed that as many as 60 percent don't comply.[20] Meanwhile, the pharmaceutical industry is pumping money into medical schools in the form of research grants for drug studies. And we're not talking chump change here: Over the next 3 years, Vanderbilt University will receive $10 million from pharmaceutical giant Johnson & Johnson to develop new drugs, with another $100 million promised if certain research milestones are met.[21] That kind of influence might eclipse a few hours of nutrition classes! So keep in mind that after reading this book, you may know more about healthy eating than your doctor does.

Medical school faculty are also on the payroll. About 1,600 of Harvard University's 8,900 professors and lecturers disclosed that they had a financial interest in businesses related to their teaching, research, or clinical care. One hundred forty-nine had financial ties to Pfizer and 130 to Merck. It's becoming hard to tell if a professor is teaching about certain drugs because they work or because the company that makes them is sending him on a golf vacation. Members of the American Medical Student Association are so disturbed by teachers taking payola from drug companies that they recently began grading medical schools' ability to monitor and control drug industry money. While the University of Pennsylvania received an A, Yale got a C, and Harvard a big fat F.[22]

I'm not saying that doctors are bad people or that *all* the information they've received is wrong. I'm just here to remind you that the pharmaceutical industry is the most profitable in the entire country and that Americans buy nearly half the drugs on the planet—spending $235 billion in 2008.[23] And when companies are chasing that kind of money, profit often trumps the truth. None of us like to think that we can't trust the institutions we've grown up with, but being a truly healthy person means exploring important issues deeply and thinking for yourself. As your body gets stronger and stronger from eating whole grains and vegetables, your intuition will get louder and louder. Remember: You were designed by nature, not by a corporation or a doctor. Thank goodness Mother Nature—being so rich herself—isn't trying to make a buck off you.

patterns worldwide. The consequences are pretty huge, including coastal flooding, drought, and severe weather events. Even the polar ice caps are melting, and they play a critical role in keeping the planet cool by reflecting sunlight. When they're gone and the sun's heat is absorbed by the dark blue water that remains, we're in for even hotter times and massive catastrophes.

Of the gases that trap heat in the atmosphere, carbon dioxide is the one we often hear about. It comes out of our cars, our heaters, and our lungs. But there is another gas, methane, that traps 21 times[24] more heat per molecule than carbon dioxide. Methane is a naturally occurring trace gas and a normal part of our atmosphere. One of its biggest sources is . . . burps. Yup. That's right. And as much as you might think your brother belches, cows standing around being over-fed and never exercised—1.3 billion of them worldwide—burp much, much more. In fact, each cow produces anywhere from 100 to 520 quarts of methane gas *daily*.[25] Not that methane is inherently bad; it exists naturally and in a balanced ratio with other gases within the atmosphere. But with all the animals we've bred for food, we've tipped the scales. Methane emitted by live-stock accounts for 19 percent[26] of the total global methane emissions. In fact, the livestock we keep—to feed us meat that hurts our bodies—produce more methane than landfills, waste treat-ment plants, and even the methane we use as natural gas to heat our homes!

By deciding not to eat that burger, you'll be reducing the numbers of cows cattlemen need to raise, thereby reducing the gases they emit. It's a straight line from a plant-based diet to a health-ier planet. Dr. Rajendra Pachauri, chair of the United Nations Intergovernmental Panel on Cli-mate Change, recently said, "In terms of immediacy of action and the feasibility of bringing about reductions in a short period of time, [reducing meat consumption] clearly is the most attractive opportunity." His specific recommendation? "Give up meat for one day [a week] ini-tially, and decrease it from there."[27]

If everyone in America were to adopt a plant-based diet, we would reduce U.S. greenhouse gas production by 6 percent virtually overnight. Six percent may not sound like a lot, but when you

Superhero: Queenie the Cow
Queenie the cow escaped from a meat market in New York City. She ran from workers and evaded the NYPD for several blocks of lower Manhattan. When she was caught and threatened with a return to the slaughterhouse, hundreds of New Yorkers spoke up for her, and she was taken to a farm sanctuary where she thrives today. GO, QUEENIE!

remember that the United States creates 25 percent of the world's greenhouse gases, it's a significant slice of the pie. And don't forget that we'd be reducing heart disease, cancer, osteoporosis, and arthritis at the same time. That, in turn, reduces hospital visits, insurance nightmares, and dependency on pharmaceuticals. The price for all this? Well, I hate to break it to you, but here goes: You must eat really yummy food and feel young, vibrant, and happy for the rest of your life.

Factory farming creates toxic sludge: The meat industry has a nasty reputation for not containing its waste very well. Not only does the poo, fertilizers, and other sludge get into the soil, it can also leach into nearby rivers and water tables. We have strict laws about the disposal of human waste but none for the animal equivalent, and according to Worldwatch Institute, U.S. livestock produces *130 times* more waste than people do! In fact, one farm in Utah with 500,000 pigs produces more fecal matter than the 1.5 million inhabitants of Manhattan.[28] All this toxic poo is doing real damage: With so many farms along the banks of the Mississippi, agricultural waste is leaching into the river at an alarming rate. There is so much excess nitrogen from fertilizer and excrement, in fact, that it has created what's called "the Dead Zone" at the mouth of the river, in the Gulf of Mexico. This dead zone, which has no oxygen and therefore cannot sustain any life, was almost 8,000 square miles in size in 2008.[29] Whoa. Next time you tuck into a juicy steak, know that it is responsible for 17 times more water pollution than a bowl of noodles.[30]

Meat wastes water: Forty-two percent[31] of the fresh water available to us in the United States is used for agriculture. Some is used to grow grain for us, some for growing grain for animals, and some for hydrating and washing the animals. It takes 441 gallons of water to produce 1 pound of beef, and that's according to what the Cattlemen's Association says. Dr. Georg Borgstrom, who chairs the Food Science and Human Nutrition Department of the College of Agriculture and Natural Resources at Michigan State University, thinks it's more like 2,500 gallons. That's not 2,500 gallons per cow—it's per pound of beef. By comparison, it takes only 33 gallons of water to grow a pound of carrots. One 16-ounce steak uses the amount of water you need for 6 months of showers! Holy cow![32]

Animals eat a lot of food: Did you know that more than 50 percent of the corn grown in the United States is eaten by animals?[33] Roughly *8 percent* of corn grown is for human food use.[34] Sixty million acres of the United States are devoted to growing hay[35] primarily for livestock, while we use only 13 million acres to grow fruits and vegetables.[36] While 1.2 billion people do not have enough to eat every day, we're bending over backward to make damn sure the 20 billion cows, pigs, and chickens are getting fatter and fatter by the minute.

The meat industry is oil-hungry: It takes more than 11 times the energy to create animal protein than grain protein.[37] When you take into account the fuel used for planting, watering, and harvesting of the grain a cow eats, its transportation, the energy used by factory farms, transportation of the cows to slaughter, and then the distribution of the meat to you . . . that Big Mac looks more like it's made of fossil fuel than beef. Because the average American eats 97 pounds of beef a year, our national burger-lust requires the energy equivalent of a mere *29 billion* gallons of gas!

Cows are cute, but they are wrecking America: The meat industry is clearly siphoning off a disproportionate share of precious resources like fuel and water, but the grazing of cattle is wreaking havoc on the land itself. Cows and other livestock are wandering around on approximately 160 million acres[38] of federally owned land leased to farmers. And their innocent grazing isn't so innocent. More than half of the topsoil of the American West has been lost since cattle started grazing 140 years ago. According to *Mad Cowboy* by Howard Lyman, it takes nature from 100 to 800 years to create a single inch of topsoil, and since the birth of this country, we've lost 6 full inches. That might just sound like a bunch of dirt disappearing, but topsoil is the incubator of life itself. Without it, no plants can grow, and without plants, all animals die. By allowing millions of cows to stomp on, poo on, and kick up precious topsoil, we are shooting ourselves in the collective hoof. When enough soil is dried or displaced, a negative spiral begins that causes rich, fertile soil to become desert. And there's no recovery from that anywhere in the near future. Desertification from overgrazing is a global problem.

Imagine if we stopped the damage now and what we could do with that real estate. We could be growing food for *people*. We could plant trees to absorb carbon dioxide and produce oxygen. We could restore natural habitats for wild animals and preserve biodiversity. Many of the world's problems could be solved if livestock were taken out of the picture.

And let's not forget what happens when wild animals start to compete with the cows for this federal land or threaten the herds. One and a half million wild animals, such as bears, bobcats, foxes, mountain lions, and even domestic pets are killed each year to protect cattle.[39] In other words, we kill one animal to protect *another* animal only to turn around and *kill* that animal to feed an appetite that is killing us and the planet! How crazy is that?

We're messing with the ocean: Once thought to be an inexhaustible source of food, the ocean today is actually being fished out. Because there are fewer fish, we're having to go deeper and deeper into the ocean to find them, and we're displacing all sorts of marine creatures and plants that are essential members of the food chain in the process. Fish farming is unfortunately

For more information visit us at: www.thekindlife.com

not the solution, since it takes 2 to 5 pounds of small wild fish to produce 1 pound of farmed salmon.[40] That formula is obviously totally unsustainable.

We're destroying the rain forest: It's one thing to damage our own country, but our lust for cheap burgers is creating so much demand for beef that the South and Central American cattle industries are clearing rain forest to make room for cattle pasture. In fact, cattle grazing is the number one factor in the destruction of the rain forest, and we're losing 2.4 acres of it *per second*.[41] That's 144 acres per minute. Seventy-five *million* acres per year! Rain forest used to cover 14 percent of the earth, but now it covers only 6 percent. You see, every hamburger requires a plot of land the size of a small kitchen to be cleared. Is that burger worth it?

Let's take a look at what we're giving up:

Oxygen: It is estimated that the global rain forests produce 40 percent[42] of the oxygen we breathe, so think of the rain forests of the world as the planet's lungs. By cutting them down, we are literally choking ourselves to death. Plus, by cutting and burning the rain forest, we are sending even more carbon dioxide into the atmosphere. Consider this: The average American car produces 3 kilograms of carbon per day. The clearing and burning of enough Costa Rican rain forest to produce one hamburger creates 75 kilograms of carbon.[43] And once that forest is gone, it ain't coming back.

Biodiversity: It is estimated that within a 4-square-mile patch of rain forest, you would find the following: 60 types of amphibians, 100 species of reptiles, 125 different mammals, 400 types of birds, 750 different trees, and 1,500 species of flowering plants.[44] Some experts believe that six plant or animal species become extinct due to rain forest destruction every hour. That's tragic enough, but biodiversity is about much more than pleasing birdwatchers and ecotourists. Our natural world is a dynamic system that has evolved over billions of years. Within this sophisticated system, every single organism has a very special job. We—the almighty humans—think these little guys are expendable, but they're not. When we destroy them, we destroy ourselves. For example, we are all totally dependent upon bees to pollinate flowers and plants, without which we would die. For all our technology, we have yet to develop a man-made substitute for the neat trick of mass pollination. Same thing with worms aerating and nourishing the soil—we can't do that ourselves! Well done, worms! Even fresh air and water—vital necessities we take for granted—are created by interlinking biosystems that we cannot reproduce. Ever tried making your own air?

Finally, more than 2,000 tropical forest plants have been identified by scientists as having anticancer properties, and 70 percent of the plants identified by the U.S. National Cancer Institute as useful in the treatment of cancer are found *only* in rain forests.[45]

So, clearly, rain forests are much more than "just" trees. That kind of rich biodiversity doesn't spring back in one generation or even a hundred. With the land being used to feed or graze cattle, who will soon turn it into desert, it may never come back at all.

Hopefully, we'll understand—before it's too late—that we can't survive in a world consisting of concrete and human beings, even if we wanted to. So if you choose to eat meat—whether it's beef, pork, chicken, or fish—know that you are stepping very heavily on the planet.

NASTY TO ANIMALS

Animals are my friends—and I don't eat my friends.
—George Bernard Shaw

Killing is a big deal: We tend to hide from this fact, but let's open our minds to it for just a moment. That was a life. Now it's dead. And it's in your body. Ever seen someone make the transition to death? It's a big deal—especially when there's suffering involved. Just for a moment, stop thinking of it as a delicious treat. Go beyond the sensory pleasure of your taste buds and consider for a moment what you're really doing when you eat meat. Could you eat your dog? Your cat? Why not? It's just an animal like a cow or a pig. What's the difference between your pet and the animal you had for dinner last night? If your answer is "I don't know," please meditate on that question for a while before eating meat again.

If your answer is "Well, I *love* my dog and he loves me—that's the difference," I ask you to consider what you're really saying. Does that mean any person I don't love is also disposable? Is "loving" the litmus test here? Or is it a matter of aesthetics? If so, who made up the rules that

---

Fish Are People, Too!

If you think that fish brains are so small they don't do much, think again. Dr. Culum Brown, an Australian behavioral ecologist, has conducted experiments with rainbow fish and found that they have longer memories than we assumed (months as opposed to seconds), the capacity to learn, and that they transmit their knowledge to other members of their school. He's even teaching fish raised in hatcheries how to respond to predators before being released into the ocean so they have a better chance of survival. So next time a fish looks at you from inside a tank at a Chinese restaurant, read his lips; he's probably yelling, "Get me out of here!"

cows, pigs, and chickens can be food, but dogs and cats are cute, cuddly things, or that squirrels are cute but rats are not? What's the difference between your dog's sweet eyes and a cow's?

If you can tell me you honestly believe there is a difference, then you've probably never hung out with a cow. I encourage you to go to an animal sanctuary and hang around with a few. They will love it, and so will you. Roll around with the pigs. Tell me that they don't love living and that they don't feel pain. Every single creature wants to live fully. That's what God designed us to do. That's our purpose. Who are we to take that away unless we have to? And these days, where's the "have to"? We used to think that slavery was okay, but we got over that. Why can't we get over the needless torture and killing of animals for our sensory satisfaction?

Meat production is downright cruel: The meat industry has also brainwashed us into thinking that we are eating happy cows from peaceful green pastures and that the mom-and-pop farms they come from are part of the great American dream. In truth, the vast majority of the meat you eat comes from corporate-owned factory farms, and even the moms and pops have to go "factory" in order to compete. Yes, there are farms that embrace more humane practices, but they are few and far between.

And it's not just the pigs and cows who suffer. Farm-raised fish are kept in cages with 40,000 other fish, enjoying the equivalent of half a bathtub of water each. Every egg has an abused chicken for a mother. People like to tell themselves that the animals have been treated decently during their lives and are then slaughtered relatively humanely, but their lives are not lives in any sense that we could relate to. From maternal separation to forced feeding of antibiotic and pesticide-laden grains to being locked in ridiculously small quarters and being pumped so full of growth hormones that they can no longer support their own weight, their lives are pure torture. But the real price is paid in a way we rarely consider; the chicken, born with wings to flap, never flaps them. Her beak, meant for pecking the earth, is cut off. The cow, meant to roam, is confined to a stall carpeted in her own waste. Sixty-five million

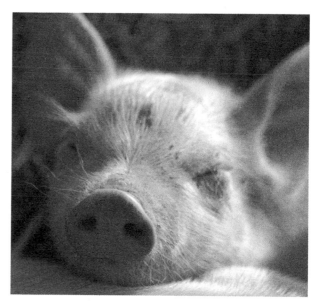

pigs are raised in confinement factories where they never see the light of day until they are trucked to slaughter. These animals experience lives tantamount to humans being strapped into straitjackets, locked in cells, abused by jailers, awaiting nothing but death. Their God-given instincts are repressed and their very beings denied.

And by the end, they know what's coming. Don't kid yourself. They can smell the blood. They can sense the fear. They can hear the other animals moaning. Wouldn't you understand, in their position? Denial would have us equate slaughter with having a pet "put down" at the vet. But that's just a comfortable delusion.

Facts:

- 90,000 U.S. cows and calves are slaughtered every day.
- 14,000 chickens are killed in the United States every *minute*.[46]
- Over 300 million male baby chicks are killed in this country per year—more than one for every person living in this country.

Although the Federal Humane Slaughter Act is supposed to keep certain practices in place, the law is rarely enforced. In 2000, a videotape was leaked out of workers at an Iowa Beef Processors (now

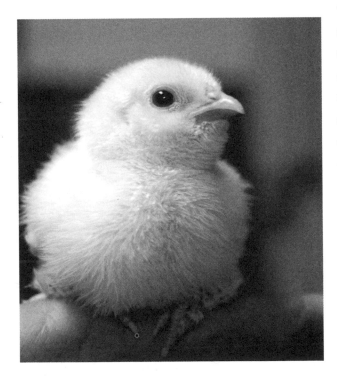

Tyson Foods) plant in Washington State. Cows were routinely "stunned" by devices that didn't work, left to experience their painful ends with sensitivity and consciousness intact. The video showed cows being skinned alive, kicking for freedom as their legs were cut off. Employees who were willing to talk estimated that 30 percent of the animals on the kill line were not properly stunned.

Also in 2000, a video showed footage of pigs at a North Carolina hog factory being kicked, stomped on, and killed by blows to the head with cinder blocks. Pigs who did not measure up to industry standards for sale were picked up by the hind legs and bashed against the floor, a practice called "thumping."

I know these stories are hard to read, but it's the reality of what goes into the food on your plate. The greatest crime being committed against these animals is not the eating of their meat, but our willful ignorance of their experience. As long as we keep our eyes closed, we can feel comfortable, and as long as we're comfortable, they will continue to suffer and die.

It's easy to get angry at the cattle ranchers and the big business that keeps meat rolling into our stores and restaurants, but I have to remember that they are just responding to market demands. If we stop the flow of money to these industries by converting to a plant-based diet, they will eventually have to convert their land and processing facilities into newer, more profitable ventures. Livelihoods need not be lost—they will just change. Likewise, as we spend our dollars on sustainable, ethical industries, we create a better world. It's simple.

When asked, the majority of Americans consider themselves animal lovers and are genuinely interested in treating animals humanely, yet we spend our hard-earned cash to support cruelty every day. We grill it up on the barbecue, add some ketchup, wash it down with a beer, and then

Eggs

More than 95 percent[47] of eggs sold in the United States come from birds confined in wire battery cages so small they can hardly move. They are virtual laying machines who are sick, abused, and often starved. After all their hard work, these birds end up so spent that the meat can only be used to make soup, chicken pies, and pet food. The rest of the hens are in such bad shape by the end that they are beaten to death, gassed, or thrown live into wood chippers.

Other victims of the egg industry are male chicks; because egg operations need many more hens than roosters, baby male chicks are routinely disposed of in one of two ways: Either they are thrown into dumpsters full of other baby chicks, left to suffocate, or they are put, live, through meat grinders to be fed to other livestock. Female chicks have their beaks ground off with a hot blade at 1 or 2 days old.

God help us all.

P.S. In terms of egg-labeling, beware of "free-range" eggs. When applied to eggs, the term "free-range" has no legal definition in this country. The term "cage-free" does not ensure any humane treatment nor does it imply access to the outdoors. Wings, beaks, and feet are still routinely clipped. Even hormone- and antibiotic-free labels mean nothing in terms of how the chickens are treated. The only certifications that pertain to animal treatment are "Certified Humane Raised and Handled" (beware of imposters; those exact words must be printed on the label) and "Certified Organic," which also upholds relatively humane standards.

take an antacid in order to digest it all! Weird. Meanwhile, the industries doing the killing—while creating images of happy cows and free-running chickens to assuage our guilt—are working overtime to push through legislation that permits them to be even more cruel and make more money.

Maybe it's time to ask the question: Is consuming all this pain and terror hurting us on levels we can't perceive? Is it cutting us off from the compassion deep within us? By not only condoning cruelty but literally consuming it, have we become desensitized to violence—against not only animals but ourselves and one another?

KICKING MEAT

When I gave up meat, I was so committed to the cause of protecting animals that I really didn't pay much attention to any physical or emotional discomfort I may have experienced, and it was such a long time ago that it's hard for me even to remember what it feels like to miss meat. Whereas I've had a handful of slips with dairy and more than a handful with sugar, I have never slipped on meat, so I'm going to lean on the experiences of my recently vegan friends who report the following challenges when kicking meat:

Cravings for meat's meatiness: Flesh has a unique texture, taste, and density. Some people say that, for a couple of months, they have a little difficulty feeling truly satisfied by a meatless

---

Superheroes: Kenneth Williams and Robert Cheeke

Think skipping meat will make you weak? At 5'11", Kenneth Williams is a professional vegan bodybuilder who knows that grains, beans, and vegetables are the perfect fuel for creating a beautiful, sculpted, and strong body. A passionate activist, Kenneth also hosts *Undercover TV*, which exposes the truth behind factory farms.

Twenty-nine-year-old Robert Cheeke lives in Portland, Oregon, but travels constantly as a bodybuilder, motivational speaker, and model. Thankfully, Robert requires no steak, eggs, or milk to keep up the pace. Robert is 100 percent vegan and looks fantastic.

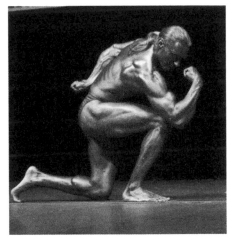

meal. It seems to take a while for the body to adjust to a whole new sense of fullness and satisfaction. Thankfully, this simply passes with time. As you make the transition, I recommend eating hearty, satisfying protein dishes, especially those containing tempeh and seitan and prepared with generous amounts of oil and seasoning. This will help your body begin to recognize a new type of fullness and satisfaction that isn't doing damage to it.

Feeling weak or experiencing a shift in energy levels: Meat is intense. As the muscle of another creature, it generates a certain type of warm and aggressive energy in us before it settles in and does its damage. Plant foods are calmer and lighter and fuel us in a very different way. It's not uncommon to experience a shift from the heaviness of meat to the lighter power of plants that feels a little strange or is misrecognized as weakness. Think of it this way: Your body, which has been accommodating meat its entire life, is now cleaning out and reworking its engine. This takes some time and is a very big deal. Be patient, and you will find that your body definitely prefers the new system and performs even better on plant power—Bruce Lee's did!

Convincing yourself that you need meat: The meat-pushers are loud. Using fear, bad science, and nutritional superstition, friends, family, or even your own mind may try to talk you into going back to meat. Don't listen. It's just old habits and misinformation creating excuses to indulge. There is absolutely no reason you need meat in order to survive or thrive. In fact, it's just the opposite: Your old friend flesh is keeping your body tired, weak, and toxic.

And anecdotal evidence from my friends bears this out. It amazes me how often I hear people say, "I stayed away from meat for a month and decided to have a hamburger one day, and I was up all night throwing up" or "I was constipated for days" or "I had horrible cramps." Some people don't really recognize how well their body is functioning until they conduct a little experiment. Although I don't recommend going back to meat for that purpose, the results always show that the body has started to hum along nicely on its plant-based diet and that adding meat back into the picture just screws it all up. When I hear this, I'm always sad that my friend has suffered, but inside I'm yelling, "Yay!" that the meat has shown its true colors.

So whether you decide to go cold turkey on meat or continue to flirt with it for a while, you will see that the body wants to be free of meat's heaviness and has the capacity to respond in swift and powerful ways. I urge you to give it a chance.

> The greatness of a nation . . . can be judged
> by the way its animals are treated.
> —Mahatma Gandhi

Nasty Food #2: Dairy

I know what you're thinking: "Dairy . . . nasty? How could that be? It's so good for you! Without milk, where am I going to get my calcium?"

I hear you. I grew up on dairy, too. My mother used to throw tea parties for her friends when I was a kid; she'd serve scones with clotted cream, and I'd drink four big cups of English Breakfast tea with milk and sugar. I believed milk was a perfect food without which I would basically collapse into a pile of splintered bones.

Dairy is one of the most difficult foods to discuss with people for two big reasons: First, we have all been hypnotized by the National Dairy Council, which has been pushing milk since 1915. It has presented itself as a protective parent, looking out for the country's health by encouraging us all to have three servings of milk or milk products per day. Well, the National Dairy Council is just a big, rich, organized group that lobbies Congress to subsidize them, funds research to support their claims, and launches incredibly expensive advertising campaigns. Remember the milk mustache campaign? So cute, right? Well, 190 million cute little dollars were spent on it, convincing us that three servings a day were a virtual guarantee of good health.[1] And who exactly pays for those 76,000 glasses of milk you drink over a lifetime? And who pockets that money? Hmmm . . .

Farmers have the right to push their products, but I encourage you to reexamine your beliefs about milk and dairy products. Are you afraid of not drinking milk? Do you see milk as a hedge against osteoporosis? A way to build strong teeth? Lose weight? Then try to reconcile those beliefs with the fact that the Chinese, throughout their long and complicated history, have never included milk or cheese in their diets. It's only in the very recent past that dairy has been introduced as a daily food, and with it has come a rapid rise in health problems like obesity and breast cancer. And how about Japan? Ever seen a glass of milk at a Japanese restaurant? The idea that human beings need milk in order to be strong or to function as a culture is simply not true.

The second reason it's hard to discuss letting go of dairy food is that it's addictive. Milk contains a protein called casein, which breaks down in the body to become caso*morphins*, as in "morphine." Casomorphins have an opiate effect[2] on your body and—like all good opiates—make you feel relaxed and happy. Casein is even more concentrated in cheese, which explains why people are very, very protective of their cheese! I can honestly say that I never think longingly about a glass of milk, but a piece of cheese? Mmmm . . . And that makes biological sense: Casomorphins were designed by nature to make a baby feel wonderful while attached to her mother. . . . How beautiful is that!? But when we get high on it as adults, we basically become milk junkies. And no junkie wants to give up her drug of choice.

So take a deep breath. No one's asking you to give it up. I'm just asking you to look at it from a different angle, to get past the hocus-pocus of the Dairy Council, and to be open to some new information.

Milk is nasty to your body: Our bodies are not meant to drink any milk except our own mother's milk, and only when we are babies! We don't drink our own mother's milk when we are 8, or 15, or 30, so why would our bodies accept another creature's milk? Did you know that we are the only animals that drink another species' milk? Pandas don't drink *gorilla* milk . . . dogs don't drink *goat* milk. . . . Even *cows* don't drink cow's milk once they've grown up—they wean themselves naturally.

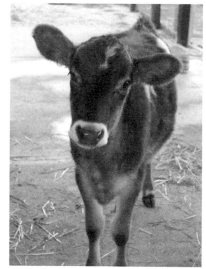

The fact is that many humans can't drink milk from other animals. In the United States, as many as 80 percent of African Americans, 90 percent of Asian Americans, and 60 percent of Hispanics are lactose-intolerant to some degree.[3] People with lactose intolerance experience gas, discomfort, and sometimes diarrhea upon drinking milk, so they wisely stay away from it. Those of us who can digest cow's milk are thought to have a genetic mutation that occurred thousands of years ago so we could survive on a herd's milk under harsh conditions.[4]

Dairy makes you fat: Remember, cow's milk is

designed to turn a baby calf into a *400-pound cow*. That, my friend, is big. And how does that happen? Well, cow's milk is made for babies, and all we really ask babies to do is get nice and fat. We're not expecting them to think, or run around, or make a living. High in protein and fat, but low in carbs and devoid of fiber, frozen yogurt seems specifically designed to turn you into a fat, slow, docile cow. Even human milk, with its greater proportion of carbohydrates, fuels energy and brain development, making it a better choice. But then, of course, *we don't drink human milk as adults*!

Eliminate milk, and you will notice your body slimming down nicely. A recent ad campaign featuring hourglass-shaped glasses of milk suggested a connection between drinking milk and weight loss. Well, the study was done by one researcher who happened to be sponsored by—big surprise—the good ol' Dairy Council, and the weight loss results came about only in conjunction with good ol' *calorie restriction*! Imagine that! Restrict your calories and lose weight! Absolutely revolutionary! Upon being sued by the Physicians Committee for Responsible Medicine, the Dairy Council was forced to suspend the advertising campaign and redact its claims. Yet we're still carrying around that hourglass of milk in our minds.

Dairy food has been linked to cancer: The medical world acknowledges that some of the biggest factors in breast cancer are fat, animal protein, and excess estrogen. Well, since milking cows are pumped full of extra estrogen to make them lactate, dairy is your best and cheapest daily source of all three. Moreover, cows injected with bovine growth hormone have higher levels of a naturally occurring hormone called IGF-1 (insulin-like growth factor-1), which is also connected to tumor growth.[5]

Superhero: Dr. Neal Barnard

Dr. Barnard specializes in helping people change their lives through diet. In 1985, he founded the Physicians Committee for Responsible Medicine (PCRM), a nonprofit organization that promotes preventive medicine, conducts clinical research, and encourages higher standards for ethics and effectiveness in research. PCRM is the loudest voice against the food and drug companies that seek to sell their wares without concern for the truth or the consumer's highest good. Dr. Barnard has written eight books on diet as it relates to illnesses such as heart disease, obesity, diabetes, and chronic pain.

Superhero: T. Colin Campbell

Growing up on a dairy farm, T. Colin Campbell believed—like most Americans—that milk was the perfect food. To that end, he did graduate research in animal nutrition in order to make bigger, better cows and pigs for us to eat. Like many, he bought into the national belief that protein derived from animal products was superior to all other types and was the key to what made America's diet the best in the world. He and his colleagues considered it their mission to help struggling nations to get as much animal protein into their diets as possible.

But Campbell's theory was turned on its head when he stumbled upon an Indian study that showed dairy protein triggering tumor growth. Skeptical of the results, he decided to conduct his own version of the experiments. The conclusions were consistent and stunning: Even when huge doses of cancer-causing toxins were given to study subjects, tumors grew *only* when they were fed casein, the protein in dairy foods. Conversely, wheat and soy protein—combined with the same doses of cancer-causing toxins—triggered no tumors.

Later, after compiling data from his monumental research project called the China Study, Campbell found more than *8,000* statistically significant correlations between various dietary factors and disease—a huge number of them pointing to the protein from meat and dairy as the bad guys.

After conducting 27 years of research funded by the National Institutes of Health, the American Cancer Society, and the American Institute for Cancer Research, Dr. Campbell emerged a strict vegan, stating:

"The diet that has time and again been shown to reverse and/or prevent these diseases is the same whole foods, plant-based diet that I had found to promote optimal health in my laboratory research and in the China Study. *The findings are consistent.*" [6]

In a study comparing the cancer rates of 42 countries, milk and cheese consumption were strongly linked to the incidence of testicular cancer among men ages 20 to 39. The cancer rates were highest in places like Switzerland and Denmark, where cheese is a national food, and lowest in Algeria and other countries with lower dairy consumption. [7] The American Dietetic Association reports that breast cancer rates are highest in places where women consume high-fat, animal-based diets. Did you know that in countries where dairy is not consumed the incidence of breast cancer is so low as to be almost nonexistent? Once women in those countries begin eating Western diets, however, their breast cancer rates increase eightfold. Even the American

For more information visit us at: www.thekindlife.com

Cancer Society recommends that we choose most of the foods we eat from plant sources and limit our intake of high-fat foods, especially from animal sources, in order to reduce the risk of cancer. More than 190,000 of our American girlfriends will get breast cancer in 2009 and more than 40,000 of them will die of it.[8] That is so, so sad. Sadder still is the fact that many of these deaths could have been prevented.

Milk does not prevent osteoporosis: This is a particularly touchy subject. This is where we—especially us womenfolk—have been completely boondoggled. We've come to believe there is a straight line between milk and strong bones despite the fact that dairy-free countries have the lowest rates of osteoporosis on Earth. In fact, the more milk a population consumes, the *weaker* its bones get. That's the *real* straight line. So why does this fallacy that milk is inextricably linked to strong, healthy bones persist so stubbornly? It's true that cow's milk does contain calcium, which is necessary for strong bones, but that's not the whole picture. Although milk offers calcium, it causes the body to *release* even more of it. It's like someone giving you $1,000 but driving away in your car! So no matter how much you're getting, you're

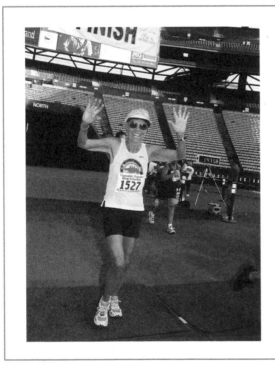

Superhero: Ruth Heidrich

Ruth was diagnosed with breast cancer at 47. After having the lump removed, further testing revealed cancerous hot spots in her bones and one on her lung. Heidrich decided to follow a strict vegan diet under the supervision of Dr. John MacDougall, who was researching the connection between diet and breast cancer at the time. Twenty-six years later, having undergone neither chemo nor radiation, Ruth not only thrives cancer-free, she has completed six Ironman triathlons, 67 marathons, and was named one of the "Ten Fittest Women in America" in 1999. She lives in Hawaii and Canada, where she writes books (*Senior Fitness, A Race for Life*), gives lectures, and cohosts a radio show called *Healing and You.*

actually losing. Meat and dairy are the chief *causes* of osteoporosis, not the cures. There are tons of sources of calcium on a meat- and dairy-free diet, and the calcium they contain is actually more readily absorbed by the body. Sea vegetables, sesame seeds, leafy greens, and beans all kick milk's butt.

Calcium Milligrams (per 100-gram serving)	
Butter	20
Whole milk	118
Chickpeas	150
Collard greens	203
Parsley	203
Soybeans	226
Almonds	234
Sesame seeds	1,160
Hijiki sea vegetable	1,400

Milk underlies asthma and allergies: This one hits home for me. As a kid, I came down with bronchitis three or four times each year. At a visit to the allergist, I was diagnosed with numerous allergies and was prescribed twice-weekly shots and an inhaler. Well, I lost the inhaler on a camping trip in my teens, but I was still getting allergy shots well into my early twenties. As far as I was concerned, I would need them forever. But very soon after becoming vegan, I stopped experiencing allergies or any asthma-type symptoms. They just disappeared.

You see, the human immune system recognizes milk from another species as an attacker—or allergen—that causes the body to go on red alert. This is why many people walk around with chronic runny, stuffy noses—even asthma and allergies—and think it's *normal*! But actually it's the body's own defense system trying to ward off a foreign invader. Dr. John Oski, chief of pediatrics at Johns Hopkins School of Medicine, believes that up to 50 percent of all children are allergic to milk, although they remain largely undiagnosed. This allergy is the underpinning of all sorts of other conditions such as sinusitis, ear infections, eczema, and even behavioral problems. Get rid of the dairy, and you should breathe easier within a week. You'll be amazed.

Dairy food has been linked to diabetes: Studies done at the University of Helsinki and the Hospital for Sick Children in Toronto showed that babies fed dairy-based formula began to develop antibodies for diabetes. As in the case of allergies, the protein in cow's milk is perceived by the immune system as an attacker. So the immune system fights back—that's its job! Unfortunately, one of these proteins is a dead ringer for a certain cell found in the pancreas, so in fighting off the perceived "attacker," the body starts to fight its own pancreas, eventually destroying its ability to produce precious insulin. The studies show that genetics may be a factor as well, but it seems that dairy is a significant trigger.

In Puerto Rico, where approximately 95 percent of babies start life on cow-based formula, the type 1 diabetes rate is *10 times higher* than in Cuba, where almost every baby begins on mommy's boob.[9]

We think of diabetes as a tragic twist of fate that pushes the sufferer into the medical system to become dependent on daily injections until death—if she's lucky! Diabetes kills 72,000 people a year in the United States (and contributes to 230,000 deaths),[10] and what we're drinking at the breakfast table plays a role. *That's* the tragic twist.

What about Eggs?

Eggs are weird. Not technically a dairy product but commonly lumped into this category, an egg is the reproductive cell of a chicken. Hmm ... We don't eat our own reproductive cells or those of most other species, so what are we doing scrambling and poaching what a poor hen ovulates?

Egg producers go to great lengths to get their product good press, and it seems to work. Whereas eggs were considered bad guys just a decade ago, nutritionists and the media are now giving them a passing grade. But the nutritional benefits of eggs ... protein, lutein, and an array of vitamins and minerals, are all easily found in plant-based sources. Meanwhile, eggs are crazy high in cholesterol; one egg contains approximately 200 milligrams of the stuff. So there's nothing magic about eggs. In fact, 95 percent of the eggs sold in the United States come from industrialized operations using antibiotics that are passed on to the eggs. If you do choose to eat eggs and are buying them from an organic and antibiotic-free producer, there's still no getting around the cholesterol issue. And remember: Conventional eggs are hiding in lots of the foods you might be ordering at restaurants: pancakes, Caesar salads, muffins, cakes ... so choose carefully.

Dairy is messing with our hormones: Dairy cows are pumped full of hormones to force them to produce up to 20 times their normal milk supply, and those hormones go straight into you. Excess hormones in dairy food are now thought to be a factor in reproductive cancers and even precocious puberty. In 1900, American girls started menstruating, on average, at the age of 14. These days, they begin at 12½, with the first signs of puberty showing up in some girls as young as 7. Some argue that the excess estrogen found in milk kickstarts the body to enter puberty earlier, and it also wreaks unnatural havoc on men's hormone levels. Yes, organic, hormone-free milk is better for the drinker with respect to the hormone issues, but it's still milk, and it still causes all the other problems mentioned earlier.

Dairy is bad for your heart: Milk, like meat, is full of saturated fat and cholesterol, which clog arteries to your heart. In study after study, incidence of heart disease increases with milk consumption. Researchers for the *Journal of Internal Medicine* write: "It is clear that saturated fats, mainly dairy fats, are closely associated with the mortality rate from ischaemic [artery blocking or constricting] heart disease."[11]

NASTY TO THE PLANET

Dairy cows create greenhouse gases: More burping = more methane = more global warming = Uh-oh.

Dairy cows produce toxic, freaky waste: These cows produce millions of tons of waste filled with antibiotics and growth hormones that seep into the earth and the water supply. Residues of antibiotics used only in animals have shown up in rivers and soil samples far from the original sites—even getting into drinking water supplies.

The hormones from dairy waste found in rivers have begun to alter the hormone balance of certain fish, causing female eggs to be found in the testes of the males. By forgoing that latte (or making it with soymilk), you will keep our soil and water cleaner and less freaky.

Pregnant cows eat a lot of food: Just like pregnant women, cows need lots of food to make a baby. All that food requires land, water, energy, fertilizer, labor, and transport we could be using for other things, like growing food for people. By saying "no" to that frozen yogurt, we can feed ourselves and others more cheaply and efficiently.

And they drink even more water: You need to drink water to make milk, so a lactating cow drinks 30 to 50 gallons of the stuff a *day*.[12] That's a bathtub full. Your eight glasses of water

Water

The planet's supply of fresh water is finite, so let's conserve it. Turn off the tap when you brush your teeth. Be mindful of saving water when you do your dishes and laundry or when you wash yourself. Flush only after number 2. Watch the film *FLOW* to learn more about the global water crisis. For more ideas about conserving and to figure out your water footprint, go to www.thekindlife.com and type in keyword water footprint.

a day is half a gallon. The average dairy farm, between hydrating the cows and washing down the facilities, uses many millions of gallons of water per year.

Making milk takes a lot of energy: Dairy farms use hundreds of thousands of kilowatt-hours of electricity per year to run the pumps that milk the cows. Not to mention the lights, filters, heating systems, and other energy-sucking devices. Since 90 percent of the electricity in the United States comes from nonrenewable sources—and dirty ones at that—the dairy industry is a big, unnecessary drain on the global light socket.

NASTY TO ANIMALS

The dairy industry is, in a word, cruel: That is why I gave up dairy in the first place. You see, cows don't produce milk all the time. I thought that, by milking them, we were basically doing them a favor. I assumed they would sort of . . . *explode* if they weren't milked! Well, they don't. Just like humans, they only produce milk when they give birth to a baby. So in order to have careers in lactation, cows are kept pregnant almost constantly.

Once she gives birth, her calf is taken away from her; baby boys become veal and girls become milkers. The separation anxiety she feels is as real to her as it would be to us. Cows have been known to escape their farms and go searching for their offspring. A farmer in England found one of his dairy cows a full 7 miles from home, suckling her biological calf.

But if we're taking the cow's milk for our use, what does the baby get? Well, for 6 months the baby boy calves are chained to little veal crates, not allowed to stand up, fed synthetic formula, and then slaughtered. And that is how we get veal. So if you use any cow dairy products, you are helping perpetuate the veal industry.

After baby is gone, mom cow is shot up with hormones to make her produce *10 to 20* times more milk than she would need to suckle her calf. This puts tremendous strain on her udders—

think of a woman with painful GGG implants hanging to her knees—often causing a horrible infection called mastitis, which makes her udders pus-ridden and bloody. To treat the mastitis, they have to give her antibiotics.

Finally she gets milked—and not by some nice pair of hands gently caressing her udders, but by a machine that is so rough it causes the blood and pus from the mastitis to go *into the milk*!

After 2 to 7 years of this (normal cows should live 20 to 25 years, but dairy cows are burned out by this torture), our cow girlfriend doesn't get to retire and live on a farm—no, no, no. She is considered a machine that has outlived its warranty, so she is sent to slaughter. Her life is miserable and painful from day one until the very end.

KICKING DAIRY

The trick to kicking dairy is to *replace it* with other yummy things, and I promise, you won't feel deprived. Okay, maybe if you are at a party and a huge tray of a variety of cheeses goes by you'll feel a twinge. Once in a blue moon I do succumb and have a bite of cheese, but it just serves to remind me of how bad I feel on dairy; it's like my body rejects it—I get gassy and fart a lot, my skin breaks out, and I get all phlegmy. And it just doesn't make me feel good . . . it's like I plugged up my engine.

Far from the perfect food we've been told it is, dairy is actually causing very serious problems, but there is life after dairy. A delicious, healthy, happy life.

I recently threw a tea party in honor of my mother. I served shortbread cookies dipped in chocolate, strawberry shortcake, scones with veggie butter, and English Breakfast tea with soy milk. Not a drop of dairy in anything, and it was scrumptious!

4

More Nasty Stuff:
White Sugar and Processed Foods

While white sugar and processed foods don't do quite the same damage to the earth or to animals as do meat and dairy, they wreak nothing less than havoc on your body and are a million miles from kind. For those reasons, I recommend you do your best to kick them out of your life.

Before you throw up your hands and declare you can't live without candy bars, let me assure you that your life will remain sweet, scrumptious, and satisfying without white sugar or your favorite microwavable snacks. In fact, natural sweets and desserts will keep you happier than you ever thought possible, and processed foods will naturally start taking a backseat to the good stuff as you fall in love with the new pantry of whole, unprocessed foods you'll be making on both the Vegan and Superhero programs. So you can relax as we discuss ditching the white stuff.

NASTY FOOD #3: SUGAR

Sugar is crack.

Like crack, white sugar lifts you up, up, up, then smacks your head on the floor, leaving you wasted and useless. And yet within minutes you're begging for more. Why?

White sugar is highly processed: Nature grows foods in their whole forms, and for the most part we're supposed to eat them that way. When we do, we get each plant's unique combination of vitamins, minerals, fiber, and carbohydrates, and our bodies know how to metabolize them perfectly. Yay, nature! But when we eat foods from which bits and pieces have been removed through processing, our bodies get confused and stressed out trying to make up for the missing elements. Instead of creating natural balance, the processed "food" creates imbalance, which in turn leads to *more* imbalance. This is how a food can affect our body like a drug. And sugar is a great example.

That's why my crack analogy is so apt. Consider these other examples. Cocaine comes from the South American coca leaf, a leaf that millions of people chew every day without getting high, dancing all night with strippers, or burning through their bank accounts. Heroin comes from the poppy flower—a beautiful red flower whose seeds end up decorating your morning bagel. It's not the plant but the *processing* that creates the intensity and imbalance, transforming the plant into a drug. So gnawing on a piece of sugar cane is fine—your body can handle it because the sugar cane comes with nature's mix of vitamins, minerals, and fiber. But eat a frosted donut, and you'll get a rush and then a crash because your body just can't handle all that sugar without the other nutrients. This imbalance creates a number of serious problems in the human body and mind.

NASTY TO YOUR BODY

White sugar leaches vitamins and minerals from your blood and bones: Because refined, white sugar is so un-whole, your body actually offers up the missing bits and pieces to help metabolize it. In other words, your precious body gives up vitamins and minerals in order to process all the sugar! "Food" is by definition something that gives nourishment, but sugar is often called an "antinutrient" because it *takes* nourishment from the body. Eventually we get tooth decay, bone loss, depression, and weak blood. Not so sweet!

White sugar suppresses your immune system: If you get colds all the time, you might want to look at your sugar consumption. When you bite into that candy bar, your blood sugar soars to abnormal levels. In order to bring it back down, your pancreas releases a hormone called insulin to handle all the excess sugar. But once all the sugar has been metabolized, too much insulin remains, and this excess insulin causes imbalances in the rest of your hormones, particularly those related to your immune system. It's a great example of one imbalance creating another. This chaotic hormonal dance leaves you weakened and vulnerable to disease. To make matters worse, sugar takes on industrial toxins during processing, and these toxins overwork the liver. When the liver has too much gunk to handle, it deposits the extra toxins in the tissue of your body, leaving a messy toxic situation that weakens your immunity as well.

Sugar puts you on a roller coaster: Sounds fun, but it's not. Beyond the sensory pleasure and the initial rush, the roller coaster takes you to extreme peaks in blood sugar, which may include nausea, headaches, and fatigue, while the roller coaster's lows (blood sugar crashing) bring on irritability, anxiety, dizziness, heart palpitations, crying, and depression. Oh yeah, and cravings for more sugar! Sugar consumption can lead to mood swings and behavior that, over years, we misrecognize as our true selves. I can personally attest that life is much happier and more balanced off the roller coaster.

White sugar is associated with cancer: As I said before, when your blood sugar soars, too much insulin is produced. This excess insulin promotes the growth of certain kinds of cancer cells, including those that attack the breasts, ovaries, lung, colon, prostate, and stomach.[1]

Sugar makes you fat: We used to think that it was only eating *fat* that made us fat. Now we know better. Because excess refined sugar converts to fat, every soda, every cupcake, and every candy bar is going *straight* to your thighs.

Sugar contributes to insulin resistance and diabetes: When you eat refined sugar, your blood sugar skyrockets to abnormal levels. In order to balance the situation, your pancreas releases lots of insulin to help usher the sugar into your cells, where it's used as fuel. However, if you're eating a steady diet of candy bars and other sugary foods, your blood is filled with sugar all the time. The insulin, designed to mop up all the sugar, stops working so well. That's bad. The sugar doesn't make it to the cells. This is called insulin resistance, and it's a doozy because your blood sugar remains high, but your cells are starving. So what do you crave? More sugar! This reinforces the horrible cycle. Over time, the pancreas can stop working, resulting in diabetes.

KICKING SUGAR

These days, I do my best to avoid sugar, but it wasn't always that way. When I first became vegan, I felt so good from giving up meat and dairy that I didn't notice how sugar was having its way with me. But that's the problem with extreme foods! You don't recognize their effects until you eliminate them.

As you change the way you eat, you will become more and more sensitive to what food is doing to you. Ultimately, giving up meat and dairy may be more important—and have a bigger impact on the planet—than giving up sugar, but there will definitely be a time when you recognize that the white stuff is not your friend. I do my best, but I'm no saint; I slip up on the sugar front quite a bit. At least every few weeks a sugary thing pops into my mouth and I really feel it.

When I eat white sugar . . .

- I get a headache. If I have sugar for a few days running, I start to feel a low-grade nausea. Not like I'm gonna throw up, just crappy.

- I end up gaining weight. Sugar is high in rapidly absorbed calories that are completely devoid of vitamins or minerals. No nourishment at all. This means extra sugar with no purpose other than to convert to fat. Sugar, like salt, can also cause you to retain water.

- After the initial rush, I feel really tired. There's too much to enjoy in life to feel tired all the time.

- The morning after eating sugar, I have bags under my eyes and feel mildly depressed. It's like a hangover without the fun the night before!

- After the sugar wears off, I feel moody and bitchy. I don't like myself much when I'm coming down from sugar, and that's no fun.

- I crave more sugar. This is how I *know* it really is a drug. Real, unprocessed foods nourish the body and make me feel whole, but sugar leaves me aching for more.

What Do You Mean by "Sugar"?

White sugar: Obviously you're familiar with sugar, but all ingredients ending in "-ose" should be considered white sugar as well: Dextrose, glucose, sucrose, maltose, and fructose are all simple sugars that show up often on food labels.

High fructose corn syrup (HFCS): Don't be fooled by the words "corn" and "fructose" here, which sound sort of innocent. Not only is HFCS as addictive as white sugar, it is in *everything* these days because corn is subsidized by the government—making it much cheaper than cane sugar for use in soda and processed foods. Worse, the corn used to make HFCS has been genetically modified (for more on genetically modified foods, go to page 65). Worst of all, because of its unique formulation, high fructose corn syrup is suspected to cause insulin resistance, believed to be a big contributor to our ever-climbing obesity rates.[2] HFCS may be even nastier than good old white sugar.

Organic evaporated cane juice: Yes, it's slightly less processed than white refined sugar, but it makes me feel almost as bad and it's just as addictive. It has a variety of sexy-sounding cousins, so watch out for Sucanat, Florida Crystals, and milled cane, as well as Turbinado, Muscovado, and Rapadura sugars.

Honey: Honey's hard to categorize. In terms of how quickly it raises blood sugar, it's very similar to the white stuff. I feel a strong sugar rush from honey, and I certainly don't use it in my cooking nor do I seek it out. From the cruelty angle, honey is an animal product, and mass honey production is not exactly kind to bees. Most vegans stay away from honey because of this. Yes, there are some groovy, kind beekeepers in the world, but they're not producing enough to make it to your grocery store.

NASTY FOOD #4: PROCESSED FOODS

Stay away from really crappy food. You know what I'm talking about: fast food; neon-colored or sparkly foods; canned, frozen, or boxed foods that have ingredient lists a mile long. Many of these processed foods contain preservatives and additives that are suspected to be carcinogens or that are contributors to obesity and heart disease. It's called "junk food" for a reason.

When convenience calls, go for healthy processed foods. Most companies who go to the trouble to make cruelty-free or organic processed foods also bother to kick out unnecessary chemicals. You'll notice on boxes of organic soups or vegan pizzas that the ingredient lists are shorter and more understandable. (See pages 84–85 for some of the convenience foods I rely on).

But don't get seduced by convenience too often. Let's face it: Anything coming out of a box is pretty lifeless. Yes, it's great for a party or at the end of a really hectic day, but your best health and deepest happiness will come from fresh, real, whole foods that you prepare yourself.

Congratulations! You've just learned some of the most important information of your life. By getting to the truth behind a mirage of misinformation, you now have the opportunity to

---

Artificial Sweeteners

Saccharin (in Sweet'N Low) and aspartame (in NutraSweet): In terms of safety, a history of controversy surrounds them both (neurological damage, bladder cancer, etc.), but I like to think of it this way: Neither of these substances was handed to us by nature. They were both synthesized in chemistry labs—one as a derivative of coal tar, and the other as an experiment to create an anti-ulcer drug. They just *happened* to be sweet and have no calories. The newest kid on the block is **sucralose** (in Splenda). This is a noncaloric byproduct of actual sugar—chlorinated sugar, to be precise—and many experts question its safety. In fact, it is following the exact path its predecessors did: failing safety tests, being approved by the FDA anyway, and now producing ever-growing anecdotal evidence of its ill effects.[3] But we're so obsessed with squeezing into that miniskirt, we don't seem to care.

My final question is, In what foods are you getting these sweeteners? Diet soda? Sugar-free gum? Pies that can sit on a shelf for a month? Chances are they are coming alongside a bunch of other chemicals, which make them even more unattractive. Remember: The closer we stick to nature, the closer we stick to good health and our true selves.

Caffeine: Would You Like Some Coffee with That Sugar?

Caffeine is the most popular drug in the world, used in every country and consumed by 87 percent of American adults and 76 percent of their children[4] every day. Whether it's from downing an energy drink, a soda, or an espresso, everyone's pretty jacked up these days. But all this speediness comes at a price. Caffeine stresses the immune system and your heart, reduces your ability to feel safe and peaceful, and can mess with your fertility! It also steals minerals from your blood and bones and dries you out, causing wrinkles! Caffeine sucks . . . literally! The one thing the coffee people will acknowledge it causes? Breast cysts. But who cares? They're just breasts!

You may be attracted to caffeine and coffee drinking for a number of different reasons:

- If you use it to stay awake or because you're just addicted, try black tea, green tea, or yerba maté instead. They're much easier on your body. Green juice can also be a good waker-upper. By the way, after a while on the Kind Diet, you shouldn't feel the need for stimulants.

- If you simply like the ritual and the smell of that morning cup of joe, go for a water-processed decaf, Teeccino (or any other grain coffee), or decaf tea instead.

- If you're just looking for that pause in the day to indulge yourself, take a real moment out of the hustle-bustle: Go for a stroll, pet your dog, or meditate for 5 minutes. I understand that indulging in a coffee break seems like self-love, but how kind are you being if you're never really at peace, never settled in your true self?

improve your health, make significant changes in the world, and live in a much more empowered way. I know some of that information wasn't pretty, but that's it. We're done. We're moving on now to the good stuff. Get ready for Kind Foods and how they will love and nourish you on every level for the rest of your life.

> He that takes medicine and neglects diet,
> wastes the skill of the physician.
> —Chinese Proverb

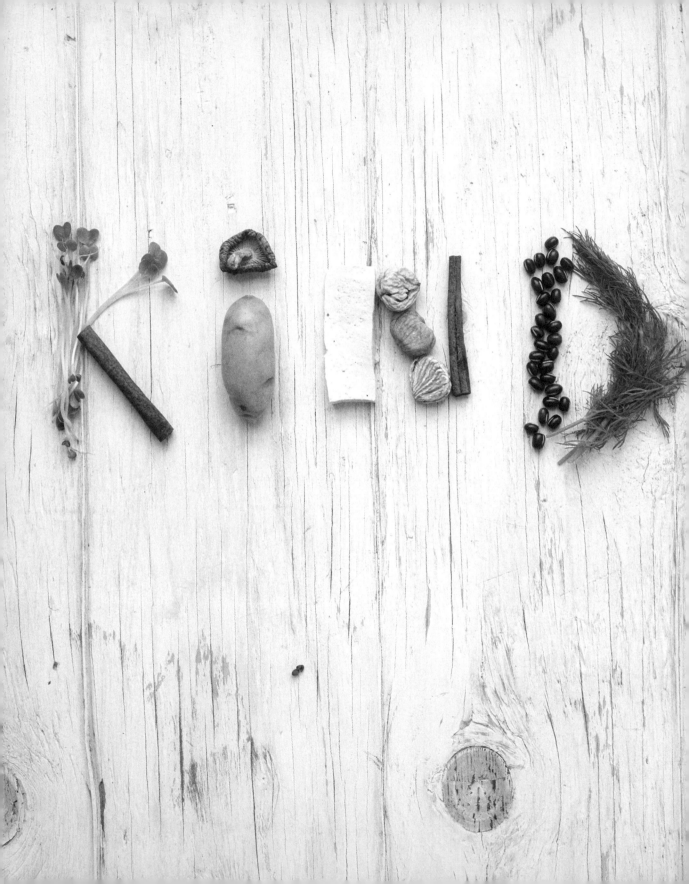

5

Kind Foods

> When diet is wrong medicine is of no use.
> When diet is correct medicine is of no need.
>
> Ancient Ayurvedic Proverb

I hope it's obvious by now that the chronic ingestion of nasty foods has gotten us into real trouble and far away from Hippocrates' sage suggestion to use foods to keep us well. Luckily, in the East, his words aren't wasted. You see, in traditional Oriental and Indian medicine, the human is considered a whole entity—body, mind, and spirit as one. Health is the beautiful, dynamic interplay of all organic systems, governed by nature rather than a stethoscope or a pill. The body is studied and treated as a whole rather than as a bunch of bits and pieces, and a fundamental life force called "chi," "ki," or "prana" is believed to run through it. Medicine is generally the practice of supporting this chi, strengthening it naturally and helping it flow when the river of energy gets stuck. Traditionally, an Eastern doctor's job was to support your inherent *wellness*—bringing you back to center as subtle imbalances arose—as opposed to fixing your illnesses. In fact, if you became ill in ancient China, you *stopped* paying your doctor because he was clearly slackin' on the job.

Furthermore, in Eastern thought, food is a big deal. It is understood that, because we eat three times a day every day of our lives, food is the biggest factor in health, or illness. If you question whether food is truly that powerful, I ask you: If you're willing to put a little pill in your mouth, trusting that it will change your whole body . . . why not a carrot? Why do you consider the carrot to be neutral or powerless over your body and mind? Maybe the things you put in your body—day after day, month after month, year after year—are a whole lot *more* powerful than the little pills you take to solve problems. Maybe Hippocrates was on to something.

If being healthy has meant, up until now, feeling "okay," let's try a new definition: What if health means feeling strong enough to do whatever you want to do, flexible enough to roll with life's blows, being peaceful inside, connected with your intuition, experiencing spontaneous bursts of gratitude, and feeling a very real sense of connectedness with all of life: nature, the universe, and all the living beings in it?

It's not difficult to achieve this new paradigm; by eating whole grains and vegetables, you will begin to feel more centered and balanced. Your blood will be strengthened, which will, in turn, support all of your vital organs. You will become more sensitive to imbalances, eventually correcting them intuitively. You will begin to experience some of the trippy, positive aspects of the Eastern model of wellness. And you will become happily responsible for your own health.

I'm here to remind you that eating is the most important thing you do. It determines how you look, how you feel, and even how you behave. Every meal drives your day in one direction or another. Food is the foundation of your life.

You are about to be introduced to an amazing cornucopia of natural foods, gems from the earth that not only taste good, but will make your body deliriously happy. And I'm not just talk-

---

In It for the Long Haul

Not only does this diet restore health and tighten waistlines, there's evidence it extends our lives as well. The U.S. National Institute on Aging did a study of the longest-lived peoples in the world and found the people of Okinawa (Japan), Sardinia, and Seventh Day Adventists are among the longest lived on earth.[1] Of course, this begs the question: Do they have common secrets? Yes, and they are:

- They eat lots of fruit, vegetables, and whole grains.
- They don't smoke.
- They are active every day.
- They stay socially engaged.
- The Adventists also eat lots of nuts and beans.

ing lentil loaf. Get ready to meet the beautiful, delicious, God-given foods that will rock your world. Welcome to the Kind Foods.

> I have become convinced that the most overlooked tool in our medical arsenal is harnessing the body's own ability to heal through nutritional excellence.[2]
> —Dr. Mehmet Oz (Yes, Oprah's Dr. Oz!)

KIND FOOD #1: WHOLE GRAINS

Whole grains are your new best friend and will be an essential part of your daily diet—ideally at every meal. These amazing little seeds are literally full of life and contain a pure, essential energy that we don't get from most other foods. Grains will keep you balanced, centered, energized, and focused in the midst of life's action. They are your new, perfect fuel. Grains will make you glow from the inside out. There is no substitute for whole grain.

Making whole grain the center of your diet may seem like a leap, but it's really not so weird. Since the dawn of modern agriculture—when people started farming, about 10,000 years ago—whole grain has been the centerpiece of the human diet. You're actually going with the flow of human history.

Correction: not *recent* human history. Although Americans have always liked their meat, grain products were not completely eclipsed by meat until after World War II, when North

For more information visit us at: www.thekindlife.com

Americans had enough money, fuel, and refrigeration devices to make meat a daily food. In fact, in many households, animal flesh started showing up three times a day: Bacon at breakfast, a ham and cheese sandwich for lunch, and a steak at dinner are considered a normal—even necessary—part of our affluent lifestyle. But all Asian cultures—elegant and sophisticated—were built on rice or millet; South and Central Americans were sustained by corn and quinoa while they built their amazing Incan walls and Mayan temples. Native Americans lived in harmony with the land on corn, wheat, and wild rice. Africa, rich with tribal history and tradition, grew up on sorghum, cassava (not a grain, but a complex carb), millet, and the tiniest grain of all, teff; while in Europe, wheat, barley, oats, and buckwheat were all traditional staples. So throughout all of modern human civilization, meat has been but a side dish to the nutritional superstar we call "grain."

Most people eat grain in the form of flour, but I'm not talking about bread and noodles when I say "whole grains." I mean wheat *before* it's ground into flour. And grains of rice *before* they're stripped of their hulls to make white rice. By eating the grain in its whole form, you get the full impact of its natural oomph and medicinal powers.

Whole grains include: brown rice, quinoa, wild rice, farro, millet, barley, whole oats, and more. You'll also find flour products made from whole grains including bread, noodles (whole wheat, quinoa, soba, and rice), and whole grain couscous. They're great to eat now and then, but you'll get the most dramatic benefits from keeping whole grains at the center of your plate.

WHAT'S WITH ALL THE CARBS?

But don't all these foods consist primarily of carbohydrates? And aren't carbs the root of all evil, especially for people trying to lose weight? Poor carbs. Diet books have given them a bad name. I'm talking about the good carbs here—the ones you *need* in your diet. All carbohydrates fall into one of two categories: simple and complex. Simple carbs—like white sugar and white flour—break down in the body really quickly, so your blood sugar spikes through the roof and then crashes. Complex carbs—like those in whole grains and vegetables—break down slowly, raising your blood sugar gently, and providing sustained energy over a long period of time, until you're ready to eat again. Complex carbs are awesome and totally necessary for your body to function.

In fact, let's get something straight: Those popular high-protein, low-carb diets are just plain bad for you. I'm not saying that you won't lose weight on them—at least for a little while—but you can lose just as much weight eating complex carbohydrates, and keep it off easily, without doing serious damage to your precious body. Ironically, a study funded by Dr. Atkins himself, a man synonymous with low-carb diets, found that, on his diet, 70 percent of people got constipated and 65 percent developed bad breath![3] You see, eating so much animal protein with so little fiber is a recipe for heart disease, cancer, arthritis, osteoporosis, and overworked internal organs; hello bad breath, constipation, dull skin, wrinkles, kidney stones, gout, and heavy energy! Yet many people have really convinced themselves that cutting back on carbs is the only way to lose weight, and plenty of new diets are happy to feed into this belief, betting you'll choose that bikini over your health. I'm here to tell you that you can have both.

So please, *please* stop freaking out about carbs.

Your body needs whole grains: These little powerhouses contain vitamins and minerals that help the body carry out its most basic functions, like metabolizing protein, secreting waste, and releasing energy from muscles. The complex carbohydrate keeps you balanced, the vitamin E protects your cells, the fiber's good for your heart . . . I could go on and on, but it's simpler to say this: Grain is our perfect fuel. Naturally complementary to the human body, it is fundamental to good health. By eating whole grains, you will break through to a new level of wellness.

Is Wheat Bad?

Wheat has gotten a bad rap lately because—like corn and soy—some form of wheat appears in almost every processed food, so our bodies have been bombarded and overloaded with wheat, often creating a mild intolerance.

Some people have a hard time digesting just the gluten found in wheat (and barley, oats, and a few other grains). True gluten intolerance is a genetic disorder called *celiac disease*, and it's relatively rare. If you think your body is not digesting grains properly, you can have your doctor order a blood test that will determine if you have celiac disease.

For most people who consider themselves "allergic" to wheat, white flour is often the culprit. Highly processed, often rancid, and commonly overeaten, white wheat flour can cause problems that *feel* like allergies. Cut out all flour for a while—to give your intestines a rest—follow the Superhero diet, and you may be able to tolerate whole wheat flour products after a few months . . . that's what happened to me!

Whole grains make you feel relaxed and happy: You will be amazed at how calm and peaceful you become as you introduce more whole grains into your daily diet. For one thing, they are chockfull of B vitamins, which relax the nervous system. Maybe that's why monks eat so much rice!

Here are more ways you'll benefit from eating whole grains:

You'll have great skin: The B vitamins found in whole grains are also necessary for making beautiful, glowing skin.

You'll feel balanced and connected with self: Whole grains make you *feel* whole. That may sound out there, but if you consider that highly refined foods can cause mood swings, hormone imbalances, and a rise in cholesterol (among other things), it makes sense that, conversely, an unprocessed food will keep us feeling balanced. Our physiology is designed to work with whole grains in their whole form, so they help us to feel *right* in our bodies and minds.

You'll lose weight easily: You never have to diet again. Low-calorie, low-fat whole grains will make you feel full, give you good energy, and nourish your body beautifully while helping you to lose weight.

You'll enjoy great poops: It's amazing how many people have a hard time on the toilet these days. You see, meat and dairy contain *no* fiber, so they are the perfect recipe for constipation. A diet rich in whole grains and vegetables, on the other hand, contains tons of fiber, and easy bowel movements are one of the first benefits people experience. No more time to read on the toilet!

Although they may be new to you, whole grains have a long history of providing stable, healthy energy to humans the world over. As you cook and eat these powerful foods on a daily basis, you will be amazed at how peaceful, smooth, and happy life can be.

KIND FOOD #2: NEW PROTEINS

The world is moving toward clean energy. Windmills, solar panels, and fully electric cars are all in our future as we move away from unsustainable, expensive, polluting sources of power. We can make that same shift in our bodies because beans are clean!

Think of meat as a funky fuel—it's heavy, contains toxins, and leaves gunk in your engine. Beans, on the other hand, burn cleanly in the body. Because they contain complex carbohydrates and fiber, beans not only supply protein to build and repair the body, they provide smooth, long-lasting energy while cleaning the engine!

Let's compare a steak to a cup of beans:

Steak	Beans
20% of calories from protein	25% of calories from protein
80% of calories from fat (mostly saturated)	5% of calories from fat (unsaturated)
0% of calories from complex carbohydrate	70% of calories from complex carbohydrate
Contains excess hormones	Helps discharge excess hormones
Raises cholesterol	Lowers cholesterol
No fiber	High in fiber
Contains steroids, antibiotics	If organic, contains no chemicals
Constipates	Keeps you regular
Unsustainably produced	Sustainably grown
Depletes the earth	Beans add needed nitrogen to soil
$5–$10/lb (1 serving)	$2–$4/lb (4 servings)

Plus beans don't require anything like the resources livestock do in order to grow—soil, sunshine, water . . . done! This simplicity makes them cheap and sustainable. If we all ate beans as our primary source of protein, we could feed the world easily.

When I still ate meat, I had a casual relationship with beans; I liked lentil soup at Shabbat dinner on Fridays, always enjoyed hummus, and topped my Sizzler salad bar creations with kidney and garbanzo beans. But I never once thought of beans as protein—that was meat's job! Now that I know how amazing and nutritious beans are, I truly appreciate them and our relationship has become committed. I love bean-based dishes like chili, split pea soup, and minestrone—to name just a few. The macrobiotic diet introduced me to a couple of wonderful new beans: the azuki and black soy. If you've had a bad experience with beans, I urge you to try some new ones . . . there is such an amazing variety that you are sure to find a few you love. Personally, I've never met a bean I didn't like.

Beans and Fartiness

Beans get a bum rap, and it's really not fair, so let's get our fart facts straight: First, we *all* do it. Each human builds up about ½ liter of gas to be expelled on the average day, which works out to roughly 14 farts. If you think you cut the cheese less than the rest of us, you're actually making up for lost stink when you sleep. Second, the majority of air that comes out your bottom was swallowed up top—through your mouth—while eating, speaking, or chewing gum. Carbonated drinks are an especially good way to build up farts as well as burps. So eating slowly and chewing your food really well are excellent ways to reduce your inner gas tank.

But back to beans: Beans and some vegetables contain special sugars that the bacteria in your gut love to munch on, and this munching produces gas as well.

Here are some other ways to break down these special sugars:

- Soak beans and discard soaking water before cooking.

- Cook beans with a small piece of kombu sea vegetable or a bay leaf. This helps to break down the beans' sugars as well.

- Bring beans up to a boil in an open pot or pressure cooker and skim off any foam that is produced in the first 10 minutes of cooking. This foam is farty. After skimming the foam, you can cover the pot and simmer the beans until done.

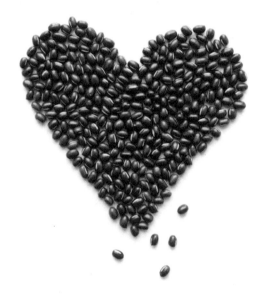

By using these cooking techniques and chewing well, you will find that beans are digested just as easily as any other food, so please, please don't let their gassy reputation get between you and the amazing, delicious, and beautiful qualities of beans. Finally, although bean farts can happen, they tend to have less odor. It's meat and egg farts, which are high in sulfur, that are the real room-clearers.

Isn't Meat a "Complete" Protein?

Chances are you've heard from your parents—or from commercials—that meat is a "complete" protein. This implies that proteins derived from other sources are incomplete, or inferior. This is a culture-wide myth.

Here's the skinny: We need protein. Protein is the basic building block of the human body. As your body goes about its daily business, old cells are being discarded and new ones are being made, and protein is the nutrient responsible for all that new growth.

So How Do We Get It?

Amino acids are tiny little acids that—when combined—make the protein in your body. As far as science can detect, there are only 20 different amino acids in nature, but together they form trillions and trillions of combinations to create all living things.

Your body can make 12 of these amino acids all by itself, but it needs to get the other 8 from food—aka the 8 "essential acids." Meat is often referred to as a "complete" protein because it contains all 8 of these essential amino acids, and that sounds great. Here's where you've been brainwashed, though: They're not telling you that (a) there are plant-based proteins that are complete, too, and—more significantly—(b) you don't need to get all 8 essential acids from a single food! Your body in its infinite wisdom knows how to put together essential acids all by itself, thank you very much! Contrary to popular belief, you don't even need to get all 8 at the same *meal*. Think about it: If it were crucial to get all essential amino acids—in the same meal—every single day, we would have to be ridiculously careful, planning every single meal with the expertise of a nutritionist in order to stay alive. But we don't. Nor do any animals, who seem to do just fine without even knowing what an essential acid is. It's just not that hard to get protein.

Will I Get *Enough* Protein without Meat?

Think of it this way: The average gorilla could lift up your whole *family*, and he doesn't eat meat (okay, a few bugs, but that's it!). Clearly he's getting enough protein. When you think about protein not as meat but as a collection of crazy *acids*, you realize that each individual creature takes what it needs from the natural world to build its body. In fact, it's downright difficult in our culture to develop a protein deficiency. (The clinical term for the disease of protein deficiency is *kwashiorkor*—ever heard of it? Me neither! Doesn't that tell you something?)

Not only does the plant kingdom supply us with abundant amounts of protein (and not just

> ### More Bean Benefits
>
> **Beans are slimming:** Because they absorb water, beans continue to expand in your stomach, keeping you feeling full. Beans are also low in fat and calories.
>
> **Abundant variety:** There are more than 1,000 varieties of beans, and they all have distinct qualities. Lentils are different from garbanzos, which are a world apart from lima beans.
>
> **Beans are versatile:** Beans are great for soups, dips, spreads, in burritos, tacos, and casseroles. They are elegant alone or in a salad and are the perfect food for every season.

in beans—almost every plant contains it), turns out we can get *too much* of the stuff because the body doesn't store it. And when there's too much, the liver and kidneys get overworked trying to eliminate it. Your liver and kidneys are the major detoxifying organs of the body, so overtaxing them just isn't a good idea. The truth is we Westerners suffer from diseases caused by *excess* protein, such as cancer, heart disease, arthritis, osteoporosis . . . the list goes on.

Many people don't need protein more than once a day, but others crave more. It depends on your level of activity and muscle mass. Especially when you're adjusting to a plant-based diet, I recommend you have a bean or some kind of protein product every day.

OTHER BEAN PRODUCTS

Tofu: Probably the most popular and well-known soybean food, tofu's origins are debated, but we know it's been around for at least 2,000 years. Tofu is minimally processed without chemicals. Tofu has the amazing ability to pick up whatever flavors surround it, so it's the most versatile food I know.

Tempeh is made from slighty fermented soybeans and originally comes from Indonesia. I know it sounds a little weird, but tempeh is *delicious*! It has a nutty, meaty, satisfying yumminess and is super high in protein. Sometimes tempeh makers combine the soybeans with other ingredients to make different styles and flavors.

Be sure to always buy organic beans, tofu, and tempeh to ensure you're not getting genetically modified soybeans. For more on GMOs, see page 65.

So explore beans thoroughly. They will support you on every level. Beans provide incredible and varied culinary possibilities and have a history as rich as whole grains'. Make sure you get to know them well.

One other protein food worth mentioning, though it is not made from beans, is seitan.

Seitan (pronounced *say-tan*): Seitan is made from the gluten of whole wheat, but it's almost pure protein. Amazing as a meat substitute because of its texture, seitan is great in a stroganoff or ground up like hamburger! Both seitan and tempeh lend themselves nicely to heartier dishes.

The Great Soy Debate

These days, many people giving up dairy are making a wholesale substitution of soy products for dairy products, eating soy milk, yogurt, cheese, ice cream, and tofu throughout the day. Plus, almost every processed food on the market contains soy or soy byproducts, so add them to the mix and the soy meter shatters.

But why is that a problem? Isn't soy good?

Yes, but too much of even a good thing is still too much. You see, one of soy's amazing qualities is that it contains plant-based estrogens called *phytoestrogens*. In small quantities, phytoestrogens have a positive effect; studies show that they are protective against breast cancer and are helpful for postmenopausal women. In moderate amounts, phytoestrogens are also fine for men. However, there is speculation that an excessive amount of plant-based estrogens may affect fertility in both men and women, interfere with reproductive development in boys, and exacerbate thyroid problems.

Before getting all crazy, keep in mind that Asian cultures have used soybeans or tofu in moderation for *millennia* without exhibiting these problems. In fact, their breast cancer rates and problems with menopause are much, much lower than ours. And let's not forget that soybeans lower cholesterol, help to prevent osteoporosis, and can alleviate problems associated with diabetes.

The answer, as in so many things, is moderation. It's good to eat tofu and tempeh a couple of times a week; and miso and good-quality soy sauce, in small amounts, are great as well. As you transition to a plant-based diet, feel free to indulge in processed soy products like soy milk, soy cheese, and soy ice cream for a while. But as you embrace whole, unrefined foods, and your body gets cleaner and more balanced, it's best to regard processed soy products as occasional treats.

KIND FOOD #3: VEGETABLES

Vegetables got a bad rap when we started packing them in cans—or freezing them in bricks to zap in the microwave! For such delicate, beautiful gifts of nature, it was cruel treatment, and for our taste buds, a modern tragedy. But when you get your hands on fresh vegetables, grown in your area, maybe even harvested that very day, you will be amazed by how good they taste. For vibrant health, tons of energy, beautiful skin, and many other bennies, vegetables need to make it to your plate every day—ideally at every meal.

Vegetables are ridiculously kind to your body. Here's why:

They are full of complex carbs: Vegetables are composed primarily of complex carbohydrates, so they deliver good-quality sugar to the blood and energy to your body.

Vegetables have tons of fiber: Not just your ticket in and out of the loo, fiber gives protection against heart disease and diabetes. Fiber also binds with excess hormones (implicated in reproductive and breast cancers), carrying them out of the body.

Veggies are alkalizing: Your blood needs to stay alkaline. That's its deal. If it becomes acidic, you get sick. Vegetables are generally alkalizing, so when you eat them, your body doesn't need to go through any acrobatics to remain alkaline. Vegetables are pure happiness for your bloodstream.

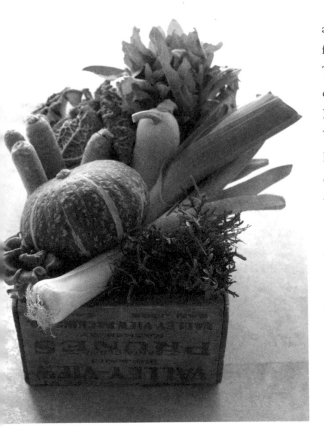

They have antioxidants: As your body goes about its daily business, cells break down and create free radicals, which are basically rogue electrons. These free radicals do damage linked to aging, cancer, and many other diseases. Luckily, Mother Nature has an amazing clean-up system in place: Vegetables and fruits contain antioxidant substances like vitamins A, C, E, and beta-carotene, which clean up all the nasty free radicals. Another reason veggie-eaters are healthier.

MY TOP FIVE VEGETABLES

Kabocha squash: To most people, squash brings to mind zucchini or maybe a winter squash like butternut or acorn squash. They're *good,* but for me none of these can touch kabocha squash. It's just so rich and sweet and melt-in-your-mouth. Steamed, roasted, added to a soup, or as a pureed soup itself, it's my favorite.

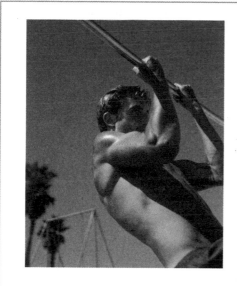

Superhero: Brendan Brazier

Brendan Brazier runs. And bikes. And swims. A lot. As a professional ultramarathoner and triathlete, he needs tons of good-quality, long-lasting energy; and he gets it . . . you guessed it . . . from a 100-percent plant-based diet. When not winning or placing in ultramarathons (at 50 km, he has won the Canadian Ultramarathon Championships twice), Brendan promotes his book *Thrive: The Vegan Nutrition Guide to Optimal Performance in Sports and Life,* addresses Congress about vegan nutrition, and has even developed a line of energy supplement powders and bars for athletes or those of us who simply need some vegan training wheels.

Leeks: Let's take a moment to appreciate the amazing leek. Although it's a member of the onion family, it's really different from your average onion. Leeks are long and elegant, with a white bottom and dark green leaves, which grow in a beautiful symmetrical fan shape. So sexy. So fancy. The French use them all the time, and they're not messin' around when it comes to food. They're great for soups and sautés, or you can braise leeks whole in the oven.

Leafy greens: You might have noticed that a lot of people drink green juice—whether it's fresh from a juice bar or in a powdered form. I've been on a few green juice kicks, but ultimately I find that eating greens themselves is much better. Any food in its whole form is better than the powdered, dried version or the juice, stripped of the fiber. Greens are packed with a mind-blowing amount of nutrients, but especially minerals like calcium, iron, potassium, and magnesium. They also include the antioxidant vitamins and tons of fiber. Greens are that rich, dark color because they absorb so much sunshine, so eating greens is like eating light.

I generally eat greens at every meal (even breakfast!). If that's not possible, I have them at least once a day. Greens make me feel relaxed, flexible, bright, and happy. There's big variety in the greens world, and what you'll find at a good health food store or farmers' market includes curly kale, collard greens, bok choy, watercress, napa cabbage, and sometimes Red Russian kale, or Lacinata kale (aka dinosaur kale or cavolo nero). Collards are my current favorite and deserve a special mention. Normally part of soul food cuisine and cooked with fatback, collards are totally delicious on their own, steamed or lightly boiled. I just keep falling in love with collards.

One more thing: When talking about greens, I am excluding spinach, chard, and beet greens. They are all high in oxalic acid, which is what makes your teeth feel funky and gritty when you eat them. Oxalic acid interferes with the absorption of calcium, so even though these foods contain lots of that lovely mineral, you're not getting most of it. I don't actively avoid spinach, chard, and beet greens, but I don't consider them my daily greens.

Daikon (pronounced *die-con*): I'd never heard of daikon until I got into macrobiotics, but now I'm a devotee. A member of the radish family, daikon comes originally from China and resembles a huge white carrot. It has amazing properties: It's a natural diuretic and also cuts through fats (that's why the Japanese serve dipping sauce with grated radish alongside tempura and other fried foods and shredded daikon alongside sashimi). But forget its medicinal properties—it is just delicious, pungent when raw, but quite mild and sweet when cooked. Christopher and I make a daikon dish using shoyu and mirin, and the daikon becomes so soft and lovely (see page 271). Daikon's also great in miso soup.

Burdock: Burdock cleanses and purifies the blood, strengthens the intestines, is anti-inflammatory and antifungal—among about a hundred other virtuous qualities. I get excited about burdock when I see it on the menu at a restaurant because it makes me think someone in the kitchen is really cool. It shows up regularly on Japanese menus and is great to add to stews and braised dishes.

Beyond my fave five, there is a world of amazing produce, exciting and elegant veggies that you should get to know on a first-name basis if you're not already fast friends (locally grown, if possible!): parsnips, dandelion, endive, scallions, watercress, artichoke, fennel, sweet potatoes, yams, lotus root. Yum!

One exception to the open-door veggie policy is any member of the nightshade family, including tomatoes, potatoes, eggplant, and peppers. For more on this, see page 99.

ORGANIC OR NO?

When you choose organic food, you are voting for healthy soil, nutrient-rich produce, clean water, and ecologically sound farming. "Certified Organic" means that the plant is:

- Grown and produced without chemical pesticides, fungicides, or herbicides
- Not genetically modified

- Grown in soil free of sewage sludge

- Free of antibiotics or hormones

Plus, most organically grown food is irrigated with filtered water, so that's pretty cool. Because organic foods are grown in richer, purer soil, they contain more minerals than conventionally grown, chemically enhanced foods, making them tastier and more nutritious.

GMOs

- GMO stands for genetically modified organism. Although nature cross-pollinates all the time, genetic engineering allows us to introduce *specific genes* into an organism in the hopes of having it develop specialized strengths. Examples include "Roundup Ready" seeds, which are engineered to withstand the pesticide known as Roundup. You see, a farmer can only spray so much toxic weed killer on a crop before damaging it. But genetically modified Roundup Ready crops can survive Roundup herbicide while it kills all the other plants around it. This allows farmers to use as much Roundup as they want on the crop. Great! Even more chemicals in my food! By the way, the company that makes Roundup herbicide—Monsanto—makes Roundup Ready seeds as well. What a coincidence!

- Once a GMO is released, we have no way of stopping it. Pollen from GMO crops has already been found infecting organic crops planted in adjacent fields. Once the pollen of a genetically modified plant fertilizes an organic host, it is no longer organic.

- By messing with natural selection, we are threatening biodiversity and doing damage we may not see for many years—after it's too late. Some people believe that the recent, massive reductions in our bee population are connected to genetically modified crops[4] and the high levels of herbicides and pesticides they are engineered to withstand. It is believed that these chemicals are getting into the pollen and being brought home to the hive, causing bee colony collapse. When the bees die, how are we going to pollinate our food crop?

- There are currently no laws in the United States requiring companies to label genetically modified ingredients in food products. Most of the corn, soy, wheat, and rice sold in this country (and in processed foods) is genetically modified, and none of it has to be labeled. The only way to avoid GMOs is by purchasing organic foods. Time to e-mail your congressman!

Organic foods outperform their conventional cousins like this:

- 63 percent more calcium
- 78 percent more chromium
- 73 percent more iodine
- 59 percent more iron
- 138 percent more magnesium
- 125 percent more potassium
- 390 percent more selenium
- 60 percent more zinc[5]

And remember, nonorganic food is not only sprayed with nasty chemicals, it comes from soil *filled* with them, so they actually get into the vegetables as they grow. There's no escaping the chemical cocktail.

Uniquely beautiful: I know that sometimes organic vegetables and fruit look a little funny or imperfect, but I love that. Organic apples are cute! And the spots won't hurt you. In fact, I think it's a shame that we have become accustomed to food that looks so uniform. I love to find the character and charm of every specimen.

If you can't find organic foods in your area:

- Ask your local grocer or health food store to start carrying them. Get some friends to ask, too, and the store should respond.
- Investigate Community-Supported Agriculture (CSA). By joining a CSA, you receive a beautiful basket of vegetables every week during the growing season. Not all CSAs are organic, but many are. To find a CSA farm near you, go to www.thekindlife.com and type in the keyword CSA.
- If the only organic vegetables you can get your hands on are carrots, onions, and maybe broccoli, don't become an organic Nazi, forgoing all variety. Eating many different foods is not only fun for your tongue, it's really important for your health. Just make sure to clean conventional vegetables well, and do your best to keep finding more and more organic veggies.
- You can type in the keyword organic at www.thekindlife.com for more information and listings about organic retailers and wholesalers in your area.

For more information visit us at: www.thekindlife.com

KIND FOOD #4: DESSERT

You may not think of desserts as health foods, but I beg to differ. By eating scrumptious, sexy, vegan desserts on a regular basis, I maintain my *mental* health, for there is no life without dessert! Desserts help me to relax and prevent me from overeating because I don't feel deprived when I know there's a yummy sweet thing in my future. To follow restrictive, calorie-obsessed diets that wag their finger at delicious desserts is not only torturous, but downright unnecessary. Let's get real: Who would want to live in a world without chocolate peanut butter cups?!

Refined carbs like white sugar and white flour are not only full of empty calories, they stimulate insulin production, which causes the body to store fat.[6] With kind desserts made from whole grain flour and sweeteners like complex carbohydrate–rich rice syrup, your body won't go into

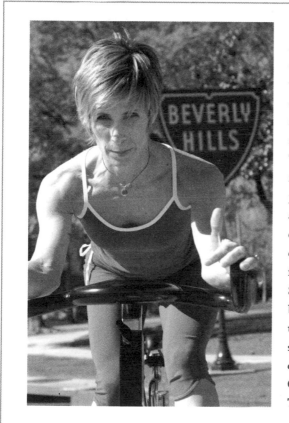

Superhero: Tevia Celli

At 41 years old, Tevia Celli began to experience blurred vision and was diagnosed with multiple sclerosis. Deciding to forgo conventional medication, she eliminated red meat, dairy, all refined sugars, and artificial sweeteners from her diet. Within 30 days, Tevia noticed a lessening of her symptoms, including what had been excruciating nerve pain in her feet. Soon, she gave up chicken and fish, and she has experienced only a few days of mild MS symptoms—usually brought on by stress or a cold—in the last 3 years. In fact, Tevia's doing great; she teaches eight Spinning classes a week and is an all-round badass athlete. Having always had a sweet tooth, she learned to bake using only natural sweeteners, oils, and flours. She started her own business, The Lil' Vegan Baker That Could, in Los Angeles. For more about MS or Tevia, visit www.thekindlife.com.

For more information visit us at: www.thekindlife.com

storage mode as quickly or easily. You will actually use the dessert's calories as useful, vital energy instead of crashing for a nap. Of course, gorging on any dessert is never the route to your skinny jeans, but enjoying moderate portions of healthy desserts will keep you happy on your way to a thinner you.

So I vote for having a healthy dessert three or four times a week. Okay, when you're trying to get into a dress for an event—like a party or a wedding—don't have the more decadent desserts that week! But when you're just living your day-to-day life, and you like the way your body looks (and after eating the Kind Diet for a while, you will), I say treat yourself like the goddess you are and indulge. It will not hurt you.

If you're accustomed to refined sugar and dairy-based desserts, your body is basically on drugs. This means your tongue is like an extremist drug addict, looking for strong hits instead of rich, deep, subtle tastes, and your brain is expecting its daily dose of opiates. Dairy actually coats your tongue in a funky white gunk that inhibits your tastebuds' ability to do their job. After giving dairy the heave-ho, your tongue will start to wake up and these desserts will taste even more amazing. These days, when I have a "normal" dessert, even at a really good restaurant, it's generally a disappointment. Of course the first bite wows me, but very soon my tongue is overwhelmed and the tastes are harsh and obvious. When I go back to my groovy desserts, the flavors of the most simple ingredients just burst on my tongue.

If you think you can't be trusted with sweets and that I'm one of those naturally skinny people who pushes away their chocolate cake after two bites . . . you're wrong. I used to go crazy with sugar, chocolate, and desserts, and truth be told, I still have nutty moments with healthy desserts. When I do, though, I don't end up sad, hung over, and mad at myself. By making whole grains, beans, and vegetables the center of my diet, my body is truly satisfied and nourished. Desserts are now the icing on my cake, not the cake itself, and that switch just happened naturally.

Here are the ingredients that are going to make your life amazing because they are kind to your body:

Brown rice syrup: I strongly encourage you to get to know brown rice syrup. It's my favorite sweetener in terms of how it makes me feel. Sweet and loyal, it brings the blood sugar up, without sending it crashing down. Brown rice syrup is made from brown rice cooked with special enzymes until it breaks down into a liquid. Because it's made up of more complex carbs, brown rice syrup delivers a mellow, gentle, yet complete sweet taste. I include it in many recipes in this book.

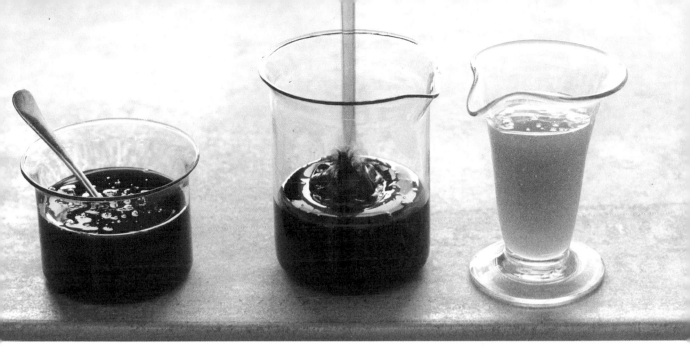

Barley malt: This dark, intense sweetener is also made from complex carbs and is as gentle to the metabolism as brown rice syrup, but with a stronger, darker character.

Maple syrup: Mmmm . . . maple syrup. Renewable, natural, and comes-from-a-freaking-tree maple syrup! In springtime, as temperatures slowly rise in the Northeast, the sweet sap of the maple tree rises as well. When the trees are tapped, this sugary water drips out, and harvesters boil it down to maple syrup. Very concentrated (it takes 40 gallons of sap to make 1 gallon of syrup), this delicious nectar is high in minerals, so it doesn't deplete yours. I love maple syrup in baking and indulgent desserts.

Agave syrup: Made from the agave succulent plant, this syrup is very sweet. Because it grows in semidesert conditions, agave is an appropriate sweetener for people who live in warmer climes, but might be weakening for people who have to make it through long winters. I find agave syrup very yummy in super sweet desserts, but for regular use, rice syrup is a smoother, calmer ride.

Molasses: Even though it's made from sugar cane or sugar beets, blackstrap molasses is processed in such a way that it retains tons of its minerals and vitamins, so the body can handle it much better. I use it sparingly in baking.

Fruit: Think of fruit as God's candy. Even if you love fruit now, once you say good-bye to white sugar and dairy products, you will really appreciate these natural treats.

It's best to eat fruit when it's in season, not only because it's more appropriate for your body, but because fruit grown out of season is rarely organic and isn't nearly as delicious.

Fruit-sweetened jam: All-fruit jams are far better for you than sugar-sweetened ones and they taste just as good or better.

Nondairy malt-sweetened chocolate: These days, chocolate is getting some really good press. It's practically being marketed as a health food, along with red wine and other questionable treats with good public relations firms behind them. Now I'm not saying that chocolate is the worst thing you can put in your body, but even the top-quality dark chocolate is sweetened with cane juice and is high in saturated fat and caffeine. I understand that we all love chocolate, and every once in a while we need a fix, but the malt-sweetened kind is your best option. Made without dairy and sweetened with corn and barley malts, this chocolate is dark but really, really yummy. You will find bags of chocolate chips made by Sunspire. They carry malt-sweetened, nondairy carob as well. To lighten them up into milk chocolate, heat over a double boiler and stir in soy milk as it melts. Try dipping a strawberry in *that*!

A plant-based diet includes such a huge variety of healthy, delicious desserts and fun foods that it puts white sugar to shame. And there's another bonus: When I choose a healthy dessert over an addictive, harmful one, I feel better not only physically but emotionally. I'm being kind to my body, the animals, and the planet. Talk about win-win.

MAGIC FOODS

Some foods are good for you, some are bad, and some are downright magical! Having grown up in a world of abundant, processed foods, you may have never thought of food as anything but yummy or filling, but nature has actually endowed certain foods with ridiculously nutritious properties designed to keep us healthy and happy. Here are some of the magic foods I encourage you to get to know:

Miso: Made from a bean (often soy but not necessarily), sometimes a grain, salt, and a special

For more information visit us at: www.thekindlife.com

bacteria called koji, miso is a salty fermented paste used in miso soup. It can also show up in sauces and condiments, but it is in soup that it is most powerful and healing. Because it is a fermented, unpasteurized food, miso is full of live enzymes that are great for digestion and bacterial flora (like acidophilus), which are basically the natural digestive critters in your gut. In this respect, miso is like yogurt without the dairy. Miso soup is great for the immune system and has been associated with longevity in Japan. In fact, studies done at Hiroshima University show that miso has a protective effect against radiation; and other studies, reported by the *New York Times* in 1993, showed that miso contained a substance called *genistein,* which blocked the blood flow to tumors. High in protein, vitamins, minerals, and alkalizing to the blood, miso keeps the body balanced and happy, so it's fine to have miso soup every day. Miso made with barley and aged at least 2 years is considered preferable to other misos in terms of its medicinal properties.

Although the miso soup served at Japanese restaurants is super tasty, the miso it's made from is extra salty, usually pasteurized, and the broth may even contain MSG (and is often made from fish stock), so don't rely on restaurant miso soup as a magic food—it's not. The same goes for packets of powdered miso, which should be reserved for travel. Fortunately, miso soup is ridiculously easy to make, so check out my recipe on page 249.

Umeboshi plums: These super-sour pickled plums are salted and pressed with shiso leaves, which gives them their pinkish red color. Incredibly alkalizing to the blood, umeboshi help to buffer excess acidity from white sugar and alcohol and are even helpful against the common cold. I learned about umeboshi when I was doing *The Graduate.* We had gone out the night before and I had a doozy of a hangover. I had just started the Superhero diet, and someone suggested I suck on an umeboshi plum to speed my recovery. I popped half a plum in my mouth, and after a few minutes, I felt much better! Umeboshi are great for digestion, diarrhea, and recovery from sugar benders. My Cure-All Tea (page 290) includes umeboshi. Superheroes might have two or three umeboshi a week in various forms. Umeboshi paste and umeboshi vinegar—byproducts of the plum-making process—are really tasty, but not medicinal like the plum itself.

Other pickles: Pickles deliver amazing digestive enzymes and are really great for your overall assimilation of food. They are also thought to strengthen the immune system, act as antioxidants, and facilitate the absorption of certain vitamins. I'm not talking dill pickles from a jar here; most supermarket pickles are not naturally fermented and are soaked in preservatives and other icky ingredients, including sugar.

I mean homemade, naturally fermented pickles made from a variety of vegetables. Try the recipe on page 276 (they're incredibly easy to make yourself) or find unpasteurized pickles or sauerkraut in good health food stores!

Most pickles can be stored in the fridge and provide a delicious, crunchy addition to any meal. The Japanese even eat pickles at breakfast . . . and so do I! Pickles generally contain a lot of salt, so don't go crazy on them; you only need about a tablespoon a day.

Sea vegetables: Unless you or your parents were born in Asia, chances are you didn't grow up eating sea vegetables. Me either. But these days, they are a delicious and truly important part of my diet. Sea veggies like hijiki, arame, wakame, kombu, and nori are simply amazing. With tons of minerals and high in protein, they are alkalizing and detoxifying to the blood. But that's not their neatest trick: Sea vegetables are considered tumor inhibitors, and researchers at both McGill University and the FDA have found that the alginate present in kombu and wakame naturally binds with and discharges scary radioactive materials such as strontium 90 and cadmium from the body! Other magical qualities: They are anti-inflammatory, antiviral, reduce blood pressure, and make for truly badass skin, hair, and nails. I totally understand that sea vegetables may sound icky, but I

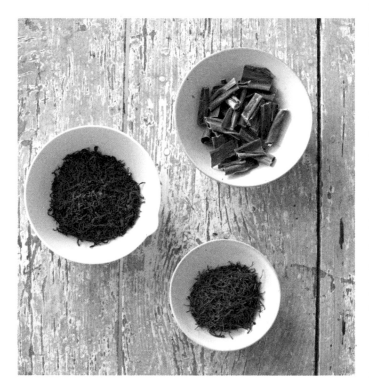

think you'll be pleasantly surprised. If you want to experience amazing health while enjoying beautiful skin, nails, hair, and strong bones, consider sea vegetables an important medicinal food to be eaten a couple of times a week. I've included some really user-friendly recipes for you to try.

Now that you've been introduced to the Kind Foods and their amazing powers, I trust you're itching to get into the kitchen and whip up some deliciousness. The recipes begin on page 137. And if you need to make, oh, a Coffee Fudge Brownie (page 181) or a Thin Mushroom "Pizza" (page 220) to eat while reading the rest of the book, go for it!

6

Nutritional FAQs

You may hear concerned loved ones urge you to be extra careful to get all your nutrients on a plant-based diet, and it's certainly true that we should be concerned about eating nutritionally sound diets—but not as vegans, as *people*.

It's not just your loved ones who have an opinion. As we've seen in the previous chapters, the food industry wants to make you feel that meat and dairy are essential to good health and that, by giving them up, you may be punching huge holes in your nutritional safety net. Funny how they forget to mention that meat and dairy create calcium deficiencies and heart disease, contribute to diabetes, are often full of industrial toxins, and that vegetarians live longer than meat-eaters. Huh!

No matter whom you're listening to, it's normal to have questions about how a plant-based diet covers all the nutritional bases. Here are the answers to some frequently asked questions that will put you and your loved ones at ease.

WILL I GET ENOUGH IRON?

Many people, especially women, are concerned about becoming anemic. Before you run out and drink some blood, it's important to understand a few things: A varied plant-based diet is not iron deficient. Although plant-based iron requires a little vitamin C in the same meal for it to be fully absorbed, that's no biggie; not only does the Kind Diet contain lots of iron-rich foods like whole grains, tofu, pumpkin seeds, lentils, and especially sea vegetables, it's rich in vitamin C–packed foods as well, like broccoli, fruits, and leafy greens (which contain both!). It's downright difficult to not get enough iron on the Kind Diet. By eating lots of fresh and delicious foods, your body will take care of its iron levels just fine. In fact, too much iron is as serious a problem as anemia,

For more information visit us at: www.thekindlife.com

causing free radicals and damage to internal organs. The chief sources of iron overload? Iron supplements and red meat.

Tips for meeting your iron needs:

- It's important to get lots of good-quality iron if you're pregnant or menstruating. Sea vegetables, dried fruit, lentils, chickpeas, and many other foods are high in iron. Use a handful of parsley or pumpkin seeds for a quick iron boost. Pregnant women also need lots of folic acid to prevent anemia. Great sources are lentils, black-eyed peas, pinto beans, chickpeas, spinach, black beans, asparagus, broccoli, and Brussels sprouts.

- Calcium, when it comes via a supplement, interferes with the natural absorption of iron. It's best to get your calcium through food to avoid messing with your iron levels. Sea vegetables, green vegetables, sesame seeds, and many beans are high in calcium.

- The tannic acid from tea interferes with iron's absorption as well. Do not drink black tea with meals.

HOW WILL I GET CALCIUM?

A varied plant-based diet is packed with calcium-rich foods, including sea vegetables, leafy greens, beans, nuts, and seeds. By eating these foods, you will get more than enough calcium. Just as importantly, you will be abstaining from foods that steal calcium from your body—namely meat, dairy, and white sugar—and it's these foods that play the biggest role in bone loss. Between adopting Kind Foods and steering clear of the nasty ones, not only will you get lots of calcium, your bones will gratefully hang on to it. For more on how nasty foods deplete calcium, go to pages 38–39.

IS A PLANT-BASED DIET HIGH IN FAT?

Fat is a nutrient and is totally necessary for the body. You need good-quality, unsaturated fat to absorb certain vitamins, make hormones, and insulate your nerves. But fat—as a food category—breaks down into two major groups: saturated and unsaturated. Saturated fats remain solid or waxy at room temperature and are found mostly in meat and dairy foods. Unsaturated fats stay liquid at room temperature and are found mostly in vegetables and vegetable oils. Saturated fats (as well as hydrogenated fats, or trans fats) are the baddies, raising cholesterol and contributing to heart disease, while unsaturated fats contain omega-3, -6, and -9 fatty acids and are believed to actually lower cholesterol. Yes, every fatty food contains both types of fat, but it's the ratio of saturated to unsaturated that matters. Here's an easy rule of thumb: Keep choosing plant-based foods and you don't have to worry about fat.

HOW DO I GET MY OMEGA-3S?

Omega-3 fatty acids are vital to the functioning of your brain and heart. These days, fish oil is a popular source of omegs-3s, but it has its problems: First, like all animal products, fish oil tends to decompose and become unstable rather quickly, producing free radicals. Luckily for us, plant-based sources of omega-3s are much more stable than fish oil and come complete with antioxidants that clean up free radicals! Second, 15 to 30 percent of the fat in fish oil is saturated, *double* the saturated fat content of plant oils. Third, let's not forget that fish contain industrial toxins, which introduce a host of other nasty problems. Finally, fish make their omega-3s from . . . drumroll . . . the plants they eat, just like we should![1]

Omega-3 fatty acids can be found in flaxseed oil, hemp seed oil, soybean oil, soybeans, and walnuts. Just a teaspoon of flaxseed oil a day will do just fine. There's flaxseed oil in the Baby Bok Choy Drizzled with Ume Vinaigrette recipe on page 265. Yum!

SHOULD I AVOID SALT?

Sodium is absolutely essential to basic, vital functions of your body like digestion, nerve connections, and the contractions of muscles, including your heart! Sodium is found in all organic matter, so we really only need a smidgen more than what we get from food. Good-quality sea salt (sodium chloride) is the best source. Because salt is a crystal that needs to be dissolved, it's best to cook salt and seasonings into dishes, as opposed to adding them at the table. On the Kind Diet, you will also get good-quality sodium in miso, shoyu, and other condiments. Too much sodium can result in water retention, high blood pressure, and bone loss, so go easy.

FYI: Avoid iodized free-running table salt because it has been stripped of its other, balancing minerals, as has the sodium present in processed foods.

DO I NEED TO TAKE SUPPLEMENTS?

Obviously, you only need supplements if your diet is lacking nutrition, so be honest with yourself: If you're currently eating crappy food, then you might want to consider a multivitamin. But please don't start to think that supplements are necessary—or even beneficial—on top of a varied, healthy diet. In fact, your body can get *too much* of some nutrients, which begins a domino effect of imbalance in your body. Over time, these imbalances can stress out your liver. Remember, vitamin pills aren't found in nature; they aren't magic. They are the processed and synthesized bits and pieces of real foods. If you are eating whole foods regularly, you are getting the nutrients in the packages made perfectly for your body to absorb. With one exception . . .

WHAT ABOUT VITAMIN B$_{12}$?

You definitely need vitamin B$_{12}$. Long-term B$_{12}$ deficiencies are extremely serious, irreversible, and affect brain and nervous system function. But we don't need tons of this vitamin—just 2 micrograms a day. B$_{12}$ is synthesized by certain bacteria, which show up in many places, including the guts of animals . . . which is why meat is a good source of B$_{12}$. Although it's true that plant foods do not contain B$_{12}$, all plant foods are grown in the soil, which is full of B$_{12}$-rich bacteria. Before the mass commercialization of agriculture, when we were all pulling vegetables from our gardens and the water wasn't purified with chemicals, the bacteria that synthesized B$_{12}$ was available to us through the soil and water. So B$_{12}$ deficiencies in vegans are not caused by the diet itself but by the hypersanitization of our modern world. Personally, I'm not a super-clean freak, so I don't scrub the vegetables from my garden like crazy, and I know that the little bits of soil that remain contain B$_{12}$. Yay, nature! To be safe, I also take a supplement—a low dose either under my tongue or in a veggie cap—every so often. Dr. Neal Barnard recommends taking B$_{12}$ once or twice a week.

DO I NEED TO TAKE ENZYMES?

In the Kind Diet, you'll get lots of amazing digestive enzymes from miso, umeboshi plums, pickles, and other fermented foods. There shouldn't be a need to take extra digestive enzymes. By chewing your grains and vegetables well, you'll ensure that your mouth releases its digestive enzymes perfectly, which helps all the enzymes in your stomach and intestines to work even better.

HOW MUCH WATER DO I NEED TO DRINK?

If you eat meat, drinking eight glasses of water a day is not a bad idea. Why? Because animal protein builds up uric acid in the body, and you need lots of fluid to flush it out. Also, your average American diet contains so much bread, meat, salt, sugar, chemicals, and caffeine that you're basically walking around dehydrated much of the time and in need of some irrigation. However, a diet composed mainly of grains, vegetables, and legumes is fluid-rich, toxin-free, and doesn't cause the body to build up so much uric acid. Therefore, you can just relax and listen to your thirst!

IS IT OKAY TO DRINK ALCOHOL?

Let's be honest. Alcohol is not a health food. Yes, some studies have shown that one glass of red wine a day (or two for men) may be good for the heart. But that's only because we're walking around with meat-battered, stress-stricken tickers, and a little booze helps to relax us, thins the blood, and contains antioxidants. However, giving up meat and dairy, eating your veggies, and getting some exercise will do all of the above. Red wine is a pretty extreme "medicine" for a condition caused by extreme foods. Remember, it's hard on the liver, dehydrates the body, and can become an addictive habit. A recent study done in England, looking at the health and habits of more than 1 million women, found that even moderate drinking (one drink a day) increased the risk of breast, liver, rectum, and upper digestive tract cancers.[2]

So we need to take alcohol out of the health category and put it where it belongs: the indulgent pleasure category. If you are used to the occasional alcoholic beverage, go ahead and enjoy it. Life is for living fully, and sometimes alcohol is part of the picture. If you choose not to drink alcohol, that's awesome. Personally, I rarely drink at home, but at a good restaurant with friends, I love a fine glass of red wine. And, well . . . there are a couple of weddings I don't remember!

Armed with all these facts, I hope you can now move forward with confidence that all your nutritional needs will be met while you remain kind to yourself and the planet.[3]

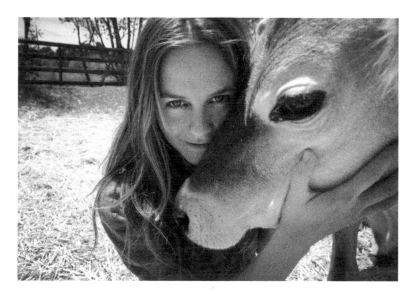

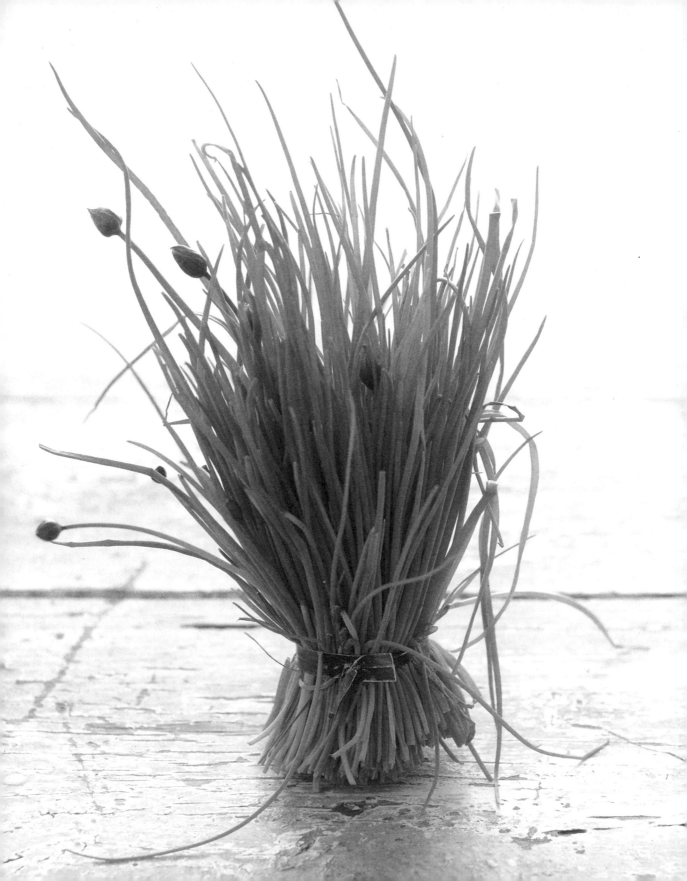

living the kind life

I'm assuming you want to be a Superhero. Who wouldn't want all the benefits of great health and to see their maximum potential in life? But I also know that Superhero status rarely comes overnight and that even Superheroes have lazy days. So I've designed this next part to help you make whatever moves are right for you in that direction.

When you make this journey in your own way, there's no such thing as failure. Maybe you'll start tonight by trying a veggie dish at the restaurant you'd planned to go to for dinner. Perhaps you'll buy some brown rice and fire it up on the stove. No matter. I believe that very powerful forces will propel you forward; first, the startling truth of the nastiness of nasty foods, and second, the mysterious, seductive quality of the Kind Foods. Once whole grains and vegetables take over your bloodstream, they will reveal how amazing you can feel . . . and that's addictive.

So I encourage you to read all three plans in order to determine your best starting point. There is no right or wrong on the Kind Diet, and you may find yourself mixing up suggestions from different plans from the get-go, or you may work through them all methodically from A to B to C, spending 30 days on each plan. It may be that you read through these plans and one of them grabs you and says, "Do me!" There's no right way. As long as you continue to make good choices, one choice at a time, you will learn, and grow, and feel better. And soon, the little choices will start to mount and your skin will begin to glow and you'll find yourself standing in the kitchen a full-blown Superhero.

YOUR FIRST STEP

Here's a little challenge: If you'd really like to experience the transformation that comes with a plant-based diet, commit to whichever plan you choose for 4 weeks.

Whether it's Flirting, Vegan, or full-blown Superhero, it's important that you follow it as faithfully as you can for those 4 weeks. If you choose to go Vegan, that means *really* staying away from meat and dairy. If you're moving up to Superhero status, it means making whole grains, vegetables, and beans the center of your diet and reducing your dependence on processed and convenience foods.

I ask for your commitment because the magical, mind-blowing changes the Kind Diet can bring about will not occur if you spread that pat of butter on your toast or add that dollop of chicken salad to your lunch. Sure, reducing meat and dairy makes a difference, but feeling the greatest benefits comes from total abstinence. It's like the difference between smoking two packs, half a pack, and no cigarettes at all. Which person has the healthiest lungs? If you're trying to quit smoking and you bum a cig off a coworker a few times a week, you haven't really quit. Your body is still processing the toxicity of smoking instead of using its energy to heal itself. Yes, you'll have made big strides, but the real freedom, the deep transformation and healing occur when you smoke no cigarettes . . . *that's* when your body switches gears. It's the same with meat, dairy, and even sugar.

So choose a plan, and do your best. And remember, it's only for 4 weeks. That's one menstrual cycle! That's two paychecks! That's four episodes of *The Bachelor*! That's it. No stress. See how you feel a month from now, and figure out your next move from there.

I have included some meal plans in the Vegan and Superhero sections, but they are merely springboards for your palate and imagination. If following a meal plan helps you, great. If not, that's fine, too. Remember we're saying hello to freedom and good-bye to rigid diets. My goal is to empower you to make good choices in your kitchen, at the grocery store, and at restaurants. The Kind Diet will give you a way of living that is flexible, doable, and yours to design day by day, meal by meal.

7

Flirting

flirting: *(verb)* to court triflingly or act amorously without serious intentions

Here's the thing with flirting: The key is that you be open. Open to being seduced. You are putting your best foot forward and looking for the best in your potential partner. So this is about making no commitments, but remaining positive and open to possibility. When you flirt, you reserve the right to walk away at any time, but you are hoping to be surprised and delighted.

The Flirting Plan contains very little pressure; in fact, it's just a bunch of suggestions you can implement for the next few weeks. By following them, you will get your foot in the plant-based diet door.

Action #1: Start dating the vegetarian restaurants in your area. (Go to thekindlife.com and enter the keyword Restaurants to find suggestions and links to the best vegan restaurant in your area.) Ask the waiters: What's the *one* thing that I must taste? What would make you sad if I didn't try it?

If there is not a veggie restaurant nearby (unlikely but possible), begin dating the vegetarian options on the menus of your favorite restaurants. Where you normally buy your lunch, get the veggie option; even chain restaurants have them these days. Subway makes a sandwich with no meat, there are veggies options at the Cheesecake Factory, even a bean burrito at Taco Bell qualifies.

Action #2: Find your nearest health food store and go. Just walk in the door and say hello. Remember: You're just flirting. Look around. Get familiar with some of the products. Run your fingers along things and laugh in a coquettish way. Browse a few books, if you like.

Go to the transitional foods chart on the next two pages and buy 10 things you want to try. Personally, I would start with Earth Balance "butter," Vegenaise "mayonnaise," and some type of frozen dairy-free dessert like the Rice Dream Mint Chocolate Frozen Pie!

Action #3: Buy some organic brown rice and unrefined sea salt. Make a pot of rice for yourself and eat it with your regular meals over the next couple of days. If you need to make a gravy for it, fry it up with some vegetables, or cover it with vegan cheese. Go for it. Just eat some brown rice and notice how it makes you feel. When it's done, make another.

Find two recipes in this book that look exciting, and buy the ingredients to make them. Go crazy with any of the recipes in the Vegan section, but don't be scared off from sampling the Superhero recipes, too. I strongly recommend the Thin Mushroom "Pizza" (page 220) or Chocolate Peanut Butter Cups (page 183).

After your little shopping spree, when you open the fridge for a snack, you will have a whole new selection of ingredients to play with. Experiment! Make a vegan grilled cheese or a PB & J with a big salad. For anything you'd make with mayonnaise, substitute Vegenaise. Go for soymilk in your coffee, and butter your toast with Earth Balance Buttery Spread. You'll be amazed at how quickly you adjust to these new foods and how light you feel with just these small changes.

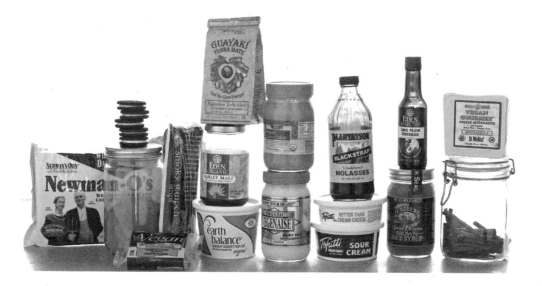

FOOD	BRAND	FLAVOR
Bacon	Light Life	Smokey Tempeh Strips & Smart Bacon
Butter	Earth Balance or Willow Run	Original
Candy bars	Luna	Chocolate Peppermint Stick
Cheese	Follow Your Heart	Cheddar, Mozzarella, or Nacho
(Parmesan)	Galaxy	Vegan Parmesan
Chicken breasts	It's All Good	Chicken breasts
Coffee alternative	Guayaki or Teeccino	Any flavor
Cookies	Uncle Eddie's	Peanut Butter/Choco Chip, Molasses
	Newman's Own	Newman-O's Dairy Free Wheat Free Chocolate Crème Cookies
Corn nuts	Grandpa Po's Nuts	Spicy, Sweet, Salty
	Gladcorn	Plain
Cream cheese	Tofutti	Any
Dog treats	Mr. Barkley's	Any
Dressing	Annie's	Goddess & Shiitake
	Brianna's	Poppyseed
Fish	Vege USA	Fish Fillets
Frozen dinner	Amy's	Macaroni & Cheese
Frozen snacks	Health Is Wealth	Pizza Munchees
Ice cream	Purely Decadent	Praline Pecan, Mocha Almond Fudge
Ice cream treats	Rice Dream	Bars & pies

FOOD	BRAND	FLAVOR
Jam	St. Dalfour	Strawberry is my favorite
Jerky	Tofurky	Teriyaki, Hickory Smoked
Juice	Santa Cruz	Hibiscus & Lemon
Ketchup	Wholemato or Heinz (organic)	N/A
Mayonnaise	Vegenaise	Grapeseed (purple label)
Meat slices	Tofurky	Hickory Smoked
Milk	Edensoy	Soy/rice blend
Milk, chocolate	Silk	Chocolate
Nondairy creamer	Silk	Hazelnut
Pizza	Amy's	Roasted Vegetable or Soy Cheese
Ribs	Vege USA	Citrus Spare Ribs
	Morningstar	Riblets
Rice Crispies Treats for kids	EnviroKidz	N/A
Sausage	Tofurky	Italian
	Field Roast	Smoked Apple
Snack bars	Wha Guru	Cashew Vanilla & Sesame Almond
Soda	Knudsen	Any
Soup	Amy's	Chicken Noodle
Sour cream	Tofutti	N/A
Yogurt	Whole Soy	Any

Transition Checklist

- Move from cow's milk to a milk alternative (see below).
- Move from white bread to organic whole grain bread.
- Move from white pasta to whole grain pasta (wheat, rice, spelt, or quinoa pastas).
- Move from canola and corn oils to organic olive, safflower, and sesame oils.
- Move from regular mustard to whole grain, organic mustard.
- Move from coffee to green tea or yerba maté.
- Move from white sugar to maple syrup and brown rice syrup.
- Move from canned and frozen vegetables to fresh, organic vegetables. Other new members of the pantry: brown rice, beans, unrefined sea salt, vegetables, fruit.

Don't forget: spaghetti sauce, tortilla chips, salsa, pita bread, tortillas, popcorn, pancake mix, veggie burgers, tofu dogs, Amy's frozen meals and burritos, marinated baked tofu, nuts, and sunflower or pumpkin seeds.

Milk substitutes: rice milk, soy milk, almond milk, hemp milk. Even coconut milk! There are so many choices. Just so you know, every type of "milk" on the market has a distinct taste—even among soy milks, there are different tastes and textures. Some are slightly sweetened. Explore and play with the choices as you find those that work best for you.

You can even make your own: Soak almonds overnight and blend in a blender with water and a pinch of cinnamon.

Superheroes: Vegetarians

The word *vegetarian* first showed up in Webster's Dictionary in 1939, and the first vegan society was formed in England in 1944. But in case you thought vegetarianism was a 20th-century trend, consider this: Vegetarianism's history goes back to ancient India and Greece; it is a tenet of major religions like Hinduism and Buddhism and has been practiced by these early and contemporary trendsetters: Plato, Ovid, Leonardo da Vinci, Percy Shelley, Voltaire, Jean Jacques Rousseau, Henry David Thoreau, Leo Tolstoy, Abraham Lincoln, Sir Isaac Newton, Charles Darwin, Albert Einstein, Mahatma Gandhi, Rosa Parks, John Lennon, Paul McCartney, Bob Dylan, Mary Tyler Moore, Oliver Stone, Alec Baldwin, Deepak Chopra, Prince, Lenny Kravitz, Kate Moss, Alanis Morrissette, Ellen DeGeneres, Shania Twain, Reese Witherspoon, Tobey Maguire, Carrie Underwood, Natalie Portman, Nelly, and Anthony Kiedis.

Energy Bars

Most energy bars contain a lot of simple sugar and—no matter how you slice it—that's not healthy. You may need that hit of simple carbs to keep you going during your Ironman race, but how strenuous is your actual daily routine? I know it might *feel* like an endless race, but energy bars are really not the answer. All that simple sugar sets you up to crave more of the same while weakening your immune system, creating new and not-so-sporty problems. Plus, it's a bar, in a package, sitting on a shelf! It's not food!

If you feel like you can't live without them or you skip meals often, look for bars that contain no white sugar and no dairy. Here are some options: Crispy Peanut Butter Treats with Chocolate Chips (page 184) or Raw Balls (page 205), Go Macro bars by Macro Treats, and Oskri sesame seed bars. If you can't find any of those, Luna and Clif make some sugar-free products as well. Try making these healthier choices as you adjust to what your body really needs to run life's races: real food.

Action #4: Take a yoga class. Start with a gentle one if you're new to the practice. Or take a dance class . . . or Spinning. Even a lazy, flirtatious stroll will do.

Action #5: Get a feel for what being vegetarian is like by going 4 weeks without beef, chicken, or pork. Alternate beans and new "meats" (soy or wheat meat substitutes such as tofu, seitan, or tempeh) with fish—one day fish, one day veggie. Fish, although it has serious issues,[1] is the easiest to digest of all the flesh foods and leaves the body feeling lighter than beef, pork, or poultry. By making this switch, you will get a better sense of what going veggie or vegan would be like.

DETOX FOR FLIRTS

If you abstain from meat and dairy completely for even a few days at a time, your body will start to discharge toxins. You may notice excess mucus, stinky perspiration, and other lovelies. Positive signs of detox include easier bowel movements and better energy, so don't miss the good stuff! With every experience of detox or adjustment, it's important just to keep moving forward, trusting that your body knows exactly what to do to heal itself. Yay, body! As long as you are getting a variety of nutritious foods, you can trust the process.

Food for thought: Any reduction in your animal product consumption is—to me—a total, unequivocal, three-way win. You win by being healthier, the planet wins for suffering less of the ecological impact of the meat and dairy industries, and an animal wins by not getting eaten!

After Flirting for a while, though, you will feel some interesting, exciting changes, and your body will naturally begin to push you to the next stage. Please follow your instincts. Although it's fine to Flirt for as long as you want, I encourage you to read through the Vegan and Superhero plans as you prepare to feel better and better, experiencing more of the benefits of a plant-based diet.

Reminders for Flirts

- Eat brown rice.
- Explore meat and dairy substitutes.
- When you feel you need meat, go for wild fish.
- Make friends with vegetables.
- Start noticing how different foods affect you.
- Keep flirting; make a new recipe from this book every week.
- Enjoy the adventure.

Eye Candy for Flirts
All of these cute boys are vegan:

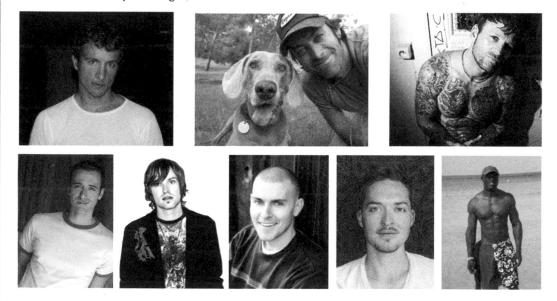

8

Going Vegan

vegan: (noun) a vegetarian who omits all animal products from the diet

Although following a vegan diet is defined by abstinence from animal products, it is much, much more than that. By committing to a new way of eating, you are investing in your health, longevity, peace of mind, and overall enjoyment of life. By giving up meat and dairy, you withdraw your support from industries that take a toxic toll on the environment and on the well-being of your fellow humans. And finally, by not eating animals, you are reducing the needless suffering that occurs in the world, on many levels. Whether or not that's a priority for you, isn't it nice to know that being good to yourself benefits others? You've arrived at the place where kindness to yourself meets kindness to the earth meets kindness to other creatures, and that's pretty cool. Abstaining from animal products is a profound act, with physical, emotional, and even spiritual benefits. Come join me and many, many others as you take this magical leap forward.

GETTING STARTED

It's helpful to cleanse your home of animal products. Start by giving away any meat or dairy products you have to friends, family, or charities. *Please* don't throw food away. I know I've labeled meat and dairy as "nasty," but to someone who isn't ready to make this change, they have real value and there is absolutely no reason to waste them.

In order to treat your body as kindly as possible (and to feel amazing), I'm going to be asking you to go a step beyond simply eliminating certain nasty foods from your kitchen and diet. I want you to *add* certain Kind Foods to your diet now rather than making the mistake of surviving on corn chips and Pepsi all day. Of course, you may be eating lots of vegan foods already, like bagels, salads, pasta, vegetables, and fruits, but I'm asking you to go one step further by incorporating some whole grains and bean products in your diet every day. I also encourage you to use the Superhero recipes as much as the Vegan ones; that way you will build a nutritionally solid center as you experience the benefits of saying "bye-bye" to meat and dairy. That's it. Simple.

LET'S GO SHOPPING

Now's the time to get serious about stocking your kitchen. Once you've given away or used up all the meat, dairy, and other nasty foods that line your shelves and fridge, it's really important that you replace them with ridiculously yummy food so you never feel deprived or likely to slip. I've organized these foods into categories, so pick liberally from each.

- **Grains:** brown rice, barley, quinoa, rolled oats
- **Bread:** whole grain breads like whole wheat sourdough
- **Other whole grain products:** couscous, noodles, mochi
- **Beans:** chickpeas, lentils, kidney beans, black beans, or any other
- **Bean products:** tofu, tempeh, seitan, and premade hummus
- **Vegetables:** leafy greens, onions, cabbage, winter squash, daikon, carrots, lettuce, cucumbers, and anything else you like
- **Fruit:** Get a good selection for snacks and desserts, but try to choose mostly from what grows in your climate.
- **Seasonings:** unrefined sea salt, shoyu, umeboshi vinegar
- **Oils:** olive, safflower, flaxseed
- **Processed foods:** See Flirting list of transitional foods (page 86) and go crazy.
- **Snack foods:** fresh fruit, figs, raisins, trail mix, edamame, toast, cereal, peanut butter and jelly, soy or rice milk smoothies, cinnamon-raisin mochi, toasted whole wheat tortillas, ramen soups, and anything else that tickles your fancy. One of my favorites is popcorn with melted Earth Balance Buttery Spread. (See the Snacks section of the recipes, pages 179–195.)

BUILDING A MEAL

Every healthy lunch or dinner is built around the same three elements: grains, beans, and vegetables. Without being super rigid about it, you should think of your meal as one-quarter grain, one-quarter protein, and one-half vegetables. It's not necessary to have a bean or protein food at every meal; once a day is really enough, though if you want to eat protein more often, that's okay, too. For meals that don't include protein, a balance of 50 percent grains, 50 percent vegetables is about right.

Of course, there's a ton of variety within these three categories, but once you understand the basic structure of a meal on the Kind Diet, meal-making becomes simple. Here are the basics:

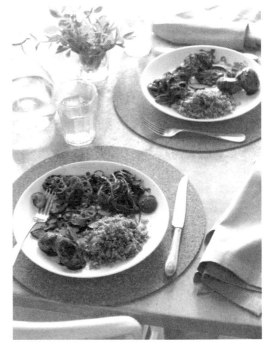

1. Start with a **whole grain or grain product** (whole grain cereal, or pilafs; noodles; bread; or tortillas).

2. Add a **protein** (beans, tofu, tempeh, seitan, or, in a pinch, any processed meat substitute).

3. Add lots of **vegetables**, some raw, some cooked. Try to get lots of variety in colors, textures, and flavors.

4. If you want **dessert**, find or make a healthy treat (rice ice cream, brown rice crispy treat, etc.) or have a piece of fruit.

Voilà! That's your meal!

Breakfast has a slightly different personality. Although Superheroes have vegetables with their grain at breakfast, you may not feel attracted to a big bowl of collard greens first thing in the morning (yet!). Just decide what grain you'll have for breakfast (oatmeal, pancakes, brown rice, cereal), add a protein if you like (scrambled tofu, tempeh bacon), and maybe a drizzle of something sweet like jam or rice syrup . . . and if you're feeling frisky, steamed greens . . . YUM!!!

As you get better and better at building healthy meals, you can keep some other elements in mind:

- Try to use as many colors as you can in a meal. This is a great way to get all your nutrients and to please your eyes as you eat.

- Vary your cooking styles; it will keep your tongue and body happy.

- Little things make a difference; a garnish of chopped cilantro, scallions, or parsley will give a dish extra vibrancy!

TROUBLESHOOTING

Variety: Don't eat the same thing every day. Variety is yummy and important. Although I have certainly gone on jags where I wanted to eat a particular food every day for weeks (Rice Dream Mint Chocolate Frozen Pie, Uncle Eddie's cookies, Tempeh Reubens would be a few examples), I'm also careful to eat a varied diet. Each food has a unique combination of vitamins and minerals. When you eat a good variety of fresh food, your body gets completely nourished, and you will never get bored!

Detox: Detox is fun. The feelings that come up as your body detoxes from meat and dairy can sometimes be a little weird, and they are often confused with the diet itself. But the problem is not the beans and grains; it's what you ate *before* them. Your body is making a big shift from one fuel to another and lots of underlying chi—or energy—is getting unblocked. This means your body is healthy, doing the moving and shaking it's designed to do. This unblocking may produce some weird stuff like rashes, headaches, phlegm, sleeplessness, constipation, diarrhea, and other fun stuff. Or not. Everyone's different. On the other side of detox, you can look forward to better skin, deeper sleep, and lots of energy. If you've been eating meat and dairy your whole life, your intestines may need some time to clean themselves out before they will be able to effectively absorb nutrition and energy from plant-based foods. It's not unusual for people to feel shaky or weak at times as their bodies and blood sugar learn to stabilize. Make sure to eat regularly and to chew your food extremely well.

Is More Really Better?

Sometimes we go crazy on things. If we hear drinking a smoothie is good for us, we drink one every day for good measure. If we hear blueberries are good, we eat a whole quart. We read an article about a certain food and get obsessed with it. We as Americans are raised on the ethic of "if some is good, more is better." But that's not actually true. When we listen only to our minds saying, "This is *good for me,*" we stop listening to our bodies. And if we don't listen to our own bodies' signals, who will? The body requires variety and has different needs within a day, a season, and a year. Luckily we have a finely honed tool to help us determine our real needs: intuition. By eating whole grains and vegetables, your intuition will become stronger and you will be more and more attracted to things that support your health. Instead of saying, "Carrots are good. I should have carrots every day," ask yourself, "Do I *feel* like having a carrot?" and really listen. Although it may not happen overnight, trust that by eating Nature, she will begin to speak through you.

Chewing

The secret to total satisfaction is in your mouth. Ahh, your mouth. In your specially designed kisser, you have the magical ability to convert a complex carb—like a grain of brown rice, or a green bean, or even a hunk of squash—into . . . glucose. That's right. Sugar. The *good* kind. You come equipped with flat molars, a jaw that moves in little circles for grinding, and a special enzyme in your saliva, called ptylin, that breaks down complex carbs into glucose. When this glucose travels to your brain, it gives you the most amazing feeling of satisfaction. You will feel nourished and centered, and your brain will be free to generate happy thoughts. And all this begins in your mouth.

So we're talking about chewing here. We're meant to chew—that's what our molars are for! Because we modern folk eat refined carbs like sugar and white flour (which break down so quickly in the mouth), we've never had to think about chewing. But I promise you the feeling of satisfaction you will get from chewing whole foods thoroughly is something you appreciate for the rest of your life. Good-bye calories! Good-bye Weight Watchers Points! Good-bye glycemic index! Hello really eating—and enjoying—food.

Truth is, when I concentrate on chewing a mouthful, my jaw aches a little, I get bored, and finally I feel like an old lady at a retirement home. But then the bliss sets in. I know it doesn't sound sexy, but by chewing thoroughly you will nourish yourself deeply, feel totally peaceful and satisfied, lose weight, and create your strongest health.

All that being said, I'm not the greatest chewer. I try hard to chew every mouthful 30 times, but I often don't meet that mark and often forget altogether. It's really about doing your best and discovering that feeling of satisfaction. Here are some chewing tips to help you practice:

Eat some meals alone: It's *way* easier to chew when you're not expected to talk.

Put your fork down between bites: This simple trick interrupts mindless gobbling.

Really taste the food: You went to the trouble to get it! By paying real attention to the food, you can relax and let each bite be chewed until it's liquid, enjoying every little bit of flavor.

Your jaw might hurt: When any unused muscle gets a workout, it feels it, and your jaw's been slackin' off for years now. Your body will soon thank your jaw because you will perform so much better on chewed food.

If you want to throw in the towel, here are some tips to keep you on track:

- Pick up this book and reread the information about Nasty Foods and Kind Foods.
- Make your favorite dish from this book.
- Eat something very rich, with lots of oil and satisfying flavors.

- Go get a great vegan meal at a restaurant.
- If you find you're struggling with cravings, see the section on Cravings on page 104.

And don't hesitate to get support. Get a couple of the books I recommend from the library to keep you inspired. Check in with the vegan world at least once a day—there are a lot of us out there! Go to my Web site at www.thekindlife.com for inspiration and to connect with others.

BE KIND TO YOURSELF

I know I said up front that staying away from all animal products is important in order to feel the full impact of the diet—and that's certainly true—but at no time is beating yourself up an option. Changing a lifetime's worth of habits can be challenging; if you fall off the wagon, just get back on. No drama. No guilt. Being vegan is a journey, not a destination. It is a gentle awakening of the heart, mind, and spirit. You'll see that there is no punishment here, just the beautiful reward of feeling better and better every day.

As you continue on this journey—4 weeks and beyond—you will experience amazing changes. Some will come quickly, some slowly, but eventually meat's hardness will melt away, leaving your body and heart soft and open. You will begin to feel more deeply. Compassion will flow from your core toward all other living beings. This is the most amazing gift of eating a plant-based diet—feeling the sacred connectedness of all living things. Enjoy.

> To become vegetarian is to step into
> the stream which leads to nirvana.
> —Buddha

Reminders for Vegans:

- Ramp up the whole grains.
- Commit to freeing your body and the planet from the grip of nasty foods.
- Dive into Vegan recipes and dabble shamelessly in Superhero recipes.
- Check in with your body; listen to its signals.
- Be proud of the choices you're making.

VEGAN MEAL PLAN

Here is a week's worth of menus using the recipes you will find on pages 141–213, with a restaurant meal thrown in here and there. Please feel free to mix and match as you like; these are only guidelines. After 7 days, repeat the menu or introduce new recipes from both the Vegan and Superhero sections. Go crazy!

DAY 1

Breakfast
   Pumpkin Bread (page 202)
   Steamed greens

Lunch
   Hot Rice with Cold Lemon, Basil, and
      Tomato (page 151)
   Sicilian Collard Greens with Pine Nuts and
      Raisins (page 176)
   Purchased squash soup (I like the Imagine
      Company's)

Dinner
   Explore a local vegetarian restaurant. Get
      something crazy like vegan nachos or a
      vegan BLT.

DAY 2

Breakfast
   Mom's Granola (page 201)

Lunch
   Restaurant veggie burger and a salad

Dinner
   Fried Rice (page 234)
   Sweet Potato–Lentil Stew over couscous
      (page 166)
   Steamed greens
   Oatmeal, Walnut, and Dried Plum Cookies
      (page 186)

DAY 3

Breakfast
   Crocodile Crunch (page 200)

Lunch
   Dolma with Tofu Cream (pages 224–225)
   Sugar Snap Peas, Radishes, and Edamame
      with Lemon Butter (page 167)

Dinner
   Waffle, Sausage, and Cheese Panini (page
      153)
   Watercress, Beet, and Heirloom Tomato
      Salad or green salad (page 173)
   Chocolate Peanut Butter Cups (page 183) or
      My Favorite Cupcakes (page 190)

DAY 4

Breakfast
   Bagel with Tofutti cream cheese or
   Toast with nut butter and jam

Lunch
   Radicchio Pizza with Truffle Oil (page 144)
   Alicia's Sexy Inspired Salad (page 174)

Dinner
   Takeout from your favorite Indian restau-
      rant: cauliflower/potato/pea dish, lentil
      soup, naan bread, or rice dish

DAY 5

Breakfast

At a restaurant:
Toast with avocado and tomatoes,
Oatmeal, or Hash browns and tofu scramble

Lunch

Your choice: Tostadas (Kinda) (page 217) or
Burrito (pages 216, 219)
Crispy Peanut Butter Treats with Chocolate
Chips (page 184)

Dinner

Rustic Pasta (page 147) or pasta with your
fave marinara sauce
Pecan-Crusted Seitan (page 154)
Steamed broccoli with Vegenaise
Garlic Bread (page 147)

DAY 6: QUICK AND EASY DAY

Breakfast

Quick Date-Apple-Cinnamon Oatmeal
(page 196)
Steamed greens

Lunch

Your choice of sandwich (see ideas on page
152)

Dinner

Chorizo Tacos (page 157)
Steamed greens
Rice Dream Frozen Mint Chocolate Pie

DAY 7: SUNDAY

Brunch

Traditional English Breakfast (page 198)

Dinner

Basic Rice (page 233, make a large pot)
Black Soybean and Kabocha Squash Stew
(page 164)
Baby Bok Choy Drizzled with Ume
Vinaigrette (page 265)
Mixed Berry Cheesecake (page 192) or
Coffee Fudge Brownies (page 181)

9

Becoming a Superhero

Superhero: (noun) a hero possessing extraordinary, often magical powers

So you wanna be a Superhero . . . great! This is one of the most exciting and life-changing opportunities you will ever have. By eating whole, natural foods, your body will cleanse itself from the inside out. You will feel reborn as you tap into the deepest energy of your being.

The Superhero plan is loosely based on the macrobiotic diet, which takes its principles from the diets of traditional cultures throughout the world—essentially fresh whole foods, grown locally and in season. In creating the Superhero plan, I have taken lots of what I love about macrobiotics—its amazing foods and its spirit of balance—and laid it gently atop my vegan foundation. Although the macrobiotic diet is not always 100 percent vegan (fish is an occasional food for some people), following it without any animal food works very well for me and many, many others.

These days, I live mostly in the Superhero plan because it makes me feel my best, but when the pressure is off or I just want to indulge in something slightly naughty, I reach into the regular Vegan recipes and make one of my favorites, like the Chocolate Peanut Butter Cups, because even Superherocs need a day off. If I had to calculate, I would say I follow the Superhero plan about 80 percent of the time and Vegan the rest.

The Superhero diet begins with selecting whole foods that grow in your region. By eating foods that grow in the climate in which we live, our bodies adapt easily to the changes going on around us, changes in weather, season, and temperature. This adaptability is fundamental to good health.

The Superhero diet revolves around whole grains, vegetables, beans, and lots of other good things. Everything should be as as fresh as possible and organic whenever that's an option. White sugar, white flour, and processed, chemical-laden garbage are to be avoided entirely. Basically, it's a return to clean, nourishing, delicious food. *Real* food.

Being a Superhero will teach you how to use food to bring the body back home when you go a little wonky. You're probably doing this already without knowing it; balancing the drowsiness of the bagel with the shot of espresso, balancing the acid stomach of the burger with the antacid pill, balancing the red wine headache with an aspirin. The problem with this balancing act is that it invites chronic problems—colds, weakness, insomnia, depression, or worse. By eating whole, natural foods, you'll find that you feel better and need fewer external aids, and you will be able to use foods to bring you home to balance when you're feeling out of sorts.

No one knows you like you know yourself, so you can become your own expert—in the field of *you*! Think about the last time you had a really bad cold. Did you visit a doctor or treat it aggressively with over-the-counter medications? Instead of throwing drugs at it, why not consider that cold an opportunity to reflect and ask yourself how you contributed to its arrival? Maybe you got run down, ate sugar or dairy. By stopping the behavior that caused the imbalance and applying a food-based remedy, you will make friends with your body, learning how to bring yourself back to balance naturally again and again.

And this responsibility means power. I love knowing that I am responsible for myself! When I have a headache, instead of asking, "Where's the aspirin?" I ask, "What caused this headache? Ah, the sugar in last night's chocolate cake. Maybe a little umeboshi tea will bring me back to balance and make me feel better." The Kind Diet is about waking up to what your body's telling you because it's your ultimate authority.

Finally, the Superhero diet is not about being restricted—on the contrary, it's learning how to play happily in a healthier world. I love eating. I always have. And I haven't given up *any* of my eating pleasure by following either the Vegan or Superhero diets. If anything, my pleasure has increased as I've become stronger and healthier, and I'm enjoying my life more than ever. It's great to know that I can take care of myself, giving my body and the planet the TLC we deserve.

Being a Superhero is really about trusting nature, which is magical and transformative. You are healthier, more powerful, and more intuitive than you know, but lousy foods have kept you stuck and weak. By embracing all the Superhero foods and letting go of everything that holds you back, you allow nature to scrub you clean to reveal your natural superpowers. It may not feel great at the beginning, but your mind will be absolutely blown as you stick with it.

The Superhero plan distinguishes itself from the Vegan plan in the following ways:

Whole grains are emphasized even more: I know I've mentioned whole grains a lot, but the Superhero plan really puts them squarely at the center of the diet. Eat whole grains at most meals, and consider bread and other flour products "fun" foods for occasional consumption.

Processed foods are reduced even further: Because the Superhero plan is about harmonizing with nature, processed foods (even vegan ones) aren't a big part of the picture. To experience the maximum Superhero buzz, cut them out altogether.

Nightshade vegetables are minimized: A handful of vegetables—namely potatoes, tomatoes, eggplants, and peppers—are generally to be avoided because they are high in substances called alkaloids, which can cause inflammation in the joints. These plants are members of a family called "nightshades" and have long been associated with arthritis.

My policy with nightshades is to keep them out of my kitchen most of the time, but I'll eat them for a treat at a restaurant. In the middle of the summer, I will definitely enjoy some heirloom tomatoes because they are one of life's great pleasures, and I want to give a shout-out to the amazing potato, which I indulge in about once a month; but as a part of my daily diet, I recognize that these veggies are not good for me. Sure, they contain lots of nutrients when broken down in a science lab, but their overall alkaloid content is too high for daily consumption, and there are definitely easier ways to get those same nutrients. By the way, although sweet potatoes are cousins to the potato, they are not nightshades. Thank goodness!

Magic foods play a bigger role: Eating miso soup, some pickles here and there, and the regular consumption of sea vegetables (one arame or hijiki dish per week, others used in cooking) are important ways to maintain Superhero powers.

Soy milk is phased out: If you want to be a Superhero, consider soy milk a treat. I use it for baking or when a recipe calls for it, but not as an everyday food. Soy milk can cause gas, is extremely processed, and is high in fat and plant-based estrogens. This is not a Superhero food, my friends! I keep soy milk in the house, but digestion-wise, I find that my body prefers rice milk. That said, I don't lean on *any* product as a milk substitute, to be used on a regular basis, other than the occasional bowl of granola. The whole idea of needing to drink a glass of "milk" of any kind is simply off my radar. Of course, plant-based milks are a million times better than cow's milk, but we really don't *need* either of them—especially Superheroes! FYI: Tofu is much less processed than soy milk, so it's an excellent, nutritious choice a couple of times a week.

Maple syrup and other strong sweeteners are used in very limited quantities: I consider maple syrup a super fun, sexy, and tasty friend, but she takes me on quite a ride, so I don't hang out with her every day. Ditto agave syrup. They are all very concentrated substances, delivering strong sweetness, and are therefore difficult to balance effectively. For example, when I eat any raw maple syrup before bed, I have a hard time sleeping and find myself waking up like a crazy person. To avoid this little drama, I stick to rice syrup and barley malt for my regular Superhero sweetening.

Fruit is an occasional treat: For your regular day-to-day eating, try to eat fruit that is grown in your climate. Fruits from the tropics are not appropriate for a body experiencing snow and sleet—they cool it off too much. Yes, on a really hot, humid Manhattan day, a slice of pineapple is amazing, but no fruit from a climate that is the opposite of yours is good for everyday consumption. Make them treats. In fact, because too much fruit is believed to weaken the blood, the ideal Superhero diet includes much less fruit than you might be used to, about one piece of fruit a day. That amount is fine, but don't feel like you *have* to have even that much; instead, focus on getting plenty of healthy greens.

Herbs and spices are used in moderation: Spices like cayenne and curries are powerful and have a strong effect on the body. If we want our bodies to come to a centered, relaxed place, it's important to use simple food—at least for a while. Many Superheroes use herbs and spices here and there to create variety, but don't get into a habit of putting them in every dish. To the Superhero tongue, simple food tastes fantastic.

Nuts are also eaten in moderation: Don't go nuts on nuts or nut butters. They're really high in fat. About a cup a week is perfect.

Salt is used with care: Excess salt can make you cranky, withdrawn, and craving sweets. It also can trigger cravings for fat or binges. Here are some good rules of thumb when it comes to salt:

- Always cook salt into dishes completely. No salt or soy sauce should be added to food at the table. Sea salt needs to be cooked into a dish for 10 minutes, and shoyu needs 5 minutes to incorporate fully.

- Develop a light touch with salt. Dishes should never taste salty—salt is there to bring the natural tastes of the food forward, not to cover them.

- If you feel like you're getting too salty (if you have a salty taste in your mouth, have dark circles under your eyes, or are always thirsty), reduce your salt intake and drink a healing broth made by simmering a dried shiitake mushroom in 1 cup of water for 10 minutes. This will help your body release the excess salt. A hot bath works, too.

YOUR SUPERHERO PANTRY

Below is a list of the foods used on the Superhero diet. Not everything here is absolutely essential, but let this be a guide, and always choose organic when available. Don't feel you need to buy everything all at once. Pick up the ingredients for some Superhero recipes (Chapter 15) that appeal to you, and cook those dishes. Next time choose different recipes that use a few other ingredients. After you've done this several times, your pantry will be nicely rounded out.

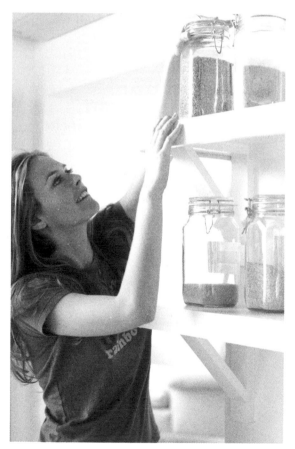

- **Whole grains:** brown rice (short grain, medium grain, long grain), brown basmati, millet, quinoa, barley, oats, wild rice, and any other grain that strikes your fancy

- **Grain products:** mochi, whole wheat, udon and soba noodles, whole wheat sourdough bread (unyeasted is best), couscous, polenta

- **Beans:** azuki beans, green lentils, chickpeas, black beans, red lentils, pinto, kidney, black-eyed peas, and any other beans that turn you on

- **Vegetables:** leafy greens (collards, kale, bok choy, napa cabbage), root vegetables (carrots, daikon, burdock), and many others: onions, broccoli, cabbage, snow peas, celery, winter squash, summer squash, cucumbers, scallions, leeks

- **Magic foods:** unpasteurized miso (aged 2 years), umeboshi plums, dried shiitake mushrooms, sea vegetables (kombu, arame, hijiki, nori, wakame, and agar agar)

- **Seasonings:** shoyu, sea salt, umeboshi vinegar, brown rice vinegar, mirin (rice cooking wine)
- **Oils:** olive, safflower (or sunflower), and sesame oil
- **Sweeteners:** brown rice syrup and maple syrup
- **Fruit:** local, seasonal fresh fruit; dried fruit like raisins and apricots
- **Beverages:** kukicha and barley teas, amazake, apple and carrot juice (best made fresh)
- **Nuts and seeds:** almonds, walnuts, pecans, sesame seeds, pumpkin seeds, sunflower seeds, tahini, and nut butters
- **Extras:** Sweet Rice rice candies, Eden rice crackers, popcorn

SUPERHERO MEALS

You'll notice that Superhero meals differ from Vegan meals in a couple of interesting ways: first, soup shows up once or twice a day (even at breakfast) and homemade pickles make an appearance every day as well. Here's a detailed breakdown of your Superhero meals.

The Traditional Superhero Breakfast

Miso soup: It makes a wonderful start to the day. Helps to gently break the fast of sleeping and prepares your intestines for the rest of the day. Don't knock it 'til you try it!

Grain: Usually leftovers from the night before, see my Breakfast recipes beginning on page 282.

Leafy greens: The chlorophyll and nutrients of leafy greens give good energy while helping your body move gently into the day.

Other: Add a little something to provide variety and flavor—maybe a tablespoon of rice syrup, a handful of toasted sunflower seeds, some almonds, or a little jam.

Building a Superhero Lunch or Dinner

The following are the basic elements of Superhero meals, but they don't always show up in neat boxes. Just consider this list a guideline for balanced eating. Sometimes you'll need to assemble several components—a vegetable dish, a grain, and a separate protein—to cover your bases, while other recipes will contain two or even three of the key elements in one fell swoop.

- **Grain:** Start with a grain or grain product. Superheroes eat whole grains in their unrefined forms more often than they do products made from whole grains. Have bread up to twice a week and noodles up to three times a week.

- **Bean:** Add a bean or bean product. And make sure to eat a good variety of beans. It's best to limit tofu and/or tempeh to a couple of servings a week; seitan to one serving a week. Recipes beginning on page 239.

- **Vegetables:** Add lots of vegetables. Make sure that you get a good variety of vegetables. Include a sea vegetable dish a couple of times a week.

- **Soup:** Have miso soup and some other kind of soup (vegetable, bean, grain, or pureed vegetable) as often as you like. If you have soup twice a day, that's great! Soup is an essential element of the diet because it relaxes the intestines, preparing them for good digestion.

- **Pickle:** Eat about a tablespoon of pickle (homemade if possible and soaked if salty) every day to help strengthen digestion.

- **Desserts:** Choose one of the Superhero desserts beginning on page 277.

Again, it's not necessary to get neurotic about it, but if you compose a meal that is one-quarter grain, one-quarter protein, and one-half vegetables, it will feel really balanced and all your nutritional requirements will be met beautifully.

MAKING THE TRANSITION

Here are a few strategies for dealing with some of the challenges you may encounter in your transition to Superhero:

Eat your evening meal early: Try to avoid eating for at least 3 hours before bed. If you're full, you spend your night digesting, which is not restful. On an empty stomach, the rest of your body can do its rejuvenation and repair.

Ramp up your chewing skills: Really good chewing can double the benefits of the Superhero diet by breaking down the foods and making all their nutrients available. The goal is not to swallow as you chew. It may seem weird at first, but closing the back of your mouth lets you use it as the digestive anteroom that it is. Keep adding saliva, which contains an enzyme, ptylin, that breaks carbs into glucose. Hardcore chewers go for 50 to 100 chews per mouthful. When it's all liquid, go ahead and swallow. You'll get better—it's a habit. Do your best. Personally, I'm a lightweight chewer, but I'm trying.

Check in with others online: You may not be the only Superhero in your neighborhood, so reach out to others who understand your journey. Go to www.thekindlife.com and find some online friends to share your story with and get support.

Detox and cravings: The Superhero diet can be intense. When you start eating such natural, whole food, your body will begin to change quickly. If, for any reason, you feel you need to ease off the diet a little bit to slow down the ride, that's fine—just don't regress all the way back to square one. Make a sexy recipe from the Vegan section. When you feel leveled off again, go back to your Superhero ways. That way you are just stretching the boundaries of Superhero as opposed to throwing in the towel. It's important to give yourself the flexibility to play between the two plans rather than impose rigid rules and unconsciously set yourself up to binge on the bad stuff.

In the first few weeks or even months, expect to experience some degree of detoxing. Your body may clean itself quickly and with some vigor, so consider detox a great adventure. By giving up most of the vegan processed foods, excess fruit, and white sugar—and by centering your diet on whole grains—your body may experience all the effects listed under vegan detox, but with greater intensity. Your menstrual cycle may go a little wonky for a few months as well. But soon you will also experience all of the benefits—giddy moods, smooth elimination, regular periods, the disappearance of old aches and pains, and much more.

Detoxing happens on an emotional level, too, so if you find that you're angry or sad, get whatever support you need. When I first followed a squeaky clean Superhero diet, I felt grumpy for a week. That's not unusual. Be sure to take care of yourself as you detoxify.

Variety is especially important on the Superhero diet because a life of only brown rice and broccoli is too limiting and intense, not to mention no fun. So make sure you're eating a wide variety of foods, using many cooking styles, and if your body is reacting in ways that concern you, please seek the advice of a macrobiotic counselor. It's actually fun to have a coach who can answer a million questions and who will empower you to continue your practice. After the initial detox, you will feel better than you have in years. Or maybe ever!

You may also find yourself experiencing intense cravings at the beginning of your Superhero journey. It's not unusual, when people change their diets radically, to experience cravings. They generally fall into one of the following categories:

Good-bye cravings: As the body discharges certain foods, we can feel a pull toward them. For instance, it's not unusual for people to crave sugar as they kick it. Same with meat and dairy. All of the nasty foods have addictive elements that can make you want them as you withdraw, but after they've really gone bye-bye from your body, you won't miss them at all. It takes from 3 to 10 days for sugar to release its grip on the body, but it can take a few months for dairy and meat to let go. It actually takes years for the body to release all the excess fats and toxins it's collected from nasty foods, but strong cravings should disappear much sooner than that.

Low blood sugar cravings: If your brain seems to flash "EAT!!" all the time, you may be experiencing low blood sugar. When making the transition to a plant-based diet, many people have a hard time absorbing complex carbohydrates and getting what they need from them in order to feel satisfied. Symptoms may also include feeling weak or shaky. Eating regularly and chewing well are the answer. By really breaking down grains and vegetables in your mouth, they convert to glucose right there in your kisser. They are then easily absorbed into the bloodstream and transported to the brain. Glucose in your brain stops the "EAT!!" sign from flashing. So if you find that you're just craving food all the time, begin to chew more carefully and you should notice a change. Your absorption will improve over time.

Naughtiness cravings: Sometimes we just feel rebellious, especially when we're changing something as fundamental as our diet. We bristle against rules and the perfect little boxes we try to shove ourselves into. If you come up against the urge to call it quits—simply out of rebellion—get the most delicious vegan dessert you can find (I recommend the Rice Dream Mint Chocolate Frozen Pie) or make the Chocolate Peanut Butter Cups on page 183 and really savor them. Oooh . . . you're so bad!

It takes a little while to get used to a new way of eating, but it will happen, I promise. When you find you're craving something that's not on your food plan:

- **Eat:** It's helpful to simply eat anything healthy—the yummier, the better. You may be having cravings simply because you're hungry. As hunger is relieved, cravings tend to be, too. And remember: Chew well. That will help to raise your blood sugar.

- **Make a substitute:** If you find you're not satisfied, make something close to what you're looking for . . . a piece of toast with soy margarine, brown rice syrup, and cinnamon makes yummy cinnamon toast! Malt-sweetened nondairy chocolate and nondairy ice creams are godsends, too!

- **Remember your commitment:** Maybe your commitment is to your health or to the planet. Remind yourself regularly of why you're following this new way of life. If I'm tempted by cheese or ice cream, all I need to do is think of the poor cow whose miserable life is behind it all. That kills the craving pretty quickly.

- **Do something satisfying:** Sometimes we think about food because we're bored or just stuck in a habit. As you make these big changes in your eating, it's helpful to have a few activities up your sleeve to give you satisfaction: calling a friend, walking your dog, taking a bath, or reading more about this lifestyle can help occupy a wandering mind.

For More

- If you or a loved one is challenged by serious illness, I strongly recommend you read Mina Dobic's book called *My Beautiful Life* and see a macrobiotic counselor. You can use the macrobiotic approach in conjunction with conventional therapies.

- For cooking classes, delivery services, and anything else you could possibly want to know, go to www.thekindlife.com.

> Leave your drugs in the chemist's pot if
> you can heal the patient with food.
> —Hippocrates

Reminders for Superheroes:

- Commit to centering your diet on whole grains, vegetables, and clean proteins.
- Chew them really well.
- Make friends with sea vegetables and other magic foods.
- Stay clear of processed foods.
- Listen to your body.
- Save the world.

SUPERHERO MEAL PLAN

DAY 1

Breakfast

Millet and Sweet Vegetable Porridge (good
for 2 days) (page 288)

Steamed kale with Ume-Sesame Dressing
(page 259)

Lunch

Fried Udon Noodles (page 229)

Dinner

Quinoa with Basil and Pine Nuts (page 224)

Hijiki-Tofu Croquettes (page 244)

Scarlet Roasted Vegetables (page 267)

Steamed greens

Plum Soup (page 280)

DAY 2

Breakfast

Leftover Millet and Sweet Vegetable
Porridge with toasted sunflower seeds
(page 215)

Steamed collard greens with Ume
Vinaigrette (page 265)

Lunch

Leftover Quinoa with Basil and Pine Nuts

Cabbage, Radish, and Cucumber Pressed
Salad (page 256)

Leftover Scarlet Roasted Vegetables

Leftover Hijiki-Tofu Croquettes

Leftover Plum Soup

Dinner

At your favorite sushi restaurant: vegetable
roll, vegetable tempura, sushi roll, house
salad with dressing

DAY 3

Breakfast

Miso soup

Hot Polenta, Millet, and Corn Cereal (page
289)

Steamed watercress with Ume-Sesame
Dressing (page 259)

Lunch

Go to a local vegetarian restaurant. Go crazy!

Dinner

Sweet rice/short grain rice (see Basic Rice
variation, page 233)

Carrot and Burdock Kinpira (page 272)

Tuna Salad Sandwich (Kinda) (page 246)

Leftover Cabbage, Radish, and Cucumber
Pressed Salad

Crispy Peanut Butter Treats (see Superhero
variation) (page 184)

DAY 4

Breakfast

Miso Soup (page 248)

Pan-Fried Mochi (page 237) with rice syrup

Collard greens

Lunch

Leftover sweet rice/short grain rice made
into a burrito or nori burrito

Leftover Tuna Salad Sandwich

Leftover Carrot and Burdock Kinpira

Fresh salad

Leftover Crispy Peanut Butter Treats

Dinner

Nabeyaki Udon (page 231)

DAY 5

Breakfast

Miso Soup (page 248)

Barley with Sweet Rice and Corn (page 289)

Cabbage and leeks drizzled with Ume
    Vinaigrette (page 265)

Lunch

Be as great a Superhero as you can be at the
    Whole Foods deli or a Mexican restau-
    rant. Get a grain, a veg, a bean, and a
    soup.

Dinner

Creamy Sweet Kabocha Squash Soup (page
    253)

Polenta Casserole with Seitan (page 223)

Fresh salad

Strawberry Kanten (page 281)

DAY 6: SUPER HEALTHY & QUICK

Breakfast

At a restaurant:

Oatmeal with fresh fruit and raisins or

Tofu scramble

Lunch

Leftover Creamy Sweet Kabocha Squash
    Soup

Leftover Polenta Casserole with Seitan

Fresh steamed greens

Leftover Strawberry Kanten

Dinner

Ginger Pasta with Zucchini (page 238)

Arame with Carrots and Onions (page 263)

Steamed greens

DAY 7: SUNDAY

Brunch

Mochi Waffles Drizzled with Lemon-
    Walnut-Rice Syrup and tempeh bacon
    (page 286)

Scrambled Tofu (page 283)

Steamed collard greens

Dinner

Rice with barley (large amount to have as
    leftovers)

Azuki Beans with Kabocha Squash (large
    amount to have as leftovers, see soup
    variation) (page 241)

Steamed greens

Candied Ginger Pears (page 279)

Make pickles (page 276; this is enough for a
    week)

Roasted seeds (page 215; make enough for a
    week)

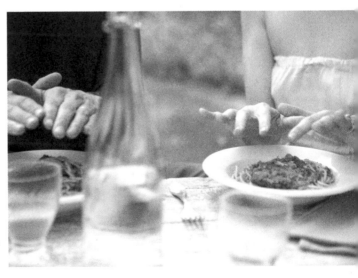

10

The Kind Kitchen

Whether you're leaving the office to go to the local salad bar, driving to the grocery store and picking through the frozen foods section, or earning the big bucks to eat at the best restaurants, you are definitely putting energy toward feeding yourself.

Perhaps you've never cooked and don't plan to. You live your life at restaurants or cafeterias, and you're pretty sure that you and cooking just don't get along. That does not preclude you from practicing the Kind Diet. Go straight to Chapter 11 to start figuring out how to do it. There are also great transitional foods (see Flirting, pages 84–85) that require little or no cooking, and they can become your new freezer goodies. You may find, over time, that you become a little more interested in putting energy into what you eat. If that happens, start with cooking breakfast, or cook one meal a week . . . take it one step at a time.

Maybe you're already an experienced cook. If so, this is just about opening your mind to new things. You are going to make delicious, life-sustaining, magical foods that will please and satisfy everyone around you.

For those of you who have some—but not tons—of experience in the kitchen, fear not. Remember, anyone can cook. There is no cooking gene that you did or didn't inherit from your grandma. If you can read, you can cook. Even the most artistic chefs in the world (and there are some truly great artists in the kitchen) had to learn the basics and practice their skills. So crack open the recipe section of this book and get started. Practice makes delicious!

Cooking can also be a family affair. When my husband and I cook together, my heart feels so full. It's a very pure joy. If you have kids, get them involved. Maybe they can shuck corn or pick some fresh cilantro from the garden. Working together to create something that nourishes your family inside and out can be a deeply powerful experience for everyone. And it's a lot of fun!

EVERYBODY HAS A SUNDAY

We all have a day in our week that is slower and more leisurely than the others. This magical day can change the energy of your whole house and your whole family.

For me and my husband, this day is Sunday and it begins at the local farmers' market.

I love the great sense of community there, and over time I've become friendly with a lot of the farmers and the other people we see each week. We don't really know one another, but every week we share our discoveries: "Hey, try this fig; you're gonna *love* it! . . . They're down there. . . . Where did you find those cosmos?" We exchange recipes and ideas. Farmers' markets are made up of family-run businesses—people who work really hard—so by shopping locally, we are supporting them and the local economy. I love knowing the person who's growing my food. There's Vicky the orange lady, Jimmy the heirloom guy . . . the mushroom dudes . . .

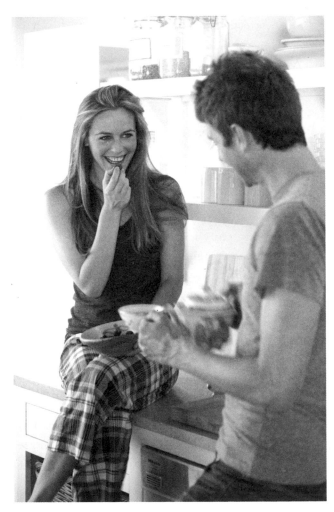

Before heading out, we take inventory of what we have left in the kitchen so we don't overshop and we don't waste food. Armed with our reusable shopping bags and grandma cart, we stroll around, discovering what's in season that week, finding foods at their peak. I feel naturally attracted to different foods at different times, and I love sensing that.

Once we're home, we unload all the goodies and begin to cook. We make a delicious lunch from all our newly bought foods and sit down to really enjoy it together. Because it's Sunday, we have the time later in the afternoon to thumb through cookbooks, getting some ideas for the coming week. We prepare some essentials to last us a while: a big pot of grain that will last a couple of days, maybe a hearty bean soup or stew, a sauce that can be used on grains or vegetable dishes throughout the week, and, of course, toasted sunflower seeds—my favorite! Although we don't freeze things, a leisurely day is a great time to make soups or stews to freeze (grains don't freeze well, but beans do). By letting our Sunday be slow and nourishing, Christopher and I start the new week feeling connected to ourselves and ready to face the world.

If it feels impossible to cook well during the week, find that one afternoon you can relax into and explore the sacred, sensual act of cooking. Don't get overwhelmed—just do the best you can! Be patient. Sometimes it will take a little longer than expected to make a meal because you're new to these foods or cooking in general. Know that once you've mastered a recipe, everything will become quicker and looser and more fun. If you're diving right in to the Superhero plan, you may need to make some extra time in the kitchen. If you really want to get into cooking, go to www.thekindlife.com for information on awesome cooking schools and online classes.

It's time to reconnect with the single most important thing you do in your day: eating! We

Planning Your Day

It takes about 5 minutes to figure out your food day. Before you go to bed, just ask yourself: Where am I going to be for breakfast? What are my options? How much time do I have? Maybe you'll have a full half hour at home, or maybe you need to eat in the car, but either way, if you give it some thought before you're in the thick of things, you can make decent choices. Every day is different; sometimes I'm at home for lunch, sometimes I'm having a meeting at a restaurant. Either way, by thinking ahead, I can make plans that ensure I make the best choices possible.

When I don't plan (and sometimes I don't), I find that my choices are made in haste, out of stress or hunger, and they tend to be less than stellar. Often, eating healthy food is not so much about desire—or virtue—but simply having access to good food! The question is: Have I arranged things so that I can get what I need? If delicious healthy food is available, I'll eat it. If it's not, I can't.

P.S.: Sometimes I plan to be naughty, and that's fine, too, because I know how to bring myself back to balance. If I'm going out to a nice restaurant that evening, and I might have some bread, some red wine, and a bite of someone's sugary dessert, I eat pretty Superhero during the day so that I can indulge happily. After the night out, I make myself a special drink to bring myself back to balance. (See page 290 for my favorite healing drink.)

eat three times a day *every single day of our lives*! It has a greater impact on our bodies and our health than anything else we do. Let's remember we have a very real and important choice: We can make ourselves sick with food or we can heal ourselves with it.

So find *your* Sunday and start cooking!

TOOLS AND KITCHEN EQUIPMENT

A few very basic tools make cooking easy and pleasurable, but if you don't have them right now, don't let that stop you from doing what you can. You will slowly figure out what you need and want in your kitchen. Let your kitchen grow as your skills grow. Ideally, choose stainless steel, cast iron, and ceramic cookware. Aluminum and Teflon, although considered safe when new, become not-so-safe after the pans have become pitted or scratched. Check out craigslist to find used or nearly new cookware and add pieces as your budget permits. These are my must-haves:

- A good Japanese-style vegetable knife is worth every penny. Its thin, straight blades make cutting a total pleasure. My favorite knife is made by a company called NHS.

- Keep a serrated knife for bread and tomatoes, but be careful not to use it on seaweed—I did that once and took a nice chunk out of my finger!

- Any kind of cutting board will do, but we love our bamboo cutting board. It also makes an elegant, practical gift for a food-minded friend.

- Stainless steel saucepans and sauté pans.

- Stainless steel mixing bowls are awesome . . . cheap and easy to store.

- A colander and strainer.

- If you cook on gas, a flame tamer (aka deflector) is really useful for spreading heat evenly under pots and pans.

- A good enameled cast-iron pot or Dutch oven is wonderful for cooking grains, beans, and vegetables.

- A blender or food processor is a great speeder-upper of things.

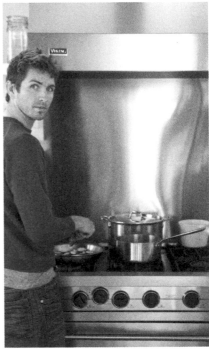

One more thing: Please consider getting rid of your microwave. In Swiss studies conducted in the early '90s, the molecular structure of microwave-cooked food was altered in ways that caused abnormal changes in human blood and immune system function. The microwaved foods also caused higher cholesterol levels than the same foods prepared using traditional cooking methods. Christopher and I chose to chuck our microwave oven completely 8 years ago, and once it was gone, we never missed it. I think you'll find that you can live without yours, too. Yes, I have to reheat things in a saucepan sometimes, but it's done in a second, it's no big deal, and the foods taste so much better!

SUPERHERO EXTRAS

If possible, cook with gas rather than electric heat. It is easier to control, tends to make the food taste better, and imparts a nice smooth energy into the food. If you're stuck with an electric range, though, don't sweat it.

Cast-iron skillet: Great for roasting nuts and seeds and for certain vegetable dishes. Also great for cooking mochi!

Pressure cooker: Weren't they big in the '40s? Yes, but pressure cookers are really great for cooking grains and beans because they squeeze them full of strong energy. They are ideal for fall and winter cooking, when our foods need that extra oomph to keep us warm and energized. If you don't have one, it's not a necessity, but if there's a pressure cooker gathering dust in a cupboard, you might want to bust it out.

Suribachi: A Japanese grooved mortar and pestle, which are great when you start making your own gomashio. They're cheap and make great gifts, too!

STOCKING THE KIND KITCHEN

These days, with budgets being squeezed everywhere, the idea of completely restocking your kitchen may feel daunting. You may be surprised to find that your grocery bill doesn't change that much. While some new foods will be more expensive, others will be cheaper. More importantly, when compared to the cost of prescriptions, workdays lost, gas to the doctor, copays . . . not to mention the incalculable cost of feeling crummy . . . good food is worth every penny.

Consider the price of what you're receiving: a beautiful body, vibrant health, a clear mind, and a longer life. Can you really put a price tag on those things? Feeling good is priceless.

That said, it's also an indisputable fact that meat, dairy, and packaged processed foods take the biggest bites out of our grocery budget. Skip those foods, load up on grains and beans, and you'll have plenty of money left over for buying the best quality produce and natural foods you can get your hands on. Yes, some of those foods are expensive—like umeboshi plums, Vegenaise, and sea vegetables—but they are well worth it. When you start cooking for yourself, you'll find that your overall food bills are about the same.

Even organic produce doesn't have to break the bank. If you shop locally—straight from the growers—it can be crazy cheap. At a recent trip to the farmers' market, I bought: 1 head of cabbage; 1 bunch of daikon; 1 bunch of scallions; 1 head of celery; 2 sweet potatoes; 2 onions; 1 head of bok choy; 1 head of Chinese cabbage; and a big handful of green beans.

Grand total? Thirteen bucks. Tell me that's not cheap. The other day I got an heirloom tomato at a grocery store for over $3, but if I'd just waited until Sunday, I'd have bought it for less than $1. A creative, delicious, healthy meal composed of brown rice, beans, and an array of vegetables could set you back a whopping $3 to $4.

If you can't make it to the market each week, check out Community-Supported Agriculture (CSA). (See page 66 for details.)

If you don't have either of these resources available, find out if there's a local co-op in your area, where you can find things in bulk or even exchange a couple of hours of labor for discounts. Thank goodness Whole Foods, Trader Joe's, and other great health food stores exist these days for all the things we can't get elsewhere. Ask your local health food store to carry things you want or need—they can order almost anything. If you have to do all your shopping at a health food store, it will be a little pricier, but the benefits are always worth it.

And don't forget, many of the priciest items on your shopping list when you were eating meat were those meat-based foods. Cheese, fish, and meat are all a lot more costly than protein sources like tofu and beans. Initially you may be investing in some new pantry staples that will add dollars to your register tape (see the list on page 101 for a complete rundown of my pantry picks), but eventually that will level off. Especially on the Superhero plan, which includes virtually no packaged or processed foods (which are always more expensive), you can eat very frugally—and deliciously.

A Shout-Out to Sunflower Seeds

Make up a big batch of seeds roasted with shoyu (see page 215), and store them in a nice jar, then use them to brighten up any meal. Toss them on *everything*! I swear you will love them!

Cooking Tips

- Try a recipe, and if you like it and it's worth repeating, think of a way to improve it. Learn from your mistakes and successes. My dogs eat my mistakes! Use your imagination and remember that—with the exception of burning down the house—nothing can go *that* wrong.

- Always read a recipe from beginning to end before diving in. In my enthusiasm, I've made this mistake several times, and it's not fun when I get to the middle of the recipe and realize I don't have flippin' fenugreek seeds! That said, it's often possible to spare yourself a shopping trip and substitute ingredients with whatever's on hand.

- When planning meals, re-create dishes you love, like spaghetti with meat sauce or your favorite Chinese dish, with new ingredients. Use a sauce you love on meat (like a BBQ, teriyaki, or piccata) and serve it over rice, seitan, or vegetables. You may love it!

- Use the herbs and seasonings from your favorite cuisines in your new healthy recipes. If you love Italian spices, use them. Ditto Mexican spices or French herbs.

- Whatever your skill level, learn to use your intuition in your cooking. Every week, I pick up collards, kale, bok choy, and cabbage at the farmers' market, so they're generally all in the fridge. When I open it up to begin cooking, I like to observe what my body gravitates toward. And it changes! My body doesn't want or need the same thing every day. Follow your intuition and let your body make some choices.

- My mother taught me never to waste food, and I think that's really important. To minimize waste, always use the stuff that will spoil the most quickly first. Great inspiration can be found in cooking what needs eating.

- Try your best to never throw away food. Someone will always want it—a friend, a neighbor, a pet. Food that's a few days old is fine for an animal. When you've exhausted all other avenues, chuck it in the compost.

- A tip: Every week, I go through the refrigerator and put the oldest produce on the top shelf to remind me to use it as soon as possible. This avoids waste and prevents me from finding old, liquefied parsley tucked away in the fridge drawers!

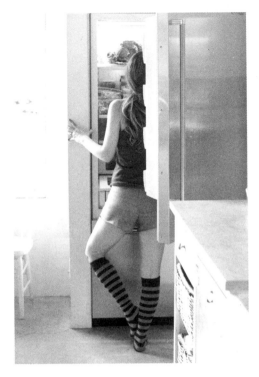

Before you shop, take inventory, make a list, and stock up for the week; a full fridge feels wonderful and will inspire you to create fantastic works of art. On the other hand, waste is not cool, so do your best to get only what you'll actually use. After a few weeks of kinder cooking, you'll have a better sense of what to buy and how much you actually cook and eat in a week.

Especially at the beginning of your transition to the Kind Diet, it is helpful to keep healthier convenience foods around, and I have listed some of my favorites in the Flirting section. You should know, though, that none of these prepared foods and packaged goods are really Superhero fare, so Superheroes should rely on them only when you're truly pressed for time, are entertaining, or would otherwise resort to something *really* naughty.

You should also make sure to have lots of homemade or store-bought treats available—for long car rides, airplane trips, or just lazy days. Healthy treats are not only delicious, they keep you balanced so that your next food choice is a good one. Keep them in your desk, your car, your home, and your purse. The office can be an especially tricky place, with Janet's big bowl of Snickers bars staring at you all day. Consider a preemptive strike by starting your own snack bowl!

My favorite store-bought treat is a creation called the Rice Dream Mint Chocolate Frozen Pie: It's a serving of mint rice dream "ice cream," packed between two oatmeal cookies, and entirely dipped in chocolate. You will love them! They live in the freezer of your better health food stores.

ENGAGING OTHER MEMBERS OF THE HOUSEHOLD

There's a good chance you're the only member of your family who's been inspired to take on this sweeping change in diet. Partners and children may want *nothing* to do with the household food changing, and that's fine. Here are a few tips to handle family issues:

- If you are in charge of the family food, there's no need to announce a "big change." Simply add delicious plant-based dishes to the family menu. The recipes in the Vegan section of this book will wow everyone, vegetarians and carnivores alike.

- Use salt, oil, and sweeteners liberally. Most tongues like salt, fat, and sugar.

- Use rice as your secret weapon. Because most people like brown rice, serve up a delicious fried rice dish a couple of times a week and you will find, over months, that it is changing people from the inside out. A more peaceful energy will begin to sneak up on your dinner table.

- Make up a big batch of seeds roasted with shoyu (page 215), and store them in a nice jar, then use them to brighten up any meal. Toss them on everything! I swear you will love them!

QUICK MEALS AND LEFTOVERS

The trick to quick meals is to double up on some dishes so you don't need to start every meal from scratch. That way meal planning becomes more a matter of assembling than actually cooking, per se, and you can get in and out of the kitchen in a matter of minutes.

- Always make extra grain and beans—enough for a couple of days. You can use this food as the base for the next few meals, adding vegetables and other extras to round out meals.

- For a quick dinner, start with a salad as your base. Just add yummy leftovers, like rice, beans, and seeds, or even a potato or tempeh . . . whatever you have around the kitchen that sounds good to you. Get creative. Throw in raisins. Go crazy!

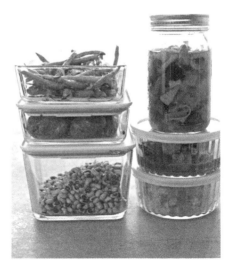

- Wrapping leftovers in nori is perfect for eating on the fly or on a roadtrip. If you have food that you're not that excited about but don't have the energy to turn it into something amazing, just wrap it in a sheet of nori and it gets a complete makeover. (See the recipe on page 219.)

- Soups are great for quick meals because you can empty the fridge into a leftover soup! Start with water or a good vegetable stock, then add grain or sweet potatoes or beans and any vegetables you haven't gotten around to using. Eat with a slice of toast. Quick, yummy, and satisfying!

- Think of baked sweet potatoes as a foolproof convenience food. Bake your sweet potato while you do a million other things, then add Earth Balance spread and salt and pepper or whatever tickles your fancy. Serve some steamed greens on the side and you're done!

- Pizza meals: I'm a firm believer in keeping premade pizzas in the freezer. In a pinch, they are easy, quick, and satisfying. Amy's makes a roasted vegetable pizza that is amazing. Also a great soy cheese pizza. Feel free to add to them whatever you fancy. Some ideas: mushrooms, tomato slices, extra basil, seitan, grilled zucchini, and more soy cheese!

- Take a hunk of French bread (or an English muffin), add some tomato sauce and veggies, drizzle with oil, and add vegan Parmesan cheese. Bake 'til crisp. Yum.

WHAT SHOULD I FEED MY PETS?

First things first: God didn't create some special, different, dried food just for animals to be dropped down from Heaven in big bags. Conventional pet food is basically junk food, only worse: It's chockfull of animal byproducts (intestines, bones, brains, and other lovelies), preservatives, chemicals, and fillers. Is it any wonder pets these days routinely die of nasty conditions like cancer and kidney failure? The only thing sadder than that collection of ingredients is the fact that your furry friend can't yell, "Stop!"

Your animals deserve real and fresh vittles—just like you—so please consider giving them a kinder diet. You guessed it: grains, beans, and vegetables! You see, a vegan diet works really well because pet dogs don't live in the wild; let's face it, they're sorta couch potatoes. They take a walk every day, maybe follow their humans around a little, and not a lot more, so a plant-based diet is just fine for most dogs' energy requirements.

All the members of Christopher's and my doggie pack are between 12 and 17 years old, weigh about 75 pounds each, and every one of them eats a 100 percent plant-based diet. I feed them Dr. Harvey's organic dog food, plus all our leftovers, so there's no waste of food or money. Because some vegan dog food, including Dr. Harvey's, doesn't have them, it's crucial to add L-carnitine and taurine supplements. Their favorite snacks? Carrots and corn cobs. Since starting to eat this way, they've stopped getting fleas, hot spots, and their coats look great. People always think they're younger than they are, so they're getting a little vain!

There are even happy, healthy, vegan cats. Check out www.vegansociety.com/animals/care/cats/ for more details.

For more information visit us at: www.thekindlife.com

II

Kind Away from Home

I eat out two or three times a week, so I consider myself an *expert* in this area. I love the adventure and the social aspect of eating out—it's a great opportunity to spend time with my husband, catch up with a friend, or have a business meeting. I also find that the convenience, luxury, and variety of eating out keep me healthy and happy.

I consider every meal potentially the best one ever, so I enjoy the quest for the world's greatest restaurant. You, like me, may choose to do in-depth research and pepper your server with detailed questions. But if that's not your thing, fear not. You can be as diligent or as relaxed as you like because these days, decent plant-based meals can be made just about anywhere. Even a steakhouse will usually carry a collection of side dishes that will generously fill you up, so there's no excuse to let your new veggie life keep you from celebrating with your friends or family.

Here are my suggestions on how to dine out well. Bon appétit!

Find a place: If you're in a new city or aren't familiar with the good health-conscious places in your area, go to www.thekindlife.com. It has listings of vegetarian restaurants all over the world, with ratings and reviews, phone numbers, and price points for each one. I tried it out in Paris and found there were so many veg places—whodda thunk? I had the best orange-chocolate cake ever! Yes, it probably had sugar in it, but it was vegan and I was in Paris, so leave me alone!

If you already eat out a lot, there may be veggie choices you've never noticed before on your favorite menus. Check the fare of all the restaurants you frequent near home or work—it may be easier to get brown rice than you think.

Check the menu online: No point wasting your time showing up somewhere that's gonna feed you nasty foods. An online menu can give you a sense of the place: the variety of its dishes, the creativity of the chefs, the overall vibe of the restaurant. I always look for dishes that sound exciting— if there's a delicious-sounding salad with chanterelle mushrooms and champagne vinaigrette, I'm there. But I also check the side dishes to make sure there's enough to put together a good meal.

Remember, the days of getting stuck with a big plate of steamed vegetables are over. Make sure the restaurant can meet your needs happily and deliciously.

Call ahead: Once you've checked the menu and gotten some information, don't be afraid to call if you have more questions. Ask if they are interested in accommodating your needs. Sometimes I just check the vibe of the person answering the phone to see how friendly the place is. I'll ask them, "What's your favorite veggie dish there?" or "Would the chef be inspired to make something new?" Just remember they are providing a service that you will pay for. If they don't want to help in a friendly manner, then hey, find a place that does because—thank goodness—a lot of places do.

Ordering: When I look at a menu, the first thing I do is determine where my grain is coming from. Do they have rice, noodles, couscous? After that's chosen, I look for a yummy protein (although I can also skip it) and finally fill out the meal with an array of vegetables. I often check out what comes with all the meat entrées. Sometimes there are amazing side dishes that aren't listed elsewhere on the menu, like roasted beets, and they are happy to let me order them à la carte. Sometimes I'll find a vegetarian dish that includes all of the above elements, and sometimes I piece them together. Either way, I find what I need for a satisfying, balanced meal. It's easy and works every time.

Here are some of the different cuisines I like that offer good, plant-based options for vegans:

Japanese: My favorite! I love sushi, tempura, noodles, and soups, and there are also yummy vegetable nori rolls, vegetable dumplings, house salads with carrot/ginger dressing, amazing seaweed salads, and that spinach dish with sesame sauce . . . mmmm. However, not all Japanese dishes are the Superhero foods they seem. For instance sushi rice almost always has sugar in it. You can ask for your sushi to be made with "kitchen rice" (without sugar), but if they can't accommodate my request, I eat it anyway. You can also ask if the tempura batter has egg in it—sometimes it does, although some places use other methods to bind the batter.

Many sushi chefs will be happy to make this awesome roll that includes avocado and a piece of asparagus tempura, or sweet potato tempura. It's delicious.

Mexican: I'm not a big Mexican food fan, but my man loves it. He lives on burritos, which you can get almost anywhere these days. Of course, picking a place that uses fresher, more organic ingredients is best, but worst-case scenario, a no-lard bean burrito without cheese or sour cream is a pretty decent vegan meal. Some places these days even offer soy cheese and tofu sour cream. Chips, salsa, guac, and a big salad round out the meal.

Italian: White pasta may not be the healthiest choice in the world, but it's a delicious, fun dish that's not too hard on your body and it's vegan. Yes, there's probably a bit of sugar in the tomato sauce, and most homemade pastas—like those used to make ravioli—are made with eggs. If so, I just let it go. Life's too short to get agitated about everything. That being said, there are tons of great Italian dishes to eat: Pasta Arrabiata or Puttanesca, risotto (ask for no cheese or chicken stock), fresh salads, and soups! Add some bruschetta and you have a great meal.

Other great choices: Thai, Chinese, Indian, Ethiopian, and Middle Eastern cuisines all feature a variety of dishes that are vegan friendly; just try to avoid sugar and MSG. Many places will make the dishes without them, so ask. I also love French food and find that I can put together a lovely vegan meal at willing establishments. If it's your first time at a particular restaurant, call ahead of time to make sure you can get something yummy and healthy.

TEMPTATION

It's not always easy to make great choices when eating out—especially when the people around you are eating nasty foods. Believe me, I understand. I experience little hiccups myself, and it's usually when I'm eating out. For instance, I *love* sushi. As a kid, I used to ride my bike to the store and spend my weekly allowance on sushi. Not candy. Not comics. Raw fish on rice.

So what's my strategy for going out with friends for sushi? First of all, I order all the vegetable rolls and other veggie dishes that look exciting. Most of the time, when I'm done with all that food, I'm stuffed and feel very satisfied. But, every once in a very long while, if I'm still tempted by the fish, I nick a piece of sushi off a friend's plate right at the end of the meal. Yes, it tastes amazing, but if I'm really honest with myself, no better than anything else I've eaten. Sometimes I just have to scratch that itch. I wrestle with guilt about eating a fishy friend, but that's my way of living in a sushi world. I hope my strategy works for you, too.

P.S. Living in a butterscotch pudding world can be hard, too! I just take one (or two) bites of a friend's pudding when it feels impossible to pass up, but then I remember, like I did with the sushi, that it's no better than the desserts on pages 180–195, and I can eat those every day!

FOR SUPERHEROES

Eating out as a Superhero may seem a little trickier, but it's really not. The biggest difference may be that as your body becomes really clean and supersensitive to extreme foods, you run a little risk of feeling pooey after eating at a restaurant, depending on where you go. Just choose carefully and come home prepared to make a little Cure-All Tea (page 290), if you think you've eaten something that your body is reacting to.

TRAVEL TIPS

Whether you are a world-weary globetrotter or simply getting away for the weekend, eating kindly while you travel can take a little effort, but it's always worth it. Here are some tips for staying balanced on the road:

Airplanes: When you're taking a long flight, try to avoid baked flour, coffee, alcohol, and strong sweets the day before and during the flight—it's even good if you can go without them the day you arrive. All these things can dehydrate you and stress your body, and both of these effects are exacerbated at 35,000 feet. If you stay hydrated and relaxed, you will arrive at your destination feeling much better and will adjust more readily.

Order a vegan or vegetarian meal for the plane. You can often do this on travel Web sites if you book your own ticket or mention it to an agent on the phone. To make sure you get your meal, call the airline 2 days before you fly to confirm. That way, you'll have something somewhat healthy on the plane. It also tells the airline that more people want healthy options these days. Plus, it puts one less dead animal on the plane that will only end up wasted (there are so many leftovers it's insane!).

Always bring your own snacks on the plane. Even if you get a vegetarian meal, airplane food is not known for its gourmet qualities, so don't depend on it.

Do a hot body scrub (see page 128) when you arrive at your destination. It will open your

---

For Students

- If you live in a dorm, ask your parents if they'll spring for a little refrigerator (some colleges will rent them to you), a rice cooker, and a toaster oven. Between those three things, you will have lots of flexibility. Just don't fill the whole fridge with beer!

- Take extra fruit and other good foods from the cafeteria for snacks.

- If your room gets decent sunlight, consider growing some herbs (legal ones!) in a window box. Basil, cilantro, parsley, and chives are good ones to start with. If you have a little space for gardening, tomatoes and lettuce are really easy to grow, too!

- Is there a vegetarian group on campus? Consider finding them to get some support and community. Have potlucks or get together for dinner at a local restaurant. There's no reason to do this alone.

For more information visit us at: www.thekindlife.com

pores, increase circulation, and make you feel very energized. All of this helps with jet lag. If you can find a patch of grass at your destination, take off your shoes and walk barefoot on it. This helps your body adjust to the new environment.

Walk as much as possible when traveling. It's good for you and helps your body acclimate better.

If jet lag is a problem for you, go to www.thekindlife.com and enter the keyword No Jet Lag to try this homeopathic remedy. I used to have really bad jet lag until I found this product and used it.

If your hotel offers them, ask for a small fridge or have the staff empty the mini bar for your use and stock up with smart breakfast and snack options. This makes life much easier, especially on long trips. If it's a really long trip, get a room with a kitchenette.

Superhero Items for the Road

- Umeboshi plums (great for nausea and an overly acid stomach)
- Sea salt
- Ramen-type noodles that can cook in a cup
- Real miso (best choice) or instant miso
- Plain, instant oatmeal (although some maple-sweetened ones are fine, too)
- Thermos travel mug
- Kukicha tea bags for Cure-All Tea (page 290)
- Homemade Crispy Peanut Butter Treats (page 184)
- Brown rice syrup candies

If you can, visit some of my favorite vegetarian restaurants. In New York, I love Candle 79, Hangawi, Teany (Moby's restaurant), and Vegetarian Dim Sum House. For Superheroes, check out Souen. For great baked goods, I go to Babycakes.

In L.A., I like Elf, Shima, Real Food Daily, and M Cafe. Superheroes should go to Inaka. For more information on great restaurants, check out my Web site thekindlife.com.

> My refusing to eat flesh occasioned an inconveniency, and I was frequently chided for my singularity, but, with this lighter repast, I made the greater progress, for greater clearness of head and quicker comprehension.
>
> —Ben Franklin

For more information visit us at: www.thekindlife.com

ENTERTAINING

I love throwing parties. I take great pride in creating plant-based menus so delicious that all my friends leave the party surprised and delighted. There is absolutely no deprivation in this way of life, and your parties will prove it. I've included some fancy menus here to show you what's possible when partying with plant-based foods.

Some of our friends have Sunday brunch parties. Guests pay a small amount, like $5, and they are served a crazy yummy brunch. Between the good food, good vibes, and nice people, it's a deeply nourishing experience. Try it yourself!

Set a time once a week for friends to gather with great new vegan dishes. Either you can trust the fates to pull together a balanced spread, or e-mail ideas about what dishes are needed. It's a great opportunity for everyone to try a whole new set of recipes and eat a great meal. It also saves cooking time and gets you out of your kitchen. Ask everyone to bring copies of their recipes to share.

There's no reason to compromise your way of eating to entertain. I can't tell you how many times my friends say, "If I could eat like this all the time, I would be veggie!" And I just smile and feel great because I know that—somewhere in their body and mind—it's registering that the plant-based food can both be delicious and make them feel good. I consider that a huge win.

Thanksgiving Menu chez Silverstone '07

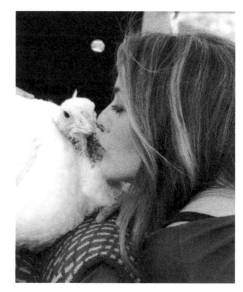

Root vegetable cassoulet with pumpkin soufflé crust

Seitan piccata with white wine and caper sauce

Cornbread, shiitake, and leek stuffing with miso gravy

Green beans with chestnuts and topped with crispy shallots

Classic garnet yams with homemade marshmallows

Classic fluffy and creamy mashed potatoes (made with soy sour cream and vegetable stock)

Butter lettuce salad with spicy pecans, grilled pears, and persimmon dressing

Pumpkin pie with soy ice cream

Pecan pie with Cool Whip!

Crispy Peanut Butter Treats

My 30th Birthday Party Menu

Ginger-pomegranate saketini

Citrus herb-marinated seitan skewers

Sesame roasted yam salad with citrus dressing

Thai spicy eggplant, squash, and coconut curry with basil and chili jam

Pappardelle nests with wild mushroom, artichokes, and truffle oil

Crème brûlée with spoons of ginger, coconut, and passion fruit

Chocolate pudding mousse with berries, mint, and cacao nibs

Cashew-pecan sandies

Vegan Cupcake Party

We recently threw a cupcake party, inspired by the book *Vegan Cupcakes Take Over the World*. Everyone brought a batch of homemade vegan cupcakes and we supplied the champagne . . . and more cupcakes!!!!

Barbecue

There's nothing like a barbecue in the summer. Toss some veggie burgers and tofu dogs on the grill along with some Gardein "chicken" breasts and skewered vegetables. Round it all out with coleslaw, potato salad, corn on the cob, chips with Guacamole (page 207), and my Artichoke Dip (page 205). Wash it down with sangria and beer, and don't forget the vegan ice cream sandwiches!

12

Getting Fit, Inside and Out

Even if the only time you leave the couch is to walk back and forth from the refrigerator, after 4 weeks on the Kind Diet, you will see significant changes in the way you look and feel. But let's face it, an entirely sedentary lifestyle isn't going to get you to your most vibrant, energetic, and healthy self. Here are my favorite ways to keep my body, skin, and brain fit and toned.

EXERCISE

On the Kind Diet, even exercise is kind. If you've thought of exercise as punishment you must inflict on yourself in order to lose weight, those days are over. If you already love your workouts, that love will deepen. Either way, it's time to start enjoying your beautiful life in your beautiful new body.

What would happen if you really listened to your body and let it go through the rhythms *it* wanted to go through? When you just exercise mechanically—raising your heart rate to a prescribed number, working out your legs because that's the regimen for Wednesday—you can lose touch with your inner self. What if you just said, "You know what? I'm tired right now! Maybe I'll actually *rest* for 5 minutes—or take a walk outside." Little decisions like those can change your whole perspective, and in those 5 minutes—resting or walking—you can get quiet inside and ask your heart, "What do I really need?" If you're too busy looking at the cardio monitor on the Stairmaster, it will be impossible to hear the answer to that question because you're just not in touch with your body. As you continue to eat whole grains and vegetables, your body will begin to tell you what it wants and needs. Your energy will lighten up, and you may not need to work as hard or sweat as much to feel the benefits of exercise.

So do what you love. I find yoga, dance classes, and walks make me feel most relaxed and energized. I want to love my *whole* life, and that includes exercise.

Here are some of the benefits of the simplest forms of exercise:

Walking: Unbelievably good for you. Great for the heart, the lymph system, and your over-all outlook on life. Take a walk every day if you can. My husband and I try to walk with the dogs every night after dinner in the summer. It's also a great way to catch up with my girlfriends (I hate talking on the phone). Looking at nature is so much better than going to the gym, and it's free—right outside your door! It's great if I can walk for half an hour, but every day is different. Doing it regularly is more important than how long you spend walking. Here's a tip: Whenever you see grass, take off your shoes and walk on it. That connection with the grass brings out your goddess and helps you connect with nature!

Yoga: Yoga is a beautiful battlefield. I breathe through the sticky stuff of my mind, the resistance in my body . . . without force or judgment . . . all on a safe little rectangle. I engage in a soft, loving battle with my stiffness and laziness in an attempt to get down to the good stuff of life. By practicing yoga, I get stronger and stronger, little by little, and I bring that strength into my life. And the best thing about yoga? You don't have to be good at it. I go to beginners' classes because there's no pressure to be anywhere but where I am.

Playing with friends: Sometimes we get together with friends and play soccer. On the pitch, we have a 5-year-old, an 8-year-old, a handful of 30-somethings, and a guy pushing 60. Together we go completely insane, running around, kicking the ball, missing the ball, and laughing our

---

Vegetarian Athletes

If you're really into working out and think that being vegan or vegetarian will compromise your strength, endurance, or athletic performance, use one of these veggie (or vegan) athletes as a role model:

- Bill Walton, John Salley, Salim Stoudamire (NBA basketball players)
- Scott Jurek (ultramarathoner)
- Carl Lewis (nine-time Olympic gold medalist)
- Bruce Lee (martial artist)
- Edwin Moses (world champion and Olympic gold medalist in track and field)
- Martina Navratilova, Billie Jean King, and Chris Evert (tennis icons)
- Mac Danzig (winner of the Ultimate Fighter, 6)

And many, many more . . .

heads off. And at the same time, it's a serious match that gives all of us a kickass workout. So find a friend and shoot some hoops, embarrass yourselves at a public tennis court, or fling a Frisbee. No gym membership required!

HOT BODY SCRUB

This technique is cheap and easy, refreshes the whole body, and makes your skin gorgeous because:

- It increases circulation.
- It helps the fat trapped under your skin to loosen up and dissolve.
- It opens the pores to release toxins.
- It helps to circulate lymph fluid.

If you're an overachiever, do the body scrub morning and night. Me, I try my best to do it every morning. I encourage you to do it for a month and see the amazing results.

Fill the sink about halfway with hot, hot water, but not hot enough to scald you. Throw in a washcloth. Remove it from the water, wring it out, and starting at your face, scrub yourself silly, continually dunking and wringing out the washcloth as it cools off. Dunk the washcloth and scrub your face, your chest, your pits, your arms, your hands, redunking whenever the washcloth cools off. Avoid scrubbing your breasts and privates, but do make sure to cover the entire groin area *except* your privates to stimulate the lymph nodes there. If you're not feeling like Miss America (yet), be sure to tell yourself nice things while you scrub; admire how cute your feet are and how lovely your curves are. For the guys, notice your manly and irresistible physique; this body scrub should be a loving experience. Whenever the water in the sink gets cool, add more hot. The whole thing should take about 5 to 8 minutes.

INNER EXERCISE

Journaling: Writing calms my mind. When I'm stressed out about something, thoughts and worries can just swirl around in my head on an endless loop. When I take the time to journal, the thoughts come out onto the page so I can really look at them and coach myself through them, asking myself, "Why are you doing that?" "What do you really want?" When I'm writing, the answers have the time and space to present themselves. We all have great stores of natural wisdom, and journaling helps to tap into them.

Meditation: If you struggle with stress or anxiety (and who doesn't?), a meditation practice can be life-changing. It doesn't have to be an elaborate ritual; just set a timer for 10 or 15 (or even 5) minutes and observe your breath (even if it means noticing you're not breathing much). Or focus on the sensations of your body, beginning at your toes and moving up your legs, torso, and so on, bit by bit. Your mind will wander, but the practice is to bring it back, again and again, gently. Eventually and with practice, the mind begins to slow down and become focused. You will then carry that peace and focus through the rest of your day. If you find meditation helpful and satisfying, try to go for 30 minutes. It's hard at first, but you will find a depth and relaxation inside that's just amazing.

Of course, life is full of opportunities to practice meditation. By relaxing when I'm stuck in traffic, waiting in line, or facing a frustrating situation, I drop my inner tension and just enjoy the moment. I'm certainly not perfect at it, but life is so much better when I am able to sink into my body and ride the waves.

LOSING MY WAY

Sometimes I forget to put myself first; all my goals and responsibilities come before basic self-care. I had one of these times recently; I was taking care of my dogs (one of them is incontinent, the other blind and unable to walk), writing this book, rehearsing a play, campaigning for our new president, advocating for the release of elephants from the L.A. Zoo, going to auditions, and trying to be a decent partner to my husband . . . not to mention handling all the random stressful surprises that pop up in life. And that's all without mentioning the endless to-do list staring me in the face. It was a real struggle; I felt like there was no way I could do it all, and yet I had to.

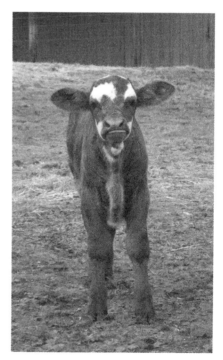

It's at times like these that I start to make shortcuts: I scarf sandwiches at the computer, eat while having stressful conversations, and make other cuckoo choices. Meditation gets the heave-ho. Exercise? Forget it. My journal gets lost under my bed as taking care of myself drops off the to-do list.

Suddenly I'm on the floor, sobbing.

I've lost my way.

But thank *God* I have a way to lose. So I remember to:

- Make clean, healthy food
- Sit down while I eat
- Take a deep breath and say a prayer of gratitude before eating
- Remember that I don't run the world, and then I cut my to-do list in half
- Restructure my time to put myself first

And I find my way again.

The second I structure my time to allow myself to eat better, I feel completely different. My whole body changes. Drastically. That's what's so amazing about this way of life—one day of clean eating and my throat stops hurting. I feel rested. I'm surprised every time it happens, and it happens *every time*.

I know you have a million excuses for not taking care of yourself. It's easy to feel pulled down by the ball-and-chain of the to-do list. But if you don't stay centered by doing the basic things, everything and everyone in your life will pay for it. I know it may feel naughty to acknowledge (even to yourself) that you are putting yourself first, but think of it this way: A mother must eat good food to produce good milk for her baby. There are no shortcuts there. So be a good mother to all the beings and creative projects in your life by taking care of yourself first. Know that when you lose your way—and you will—you will always be able to come back home.

Our lives are not in the lap of the gods, but in the lap of our cooks.
—Lin Yutang

13

We Are All Activists

Eating a plant-based diet is the most ecologically friendly thing you can do. But there's always more to be done to help our collective home—the environment—so please don't stop there.

Each and every one of us can be an activist for change, and you don't have to pick up a sign or march at a rally to do it. Just start to think about your choices and vote with your dollar. For example, every time you shop at a farmers' market—or buy organic food—you are supporting your community. Every time you purchase organic plant-based food, you are protecting the quality of the soil and participating in a more equitable distribution of resources. Conversely, every time you buy a mass-produced steak—packaged in Styrofoam and plastic—you are feeding a huge, unsustainable, toxic death machine. This may sound harsh, but it's the truth! There's a whole world of consequences behind every decision we make.

I consider every choice an opportunity to make positive change, and every change matters. Yours, mine, and the queen of England's. Throughout the course of your daily life, you have the power to make real and important changes in the world just by being mindful of your choices.

And it's easy. For example, when I need to dispose of something, I can choose whether to throw it in the trash or in the recycling box. One choice makes more landfill while the other keeps resources circulating. Just deciding which box to throw my trash in is a little choice with enormous consequences. Little choice; big impact.

If I have to go a 7-Eleven, chances are there's not much there that I want, but I can walk out of there making the best choice possible: maybe sunflower seeds and apple juice. Yes, I'm bummed about the packaging and that they're not organic, but it's my best 7-Eleven choice. I walk away being kind to my body instead of hurting it. I did the best I could under the circumstances, and that's what we're looking for: the best choices under any circumstances. And those little daily choices can turn a lot of things around.

The world is changing very quickly. Because I've been paying attention to the food/animal/environment issue for a while now, let me tell you that there has been *enormous* movement in this area. Organics is the fastest-growing sector of the food industry. Vegetarian joints are opening up every day and thriving. Suddenly it's not only cool but also financially savvy to be green. In 10 short years, it's like the whole world has awakened. So, making what used to be radical choices is now just plain smart and the right thing to do. How great is that?

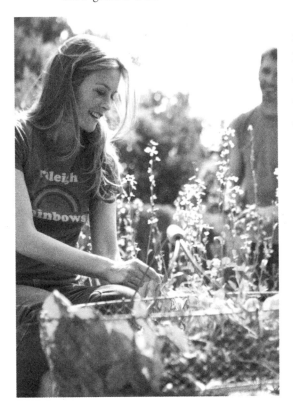

Sometimes it's hard to get perspective on the really big shifts, but as time marches forward, the little things can show us the impact we are having. Christopher and I started our compost heap about 6 years ago with a handful of worms. As time went on and we threw scrap after scrap onto the compost, they multiplied. Well, now it's a freakin' worm factory! They're so vibrant and amazing, doing their noble work. And because of them, there are new types of birds coming to our house as well as little lizards, and butterflies, and hummingbirds, and other animals. Nature is smiling on us because of the little choices we make every day. It's amazing to watch the earth bounce back.

Of course, there's more to do. Go ahead and volunteer to help dig wells in Africa. Please give your extra money and time to worthy charities. Yes, write your senator and march on Washington. I need you, the animals need you, and all the people who have yet to be born need you. But remember that simply by abstaining from meat and dairy, you are doing so much. Making that vital choice supports every form of life on the planet, from microbes in the soil, to your fellow human beings, to our precious atmosphere. And as you continue to eat whole grains and vegetables, saying good-bye to crazy, toxic foods, you will become stronger and stronger, more and more powerful; and protecting the earth will feel like second nature.

LIFESTYLE TIPS

Here are some simple and super-easy steps that you can take to truly help our planet! You can find more info about these lifestyle choices, and many other small changes that you can make in order to be kind to the planet, by going to www.thekindlife.com. Just type in the keyword lifestyle and you will find loads of info, programs to get involved in, and links to other helpful Web sites.

- Reuse things: Save both money and resources by reusing stuff like paper, jars, and containers. Paper especially is everywhere. Used paper is great for shopping lists or your kids' artistic creations. Print and fax on the back of used paper, too.

- Buy secondhand: There's almost nothing you can't find secondhand these days. I buy most of my clothes at vintage stores and always cruise the Internet for other necessities to avoid creating more stuff. Look for furniture, books, appliances, bikes, and cars second-hand. I just bought the cutest purple kettle from craigslist! Be sure to watch an amazing video by Anne Leonard at thestoryofstuff.com.

- Give stuff away: When Christopher and I are done with something, we put it out on our street with a big sign that says "FREE." It's always gone within the day. I believe there is a happy home for every unwanted or unneeded possession. Do the work to find that home, and you've slowed the creation of a landfill. And you will benefit, too; lightening your material load frees you up on all levels. To give stuff away via the Internet, go to freecycle. com.

- Recycling is great, but it requires a *lot* of energy, so try to reuse before you recycle. That said, recycling is better than making landfill. Live by the adage "Reduce, reuse, recycle."

- Use natural materials whenever possible: Modern products can be toxic; between plastics, vinyl, flame retardants, and pesticides, furniture and clothing can leave a dangerous mark on you and the environment. When you're buying new things, try to find items made as naturally as possible; for outdoors, it's good to buy used items or products made from recycled materials. That way, you're delaying waste, and any remaining funkiness can be released into the open air and not inhaled by you!

- Use natural cleaning and personal products: Household items such as all-purpose cleaners, laundry detergents, and even feminine products are now made with biodegrad-able, nontoxic ingredients. For an in-depth look at keeping a green home, read *The Eco Chick Guide to Life: How to Be Fabulously Green* by Starre Vartan.

- Use nontoxic, biodegradable beauty products: There's no reason to trash your health or the planet just to get gussied up.

For more information visit us at: www.thekindlife.com

- Give thoughtful, practical gifts: I love to give food, kitchenware, books, and beauty products as gifts. I love the thought of my friend actually *using* something I've given her.

- Get a good water filter for your tap. Stop buying bottled water.

- Stop using plastic bags and invest in a canvas bag for shopping. Americans use 380 *billion* plastic bags per year. We can put a dent in that number, one bag at a time.

- Reduce your electricity use by unplugging appliances when they're not being used. Get compact fluorescent light bulbs. Turn off lights when you're not using them.

- Burning candles is a sexy lighting choice, but use soy candles. Conventional candles are made from toxic petroleum byproducts, the palm wax industry is responsible for destroying orangutan habitat, and beeswax—unless you're getting it from a local, groovy beekeeper—is bad for bees.

- Walk or ride your bike when you can.

- Reduce paper waste by getting your news online. Reduce junk mail by signing up at mailstopper.tonic.com.

For more information on saving the planet with style, go to my Web site at www.thekindlife. com, where you can check out my favorite ecofriendly designers, makeup companies, household products, plus all my newest and latest groovy finds.

For more information visit us at: www.thekindlife.com

FINALLY

I believe that following the Kind Diet can lead to world peace. That might sound naïve, but consider this:

World peace begins inside you—literally. In your body and mind. Global peace can only be achieved when the individuals living in the world recognize peace within themselves.

And food plays a big role in that. Food affects how you perceive the world, how angry you get at other drivers, how ossified your resentments become, how much your joints ache at the end of the day. Those things can make or break your inner peace. Luckily, we're seeing that a varied plant-based diet will make your body more flexible, your mind more open, and your day-to-day experience of life more peaceful.

And to believe otherwise? *That* is naïve.

Yes, some of our problems need to be picked at in a laboratory, others must be hashed out in the halls of government, but what shows up on the dinner table is the foundation of our lives— the base—and it's the most fertile soil in which to sow the seeds of peace. We *all* need good food, clean air, and clean water. Unless we can breathe and eat and live well, how can we expect to live together peacefully?

I'm not saying that by changing your diet the world is going to change overnight. But by taking care of your body and consciousness, you will impact everyone in your life —whether you see it or not. By choosing kindness as your creed, in how you treat yourself, the planet, and other creatures, you are expressing the greatest power you have. Instead of trying to *achieve* peace, you *are* peace. And that, my friend, is big.

And who knows? Maybe the whole world *will* start the Kind Diet. I'd love to see what would happen if the whole world were vegan for even a month. Eating in a way that supports us on every level, without the industrial toxins, excess hormones, the adrenaline and cruel vibes of meat running through our veins—how might we behave?

But let's begin with you. And me. And express the lovely peace we feel inside. As we relax and enjoy this beautiful journey called life, we can laugh and wink and play and bring yummy food to our friends' parties and feel good on every level until the world comes knocking on our doors, asking, "Can I taste that?"

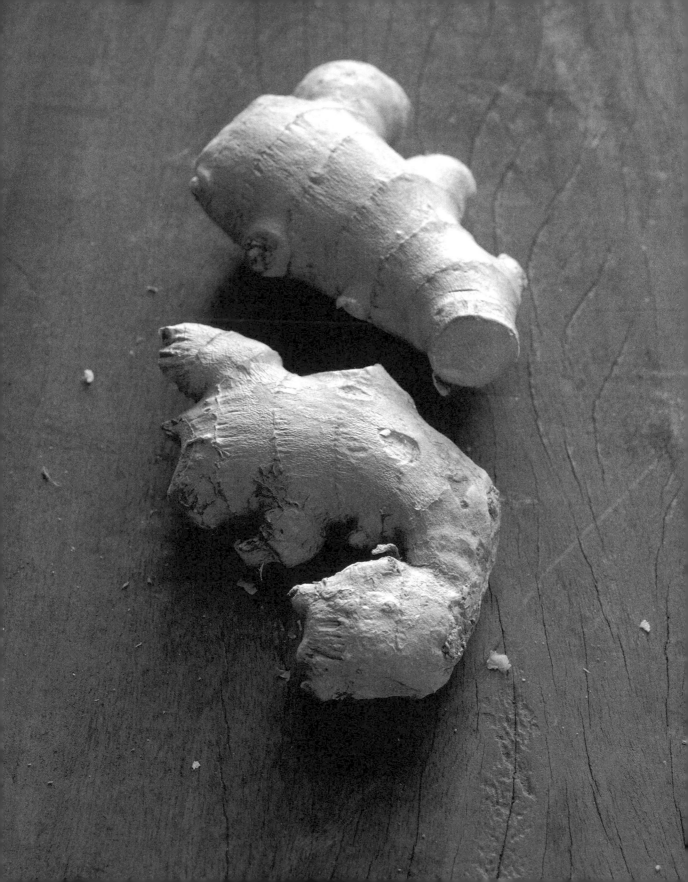

PART III

the recipes

Here's where the magic begins. In using these recipes, you will transform your kitchen into a powerful place of health and happiness, one dish at a time. You will see your skin begin to glow, your body begin to relax, and your mind settle into peace.

I've divided the recipes into two groups, one for Vegans and another for Superheroes, but if you are just starting out on your vegan path, please don't consider the Superhero recipes off limits. To the contrary, I invite vegans to eat as many of the Superhero dishes as possible as often as possible. Some of them are so good, I would be devastated if you didn't get to try them. (Try the Maple-Roasted Lotus Root, Sunchokes, and Leeks dish on page 269 or the Arame Turnovers on page 260 if you have any doubts about how delicious Superhero food can be.)

If you are really striving to attain Superhero status, on the other hand, vegan dishes should be an occasional indulgence (see page 141 for more on balancing Vegan and Superhero diets), but you can indulge in any of the Superhero dishes as often as you like. If losing weight is your priority, I've begun this section with tips for quicker weight loss that you can apply while you eat your way to absolute nirvana. So let's get started . . . now!

TIPS FOR QUICKER WEIGHT LOSS

- Follow the Superhero plan 6 days a week and regular Vegan 1 day a week. You will see amazing results. You will not only get all of your nutritional needs met, your cholesterol will go down, your blood pressure will drop, and you should lose a couple of pounds a week! Add exercise to the mix, and your body will respond even faster. If you don't want to go 6 days Superhero/1 day Vegan, just allow yourself 3 regular Vegan meals over the course of the week.

- Eat as many whole grains and vegetables as you like. I mean it. Go crazy. And when I say whole grains, I mean the grains themselves, not the bread or noodle products. It's the whole grains that will get your skinny on.

- Drink the Weight Loss Tea (Carrot-Daikon Drink) every day on an empty stomach for 10 days. After 10 days, drink it three times a week for 3 weeks. If you want to continue, a couple of times a week should do the trick; do *not* drink it every day after the initial 10 days. Too much can make you weak and demineralized. Wait 3 months before repeating the intensive 10-day program again.

- That being said, it's okay to make friends with daikon. It is a natural diuretic, and you can use it in soups, stews, and other vegetable dishes. It's fine to eat a little daikon every day as a part of your regular meals.

- Chew your food extremely well. The more you chew, the more energy you will get from the food and the more satisfied you will feel.

- Do your best to eliminate white sugar from your diet completely. It's fine to eat some natural sweeteners, but white sugar is truly addictive and just makes you crave more. That addictive cycle can slow down weight loss and hijack sanity. Transition to sweeteners like brown rice syrup to break your white sugar habit.

- Keep truly indulgent vegan foods out of the house. Yes, you can have a piece of agave-sweetened chocolate cake every once in a while, but having the whole cake staring you in the face every time you enter the kitchen is just cruel. If your focus is on losing weight, choose at-home desserts from the Superhero plan.

- Consume salt, shoyu, and miso in moderation. Seasoning should taste mild. Too much salt can set you up to overeat or crave strong sweets.

Weight Loss Tea (Carrot-Daikon Drink)

SERVES 1

½ cup grated (into a pulp) carrot
½ cup grated (into a pulp) daikon
¼ umeboshi plum

1–2 drops shoyu
¼ sheet nori, ripped into small pieces (optional)

Bring the carrot, daikon, umeboshi plum, and 1 cup of water to a boil in a small saucepan. Reduce the heat, and simmer for about 3 minutes. Add the shoyu and simmer for 2 to 3 minutes longer. Add the nori, if using. Drink hot, eating the carrot and daikon pulp along with the tea.

- Balance begets balance and crazy begets crazy. Start your day with a nutritious, satisfying breakfast and you will eat better the rest of the day. Skip breakfast and you will go to the opposite extreme of overeating or eating crazy food later in the day.

- It's okay to start your day over if you've made some wacky choices. Just sit down, chew some whole grains and veggies, and you will feel fine.

- Stop eating 3 hours before you plan to go to bed.

- Do some kind of fun exercise three to five times a week. See pages 126–129 for suggestions.

- For bonus points, do a hot body scrub every day. See page 128.

And while the Kind Diet is amazing for losing weight, don't think you can't keep your curves or build muscle on a plant-based regime. If you're looking to gain weight, simply eat a balanced diet and give yourself permission to really enjoy flour products like bread and noodles; oils, tahini, and nut butters; and tempeh, seitan, and hearty bean dishes.

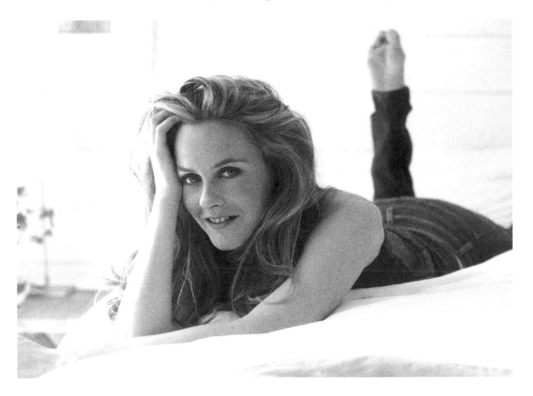

14

Vegan Recipes

On the following pages you will find some of my very favorite recipes to get you started on your journey. These are recipes I like to serve to people who may be skeptics; they're easy to make and easy to love, and none of them screams, "Meatless! Vegan!" I think they are all amazing, and when I entertain, they always go over well with our guests.

I want to mention, though, that you can easily perform vegan makeovers on many of the recipes you already have just by making simple substitutions: soy, rice, or nut milk for regular milk; Earth Balance buttery spread for butter; water or vegetable broth in place of chicken or beef stock. And you can make lots of simple meals without referring to a recipe at all—just remember to build your meal around a serving of grains (rice, quinoa, whole grain pasta, and so on), add some protein (some yummy beans, or tofu, maybe tempeh or seitan), then go crazy with as many greens and veggies as you like, either lightly dressed with a vinaigrette or brightened up with a bit of gomashio—so easy to put together and so delicious.

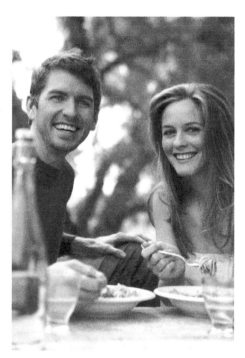

Remember, too, that you can cook from the Superhero section (Chapter 15) whenever you like. In some ways it breaks my heart to separate them from the Vegan recipes because I don't want to give you the impression that vegans shouldn't be eating from the Superhero menu regularly. To the contrary, please eat *lots* of Superhero foods. It's all vegan, too, just a little simpler and more strengthening. Likewise, when Superheroes need a little break, they can sample from the richer Vegan dishes. So although the recipes are separated, they're not . . . dig?

Lastly, please don't regard these recipes as written in stone; let them serve as a springboard to your brilliant inner chef, and when you make something new and fantastic . . . send me the recipe!!!

A note about the recipes and some of the ingredients I use most frequently:

Salt: The best salt to use is unrefined sea salt. I refer to it in the recipes as "fine sea salt" because it's not the big, chunky salt crystals, but the finer white crystals. Sea salt contains 80 minerals needed by the human body, and it reflects the natural mineral composition of our blood. Table salt has had most of those minerals removed and can lead to all sorts of nasty problems like high blood pressure. The brand I use is called Si Salt and it's naturally sun-dried in Mexico. If you can't find Si Salt, be sure to choose a sea salt that is unrefined.

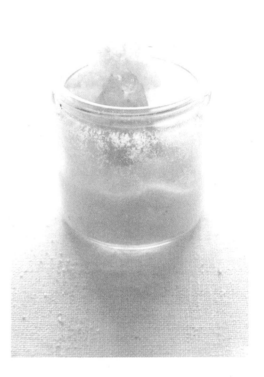

Shoyu and tamari: Shoyu is the Japanese word for soy sauce, and it's how most soy sauce is labeled in the health food world these days. Shoyu is made from soybeans, salt, and wheat. Tamari is also made from soybeans, but contains no wheat. If you have a wheat intolerance, go for tamari, but I use shoyu in these recipes. It's important to use a shoyu without sugar, alcohol, or chemical preservatives. I like Nama Shoyu ("nama" means raw) made by Ohsawa brand, and Mitoku and Eden are other good choices. The shoyus that show up at most Japanese and Chinese restaurants are not of good quality and contain added sugar and other nasty ingredients, so make the effort to source out a good one to use at home. A better shoyu can be a little pricey, so try to order it in bulk.

Butter: There are a few different vegan or soy-based margarines out there, but my favorite is Earth Balance organic buttery spread. In any of my recipes where a butter substitute is called for, I use this organic buttery spread and refer to it as Earth Balance butter. I've experimented with a lot of brands, and it's my hands-down favorite. It comes in tubs and sticks, so it's versatile, and it's widely available at supermarkets, health food stores, and the big natural food chains. If you prefer another brand, then go for it, but avoid any with hydrogenated oils.

Mayonnaise: Whenever a recipe calls for a mayonnaise-y type taste, I use Vegenaise. Again, there are a few faux mayos on the market, but I like this one the best. It is made by a company called Follow Your Heart and sweetened only with brown rice syrup. Unlike the other brands, which sit on the shelf, Vegenaise lives in the refrigerated dairy section of the health food store.

Cheese: The vegan cheese I use is made by Follow Your Heart as well. They make jalapeño, mozzarella, and Cheddar flavors. Of all the vegan cheeses I've tried, I find it tastes and melts the best.

Sour cream: Whenever I use sour cream, it's vegan sour cream made by Tofutti. FYI: They also make the best cream cheese.

Tofu: You can buy tofu in different textures; soft is great for sauces and dessert toppings. Firm is fine for most cooking and extra-firm makes nice, chunky, solid pieces perfect for stir-frying and creating meat substitutes. You can also buy it baked or premarinated.

Seitan: Seitan is now made by a few companies and generally comes in a plastic tub like tofu or in a vacuum-packed bag in a box. You can find it near the tofu and tempeh. Although all seitan is seasoned with shoyu, some are specially seasoned to taste like chicken, barbecued beef, and so on. In this book, when I call for seitan, I mean regular, unflavored seitan.

Maple sugar: Many of the dessert recipes call for maple sugar, which is crystallized maple syrup. When using maple sugar for baking recipes, crush and sift it a little to reduce big crystals to smaller ones. You'll find that maple sugar is expensive, so if you're making yummy vegan desserts on a really regular basis, you might want to consider an alternative such as vegan cane sugar, which is available at Whole Foods. But before you make that decision, I just want to remind you that maple sugar is a *much* healthier choice, and that's what you're paying for—no headache, no hangover, no addictive craving, and no health issues. I can't, with a clean conscience, recommend that you use white sugar, but I understand if your budget won't make room for the expensive stuff all the time.

Organics: In order to avoid writing the word "organic" before every single ingredient, I've just assumed it. Whenever possible, I use organic ingredients.

GRAIN AND PASTA DISHES

Get ready to fall in love with grains in a whole new way—not just in the form of refined flour products, but in their earthy, hearty, natural whole state. A grain dish should be at the center of every meal. They give you loads of energy, are filling, and are extremely nourishing, with all kinds of great minerals. Whole grains and products made from whole grains are simple to cook and can be made into elegant dishes to serve family or friends. Once you've mastered the basics, like brown rice, try your hand at barley, farro, amaranth, or millet; and when you are comfortable cooking them, experiment and get creative. With the addition of some chopped veggies and herbs, and maybe a bit of oil and lemon juice or vinegar, cooked grains make great salads, fillings for stuffed vegetables, or pilafs. To keep your palate deliriously happy, pastas are also really easy and versatile, and you can probably adapt many of the recipes you are already making. Try whole wheat and rice pastas, but don't rely on the package instructions for cooking times. Keep checking to ensure the strands stay separate and don't overcook.

Radicchio Pizza with Truffle Oil

When my friend Liz first taught me how to make this pizza, she used an organic, sourdough spelt crust, but really any whole grain crust will do. This pizza is perfect for dinner parties or just a cozy night at home.

SERVES 2 TO 4

1 large head radicchio

Olive oil

Fine sea salt and freshly ground black pepper, to taste

White truffle-infused oil, to taste

1 pizza crust, fresh or frozen, preferably a healthy, whole grain variety

Cut the radicchio in half, then slice each half crosswise into thin ribbons (as thin as possible!). Dress with olive oil, salt, pepper, and a few dashes of white truffle oil to taste.

Preheat the oven to 415°F. If using a fresh pizza crust, toast in the oven for 7 minutes or until it is heated through and slightly golden but not crunchy; if using a frozen crust, bake according to package directions. Scatter the dressed radicchio over the pizza crust and return to the oven for another 3 to 5 minutes, until the radicchio is warm and just starting to wilt. Serve immediately.

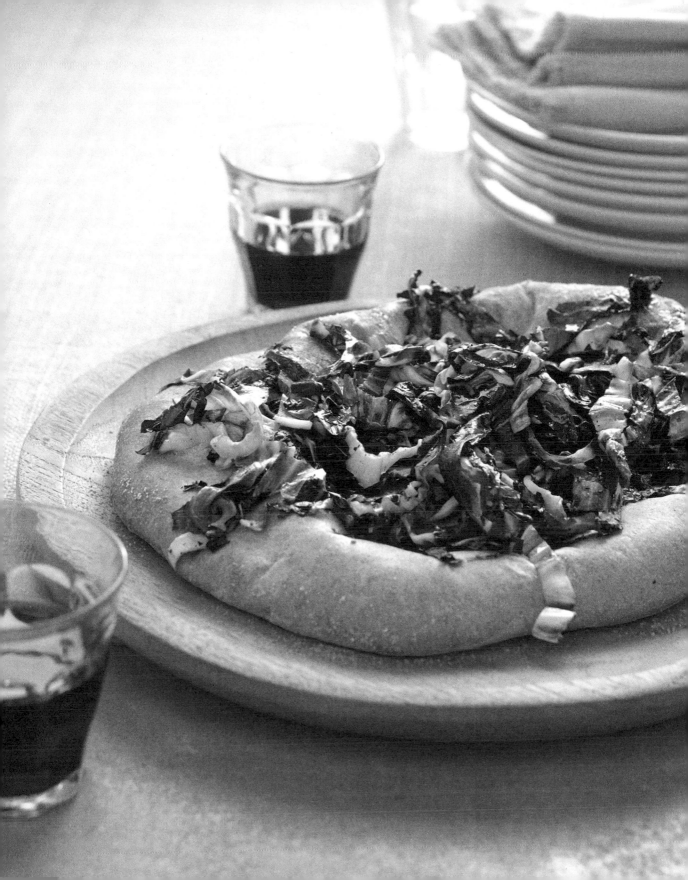

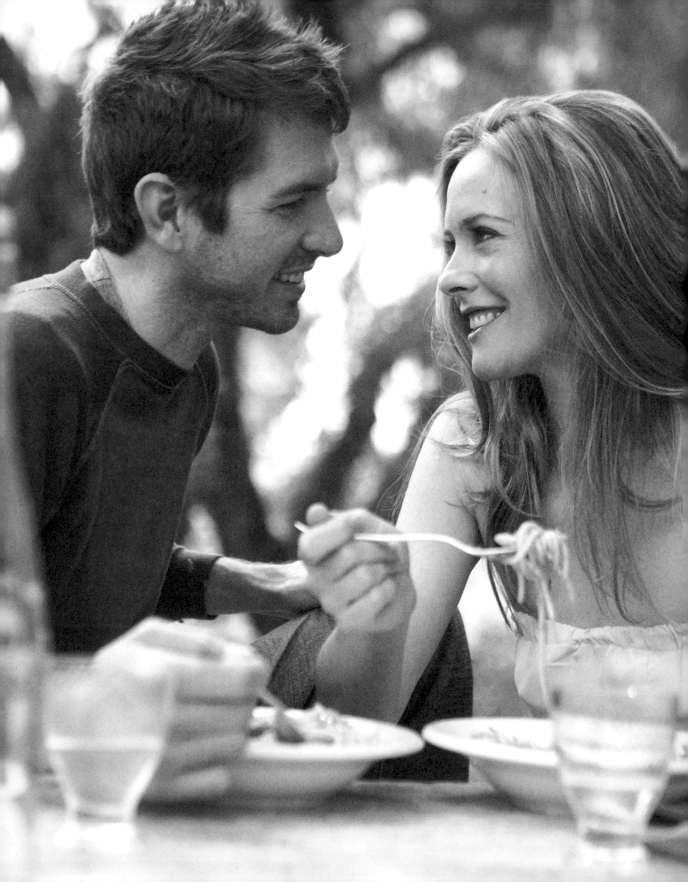

Rustic Pasta

This hearty, manly dish is a perfect complement to the Pecan-Crusted Seitan, but don't hesitate to serve it on its own or with a big fresh salad. You can also top it with packaged "meat" balls or stir in Yves brand Meatless Ground.

SERVES 4 TO 6

½ pound pasta, long or short shape, as you prefer

2 tablespoons olive oil

2 large onions, thinly sliced

2 garlic cloves, finely chopped or thinly sliced

2 celery stalks, diced or thinly sliced on a diagonal

¼ cup shoyu

½ teaspoon fine sea salt

½ teaspoon garlic powder

1 head green cabbage, thinly sliced

5–6 tablespoons marinara sauce

Bring a large pot of water to a boil for the pasta. Salt the water and add the pasta; cook just until al dente. Drain the pasta well.

Meanwhile, heat the oil in a large skillet over high heat. Add the onions and cook for 7 minutes until softened, then add the garlic and sauté for 3 minutes longer, until the onions are transparent and turning golden.

Add the celery to the skillet and sauté for 3 or 4 minutes. Stir in the shoyu, salt, and garlic powder, then add the cabbage; sauté for 4 minutes. Reduce the heat to a simmer and cook for 5 minutes longer.

Add the pasta to the skillet with the sauce and toss together. Cook over medium-high heat for a minute or two and serve.

Note: Garlic bread is delicious with pasta. Make your own!

Cut off the top of a garlic head, coat with olive oil, and season with salt and pepper.

Wrap it in foil, and roast it at 350°F for 30 to 50 minutes or until golden and tender. Turn it over halfway through cooking. Squeeze out the garlic from the skin and smear it onto toasted bread sprinkled with olive oil. Delicious!

Another version: Pan-fry pieces of bread in sesame or other oil for a couple of minutes on each side, until golden brown. Cut a garlic clove in half and rub onto the fried bread slices.

Moroccan Couscous with Saffron

I adore couscous, and this is a wonderful way to prepare it. Not only is it tasty, it looks gorgeous on a big serving plate as the centerpiece of a meal. You can complement it with a simple salad or let it be the beginning of a feast that includes soup, hummus, and veggies.

This recipe serves six, but you can halve it or just make a big batch and keep leftovers in the fridge.

SERVES 6

2 cups peeled butternut squash, cut into ¼" to ½" cubes

2 cups yellow onion, large dice

1½ cups carrots, cut into ¼" to ½" cubes

1½ cups zucchini, cut into ¾" cubes

2 tablespoons extra-virgin olive oil

Fine sea salt

1½ teaspoons freshly ground black pepper

1½ cups vegetable broth

2 tablespoons Earth Balance butter

¼ teaspoon ground cumin

½ teaspoon saffron threads

1½ cups whole wheat couscous

2 scallions, white and green parts, chopped

Preheat the oven to 375°F. Place the squash, onion, carrots, and zucchini on a baking sheet and toss with the olive oil, 1 teaspoon salt, and 1 teaspoon pepper. Roast for 25 to 30 minutes, turning once with a spatula about midway through.

While the vegetables roast, bring the vegetable broth to a boil in a saucepan. Remove the pan from the heat, and stir in the butter, remaining ½ teaspoon pepper, cumin, saffron, and salt to taste. Cover the pan and steep for 15 minutes.

Scrape the roasted vegetables and their juices into a large bowl, and add the couscous. Bring the vegetable broth back to a boil, and pour over the couscous mixture all at once. Cover tightly with a plate and allow to stand for 15 minutes. Add the scallions, toss the couscous and vegetables with a fork, and serve.

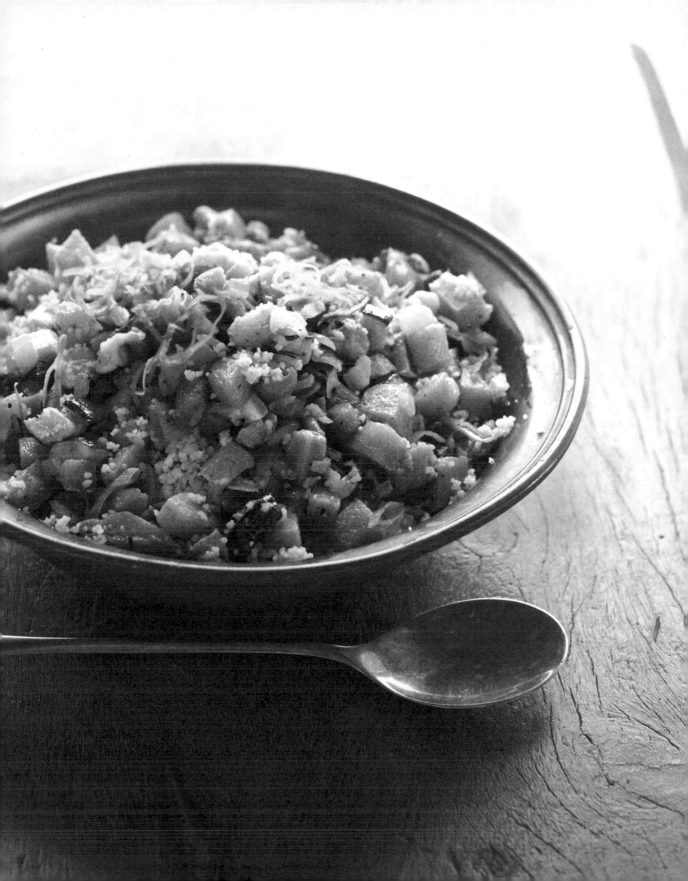

Barley Casserole

Get out your Birkenstocks! This casserole is hearty, tasty, and deeply groovy. Perfect for a family meal or to bring to a hippie potluck, this recipe makes a lot, so keep leftovers in the fridge to serve later. Hulled barley (also known as whole barley) is great in this dish, but if you can't get your hands on it, use pearled barley instead.

SERVES 6 TO 8

2 cups hulled barley	5 tablespoons shoyu
2 tablespoons olive oil	¼ teaspoon fine sea salt
1 large onion, sliced	¼ teaspoon dried basil
3 garlic cloves, finely chopped	¼ teaspoon dried oregano
2 carrots, grated	¼ teaspoon garlic powder
2 celery stalks, diced	¾ cup Tahini Dressing (recipe follows)

Preheat the oven to 350°F. Bring 3 cups of water to a boil in a large saucepan; add the barley, and cook for approximately 55 to 60 minutes or until tender. Drain off any remaining water, and set cooked barley aside.

Heat the oil in a large skillet over medium-high heat. Add the onion and garlic, and sauté until the onion is tender, about 5 minutes. If the onion starts to stick or get too brown, add a bit of water to the pan. Add the carrots, celery, shoyu, salt, basil, oregano, and garlic powder and cook for 5 minutes, stirring often, until the vegetables are tender. Add the barley, and stir over medium-high heat for 3 minutes. Taste the seasonings and adjust if necessary.

Transfer half of the barley mixture to an 8" × 12" baking dish; drizzle half of the Tahini Dressing on top. Add a second layer of barley mixture and the remainder of the dressing. Bake, uncovered, until heated through, about 35 minutes.

Tahini Dressing

¼ small onion, diced	Pinch of paprika
½ cup tahini	⅛ teaspoon crumbled dried basil or ½ teaspoon chopped fresh basil
1 tablespoon shoyu	
Pinch of garlic powder	Pinch of dried oregano

Combine the onion with 2 tablespoons water in a small skillet, and sauté over medium-high heat until softened, about 4 minutes. Add more water as needed if the onion begins to stick or brown.

Scrape the onion into a blender and add ½ cup water and the remaining ingredients. Blend for 1 minute or until creamy.

Hot Rice with Cold Lemon, Basil, and Tomato

One of my favorite snacks has always been rice covered in chopped tomatoes and topped with a generous sprinkle of salt. This recipe evolved from that snack. It's a great way to serve grain, and the vegetables make the whole dish light and refreshing.

SERVES 2

1 cup Arborio rice

2 tablespoons extra-virgin olive oil

3 tablespoons fresh lemon juice

3 pinches of fine sea salt

2 pinches of freshly ground black pepper

½ cup (or as much as you want) fresh tomato, large dice

2 tablespoons chopped fresh basil

Place the unrinsed rice in a saucepan with 3 cups water. Bring to a boil, reduce the heat, cover, and simmer 10 to 15 minutes or until mostly tender but still a little firm in the center of the grain. Drain off any water that was not absorbed, and transfer the rice to a mixing bowl.

Add the olive oil, lemon juice, salt, and pepper to taste (it's better to start off with a tiny amount of salt and pepper and add more if you need it). Mix well, add the tomatoes, and sprinkle with the basil. Toss to combine, and serve.

PROTEINS

In this section you'll find delicious ways to serve your new key protein foods: beans and seitan. No time to cook? Here are some delicious, filling, and super-easy ways to feed yourself in a hurry.

Burgers: Great for summer barbecues, pool parties, or just a quick lunch at home. Many people love Boca burgers, so they're a great place to start as you explore the big ole world of vegan burgers, but there are loads of interesting options out there.

Start with a healthy bun. Although my favorite burger bun is two pieces of chewy, toasted sourdough bread, many companies make great whole wheat buns. All good health food stores should carry some.

Add extras like fresh heirloom tomatoes, sautéed mushrooms, sautéed onions, vegan cheese, ketchup, whole grain Dijon or stone-ground mustard, Vegenaise, lettuce, avocado, and pickles. Tempeh bacon is also a great topping—just fry it up like real bacon and enjoy!

Hot dogs: Another easy, yummy food. There are great veggie dogs made by Morningstar, Tofurky, and Lightlife. Just follow the directions on the package and serve on a healthy, whole grain bun. Top with ketchup, mustard, relish, sauerkraut—you name it.

Sausages: Although the hot dog companies above also make good sausages, I recently discovered an apple-smoked vegetarian sausage by a company called Field Roast. It's amazing.

Sandwiches: Ahhh, the glory of sandwiches—where yummy meets quick meets easy! I consider the sandwich sorely underappreciated.

Use a great sourdough or other whole grain bread from the farmers' market, toasted or not, as you prefer. Some of my favorite sandwich stuffers include Vegenaise (a must), avocado, hummus, thinly sliced baked tofu (you can find it in a bunch of great flavors at the health food store), sprouts, heirloom tomatoes, whole grain Dijon mustard, cucumbers, chives, freshly ground black pepper, and Tofurky (or any other vegan lunch meat). Even stuffed grape leaves taste great in a sandwich. Incorporate anything that makes you happy, and arrange your sandwich to suit your fancy.

Waffle, Sausage, and Cheese Panini

Okay, this dish is really decadent. If it were made from the animal-based versions of these foods, I'd be setting you up for a heart attack (but of course it isn't, so I'm not!). That said, it does contain a lot of processed foods and therefore shouldn't be a daily treat. Oh, what the heck: If you're just getting off meat and dairy, eat this messy, fun, scrumpdiliumptious dish as much as you want!

SERVES 4

4–6 (1- to 1.5-ounce) Italian-style soy sausages

⅓ cup fruit-sweetened apricot jam

¼ cup Vegenaise

1½ teaspoons chopped fresh thyme or ½ teaspoon dried

¼ teaspoon freshly ground black pepper

8 frozen whole grain waffles, toasted

4 tablespoons oil-packed sun-dried tomatoes, drained and chopped

1½ cups arugula

4 slices vegan mozzarella

Cook the sausage according to package directions until browned in a large skillet. Transfer the sausage to a cutting board, and when cool enough to handle, slice each sausage in half lengthwise and then in half crosswise.

Stir together the jam, Vegenaise, thyme, and pepper in a small bowl.

Wipe out the skillet you cooked the sausages in and place over medium heat, or preheat a panini press or countertop grill. Spread each waffle with 1 tablespoon jam mixture. Sprinkle sun-dried tomatoes over 4 waffles and layer each sandwich with arugula, 1 cheese slice, and one-quarter of the sausage slices. Top each sandwich with the remaining waffles.

Brush the heated pan, panini press, or grill with oil. Add the sandwiches, and cook 3 to 5 minutes or until the cheese is melted, making sure to turn the sandwich once if you are using the skillet method. Cut the sandwiches in half, and serve.

Note: Use a second skillet weighted with a heavy can or two to press the sandwiches as they cook to re-create the panini press effect in your skillet.

Pecan-Crusted Seitan

This recipe was created by my dear friend Joy and is published in *The Candle Café Cookbook*. It's a real crowd-pleaser—perfect at a fancy dinner party or at a Thanksgiving feast to replace that big dead bird.

SERVES 4 TO 6

Marinade

¾ cup tomato paste

¼ cup umeboshi vinegar

¼ cup dry red wine

½ cup freshly squeezed orange juice

¼ cup shoyu

¼ cup minced garlic or less to taste

¼ cup chopped fresh parsley

2 tablespoons minced fresh tarragon or 1 tablespoon dried

2 tablespoons minced fresh rosemary

8–10 pieces plain seitan (about 1 pound)

2 cups all-purpose flour

½ teaspoon fine sea salt

½ teaspoon freshly ground black pepper

1 cup ground pecans

2 tablespoons finely chopped fresh rosemary

¼ cup extra-virgin olive oil

Combine the tomato paste, vinegar, wine, orange juice, shoyu, garlic, parsley, tarragon, and 2 tablespoons minced rosemary in a blender and blend until smooth. Transfer the marinade to a shallow dish, add the seitan, and turn to coat on all sides. Cover the dish and marinate in the refrigerator for at least 3 hours or overnight.

When ready to serve, mix together the flour, salt, pepper, pecans, and chopped rosemary in a shallow bowl. Dredge the marinated seitan in the flour mixture.

Heat the oil in a sauté pan, and add the cutlets to the pan. Sauté until golden brown on both sides, 2 to 3 minutes per side. Serve immediately.

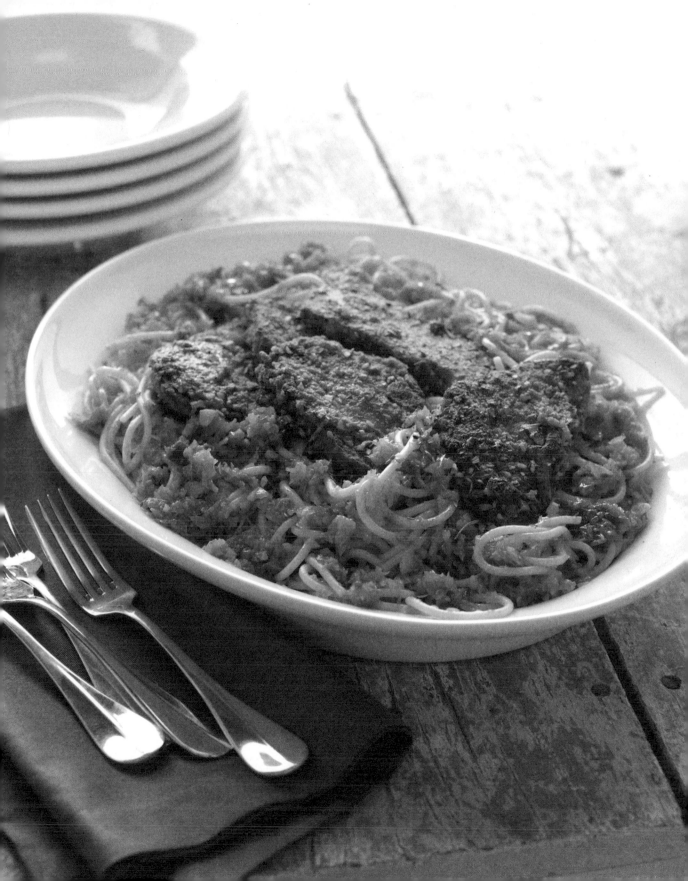

Seitan Piccata with White Wine and Capers

Adapted from *The Candle Café Cookbook*, this recipe is also great for carnivores. The wine sauce gives this dish a creamy, chicken-y character, making it an elegant entrée for a dinner party. We served this at my 30th birthday bash, and it was so good we made it again at Thanksgiving! I order it every time I go to Candle 79 in New York City. That place is so full of love. If you go there, give Joy a hug or rub Bart's belly, and tell them Alicia sent you.

SERVES 4 TO 6

1 pound plain seitan, preferably in large pieces

Whole wheat flour for dredging

¼ cup extra-virgin olive oil

½ cup diced shallots

½ cup diced onions

1 teaspoon chopped garlic

¼ cup drained capers

1 cup dry white wine

¼ cup fresh lemon juice

1 cup vegetable broth, preferably homemade

2 tablespoons unbleached flour

4 tablespoons soy margarine

1 cup chopped fresh parsley

½–¾ teaspoon fine sea salt

½ teaspoon freshly ground black pepper

Slice the seitan horizontally into thin cutlets if very thick. Dredge the seitan in the whole wheat flour, shaking off any excess. Heat 2 tablespoons olive oil over high heat in a large skillet. Add the seitan pieces, and sauté until crisp and golden brown, about 30 seconds per side. Transfer the seitan to a serving platter or individual plates.

Heat the remaining 2 tablespoons oil in the same skillet. Add the shallots, onions, garlic, and capers and sauté, stirring frequently, until softened, 1 to 2 minutes. Add the wine, and cook, stirring frequently, until reduced by half. Whisk in the lemon juice, and cook until the sauce has reduced a bit more, 1 to 2 minutes longer.

Whisk in the broth and the unbleached flour, and bring to a boil. Reduce the heat, and simmer for 1 minute to thicken. Whisk in the margarine, parsley, salt, and pepper. Pour over the seitan, and serve immediately.

Chorizo Tacos

These tacos are perfect for your meat-eating friends. For my 25th birthday, we held a party at a farm animal sanctuary. It was unbelievably fun sharing that day with friends, family, and the pigs! Christopher ran a taco stand and served these tacos to 150 people! They were fantastic.

SERVES 2 OR 3

1 tablespoon olive oil

8 ounces sliced vegan chorizo or taco crumbles

4–6 corn tortillas, soft or hard as you prefer

½ cup diced onions

1 cup shredded lettuce

½ cup chopped tomatoes

Prepared salsa

1 cup tofu sour cream or Tofu Cream (page 225)

⅔ cup shredded vegan Cheddar cheese

Hot sauce (optional)

Heat the olive oil in a medium skillet over medium-high heat. Add the chorizo or taco crumbles and cook, stirring until heated through, 3 to 4 minutes. Transfer to a small bowl.

If using soft tortillas, wrap in a slightly damp kitchen towel and heat in a 350°F oven or toaster oven for 5 to 6 minutes or until warm and pliable. (Hard taco shells don't need to be heated.)

Arrange the onions, lettuce, tomatoes, salsa, tofu sour cream or Tofu Cream, and cheese in small bowls alongside the chorizo. Pass around the tortillas so everyone can fill their own tacos and add hot sauce to taste.

Crispy Tofu Slices with Orange Dipping Sauce

This recipe was invented one day while I was tidying the kitchen and trying to use up some odds and ends. Perfect as dinner party appetizers, these tofu slices taste just as good as they look. As a meal, serve them with Hot Rice with Cold Lemon, Basil, and Tomato (page 151) and a side of Baby Bok Choy Drizzled with Ume Vinaigrette (page 265). If you don't have the corn and brown rice flours on hand, just use an all-purpose or whole wheat flour.

SERVES 2 OR 3

1 (8-ounce) package savory-flavored baked tofu

½ cup corn flour

½ cup brown rice flour

Safflower oil

⅔ cup fresh orange juice

⅓ cup maple syrup

Cut the baked tofu into slices about ¼" thick. Mix the flours together in a shallow bowl.

Pour enough oil into a large skillet to cover the bottom of the pan with a thin layer, and heat over medium heat. Dip each of the tofu strips into the flour mixture, coating well on all sides. Place the tofu strips in the skillet, and cook until lightly browned on both sides, about 3 minutes per side. Transfer the fried tofu strips to a plate lined with paper towels (or a piece of paper grocery bag) to drain.

Stir together the orange juice and syrup in a small bowl. Serve the tofu strips with the dipping sauce alongside.

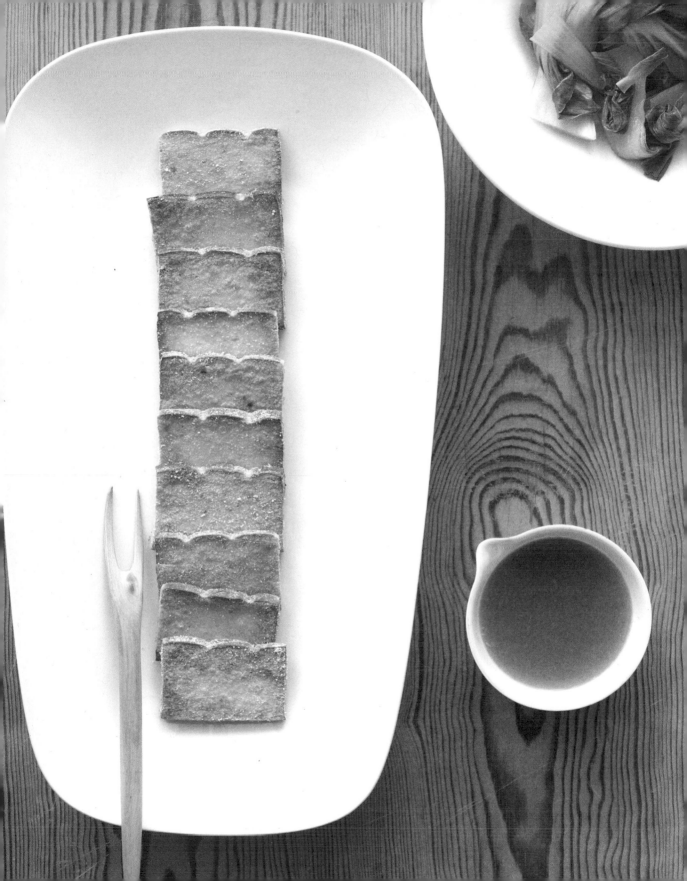

Ginger-Baked Tofu

There's something about the combination of ginger, garlic, and shoyu that makes this dish truly elegant and exotic. The tofu emerges from the oven slightly browned but still soft. I think it's the best tofu dish I've ever had, and I challenge anyone—even meat-eaters—not to like it.

SERVES 2 TO 4

1 pound firm tofu

⅓ cup shoyu

1 tablespoon toasted or untoasted sesame oil

2 tablespoons minced fresh ginger

1 tablespoon finely chopped garlic

¼ cup brown rice vinegar

2 tablespoons umeboshi vinegar

½ teaspoon crushed red-pepper flakes (optional)

1 teaspoon brown rice syrup (optional)

Finely chopped scallions for garnish (optional)

Cut the tofu in half width-wise, and place each half on its side then slice in half again. You will be left with 4 tofu "steaks."

Pour ¾ cup of water into a bowl. Whisk in the shoyu, oil, ginger, garlic, vinegars, red-pepper flakes (if desired), and rice syrup and pour over the tofu, covering it. An 8" × 6" Pyrex dish works perfectly. Marinate for at least 1 hour.

Preheat the oven to 375°F. Either drain the baking dish of the majority of the marinade, or place the tofu on a baking sheet and baste with the marinade. Reserve the remaining marinade.

Bake the tofu for 15 to 20 minutes. Turn the tofu pieces with a spatula, baste again with the marinade, and bake for 10 to 15 minutes longer. Garnish with scallions, if desired, and serve warm.

Note: Without the crushed red-pepper flakes, this is a full-on Superhero dish.

Thanksgiving Tofu

Thanksgiving is my favorite holiday, but that wasn't always the case. I was bummed out by its history and the big carcass in the middle of the dinner table. These days, by cooking delicious vegan foods, I make it a Kind Thanksgiving: one that includes no suffering to human bodies, turkeys, or the environment. And for that, I can give sincere thanks. I served this tofu dish at a Thanksgiving dinner for 27 people and it was a big hit. It feels like a holiday dish because it contains stuffing, but it can really be served any time of year. It's very filling, so be sure to balance it with a big, fresh salad. If you're a gravy lover, Tofurky makes a great gravy that nicely complements this dish.

SERVES 4 TO 6

2 (18-ounce) packages firm tofu

Cornbread Stuffing

1 cup diced onion

1 cup diced celery

1 tablespoon sesame oil

½ teaspoon dried sage

½ teaspoon dried thyme

1 teaspoon dried parsley or
   1 tablespoon fresh

Fine sea salt and freshly ground black
   pepper, to taste

3 cups cubed whole wheat bread
   (crusts included)

2 cups cubed Cornbread (page 163)
   or just use an additional 2 cups
   bread cubes if pressed for time

1–1½ cups vegetable broth

½ cup chopped pecans or walnuts

Basting Liquid

3 tablespoons sesame oil

2 teaspoons shoyu

One hour before cooking, mash or crumble the tofu and pack it into a medium, rounded colander lined with cheesecloth or a clean dish towel. Place a small plate on top of the tofu and weight it with a heavy object such as a can or jar. Place the colander on a plate or tray to catch the draining liquid and set it aside for 45 minutes.

While the tofu drains, combine the onion, celery, and sesame oil in a large skillet and sauté over medium heat for 3 to 4 minutes. Add the herbs and salt and pepper, and sauté 1 minute longer or until the onions are translucent. If the pan becomes dry, add a little water. Combine the sauté with the cubed breads and enough vegetable broth to moisten. Stir in the nuts.

Preheat the oven to 400°F. Using your hands, press the tofu onto the bottom and sides of the colander, creating a hollow space for the filling. Pack the stuffing mixture into the tofu shell, and press down firmly.

For more information visit us at: www.thekindlife.com

Oil a baking sheet and place it over the colander. Quickly invert the baking sheet and colander, then carefully lift off the colander and cheesecloth. Stir together the basting liquid ingredients, and use a pastry brush to baste the entire tofu dome with the mixture (see Note). Cover the tofu with foil, and bake for about 1½ hours. After 1 hour, remove the foil, baste again with the remaining basting mixture, and return to the oven for 20 to 30 minutes longer or until golden. Watch to make sure the tofu does not burn. Use 2 large spatulas to transfer the tofu dome to a serving platter. Cut into wedges, and serve.

> Note: If you need more basting liquid, add more oil and shoyu; just be careful not to use too much or the tofu can end up a little oily.

Thanksgiving Options:

These also make good entrées for a Thanksgiving feast: Pecan-Crusted Seitan (page 154), Seitan Piccata with White Wine and Capers (page 156), and Gardein Veggie Chick'n Breasts.

Cranberry Sauce

I am a sucker for maple syrup, so I use it to sweeten my cranberries, but feel free to experiment with agave syrup or rice syrup to see what you prefer. This recipe is so quick and easy that you'll never buy premade cranberry sauce again.

MAKES ABOUT 3 CUPS

4 cups raw cranberries

½ cup maple syrup

Juice from 1 orange

Rinse and clean berries well. Transfer to a large saucepan, and add the syrup, orange juice, and ¼ cup of water. Bring to a boil over medium-high heat, stirring often. When the mixture comes to a boil, reduce the heat, cover, and boil gently until the berries pop, about 10 minutes. Chill for 1 hour before serving.

Cornbread

Everyone needs cornbread in their life; it goes great with soups, stews, or just by itself. This recipe is my personal favorite. It uses sorghum, which is a type of molasses, and I think it tastes great. You can bake it in a pan to cut into cubes for stuffing, or bake in muffin tins and serve as corn muffins with Earth Balance spread. Mmmm . . . Either way, this cornbread recipe comes out golden brown and slightly sweet. You will love it.

SERVES 12

1 cup sorghum *or* ½ cup sorghum plus ½ cup maple syrup

1¼ cups soy milk (or soy/rice blend)

¼ cup safflower oil

1½ cups cornmeal

½ cup whole wheat pastry flour

1 teaspoon baking soda

½ teaspoon fine sea salt

Preheat the oven to 400°F. Oil a 9" × 9" (or similar size) baking dish or 12-cup muffin tin. Combine the sorghum, soy milk, and oil in a medium bowl and mix well. In another bowl, stir together the cornmeal, flour, baking soda, and salt. Add the dry mixture to the wet mixture, and mix just until well combined.

Pour the batter into the prepared pan, and bake for 25 to 30 minutes or until a toothpick inserted in the center of the cornbread or a muffin comes out clean. They will be golden brown and crazy delicious.

Muffin Notes:

- Stir the batter just enough to combine the ingredients. Muffins can become heavy and tough if the batter is overmixed.

- Work quickly with muffin or cake batter. Baking powder will lose its effectiveness if it sits for too long in the batter.

- Make sure your baking powder is fresh. Obey the expiration date on the tin, as old powder will no longer be able to leaven your breads and muffins properly. You can test your baking powder by putting 1 teaspoon in half a glass of hot water. Fresh baking powder will bubble vigorously.

- Restrain yourself from peeking at your baked goods in the oven. Opening the oven will cause the temperature to fluctuate, which messes with the baking process. Even if it means sitting on your hands, wait until the end of the recommended cooking time.

- Muffins can become gummy in the refrigerator, so store them at room temperature for the first couple of days. After 3 days, I recommend you freeze them.

Black Soybean and Kabocha Squash Stew

I've never served this dish to anyone who didn't freak out about how delicious it was. Warm, nourishing, and great for winter, serve these beans with a simple bowl of rice and steamed greens. If you can't find kabocha, butternut squash will do, but kabocha is just *so good*. This also tastes great the next day.

SERVES 4

1 cup dried black soybeans

1" piece kombu seaweed

About 2 tablespoons extra-virgin olive oil

2–3 garlic cloves, thinly sliced

1 red onion, diced

1 teaspoon chili powder

Fine sea salt

Generous pinch crushed red-pepper flakes

1 teaspoon ground cumin

2½ cups canned diced tomatoes

½ kabocha squash, halved, seeded, and cut into 1" pieces (peel only if the kabocha squash is not organic)

1 cup mirin

2 teaspoons white miso

2 celery stalks, diced

3–4 fresh cilantro sprigs, chopped

Rinse the soybeans, then turn them out onto a kitchen towel and rub to remove as much moisture as possible. Place the beans in a dry, medium skillet, and pan-toast them over medium-low heat for 5 to 10 minutes, until they puff up a little and their skins begin to split.

Transfer the beans to a large pot, and add the kombu and 3 cups of water. Bring to a boil, then cover, reduce the heat to low, and cook for 90 minutes or until the beans are tender.

While the beans cook, combine the oil, garlic, onion, and chili powder in a large skillet over medium heat. When you hear the onion start to sizzle, add a pinch of salt, red-pepper flakes, and cumin and cook, stirring frequently, for 2 to 3 minutes. Add the tomatoes, squash, mirin, and 1 cup of water. Bring to a boil, cover, and reduce the heat to low. Cook until the squash is tender, about 35 minutes. Remove a small amount of the broth from the skillet and use this to dissolve the miso. Once dissolved, stir the miso into the vegetables.

Once the beans are fully cooked, drain them of any leftover liquid. Add the beans to the vegetables, and simmer over low heat until all remaining liquid has been absorbed. Turn off the heat, stir in the celery and cilantro, and serve hot.

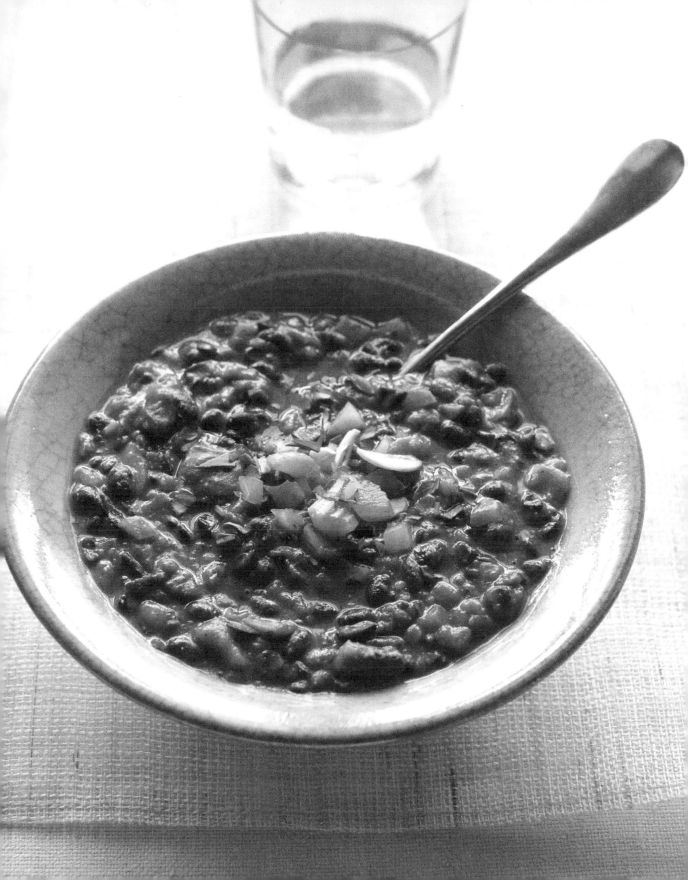

Eggplant Chana Masala

Because it uses canned beans and chili, this recipe is quick and convenient. It tastes so good it's downright *dirty*!

SERVES 8

3 large onions, roughly chopped

4–5 garlic cloves, minced

1–2 tablespoons olive oil

1 teaspoon curry powder or to taste

1–2 teaspoons cumin or to taste

1 large eggplant, peeled and chopped into ½" pieces

2 (15-ounce) cans chickpeas, drained

2 (14-ounce) cans peeled tomatoes, drained

1 can vegetarian chili (Health Valley and Amy's make good ones)

1 large handful chopped fresh cilantro (about ½ cup)

Sauté the onions and garlic with the oil, curry powder, and cumin in a large pot until the onions are soft or translucent, approximately 5 minutes. Add the eggplant, and sauté for 5 minutes longer, until lightly browned and softened. Sometimes the eggplant will absorb a lot of oil, so you might need to add more to prevent sticking. Add the chickpeas, tomatoes, and chili. Simmer for 20 to 30 minutes. It will get watery, but then reduce to a thick, stewy chana masala. Add more spices to taste. Stir in the chopped cilantro and serve.

Sweet Potato–Lentil Stew

Served on its own or as a soupy stew over brown basmati rice or couscous, this dish is hearty and filling. It's also great with steamed collard greens and a corn muffin (page 163). If you worship sweet potatoes like I do, add another half or whole potato.

SERVES 4 TO 6

¼ cup safflower oil

1 medium onion, diced

2 small tomatoes, diced

1 teaspoon minced fresh ginger

1½ teaspoons turmeric

1 teaspoon cumin

1 teaspoon ground coriander

½ teaspoon ground cinnamon

⅛ teaspoon cayenne

Fine sea salt

2–3 medium sweet potatoes, peeled and cut into ¾" cubes

7 cups vegetable broth

1 cup brown lentils

Heat the oil over medium heat in a large, deep pot. Add the onion and cook, stirring frequently, for 2 minutes or until the onion starts to soften. Stir in the tomatoes and ginger and cook for 3 minutes. Stir in the turmeric, cumin, coriander, cinnamon, cayenne, and a small pinch of salt. Cook and stir for 2 minutes, then taste for seasonings; try to use only enough salt to heighten the flavors.

Add the sweet potatoes, broth, and lentils. Stir well, and bring to a boil over high heat. When the mixture comes to a boil, reduce the heat, cover, and simmer for 40 minutes or until the lentils and sweet potatoes are soft.

Sugar Snap Peas, Radishes, and Edamame with Lemon Butter

This pretty, sophisticated spring dish is perfect for a ladies' luncheon or a light supper. Leave out the Earth Balance butter and it qualifies as a Superhero recipe. This is lovely made with fresh English peas when they are in season; substitute 2 cups of shelled peas for the sugar snaps.

SERVES 6

2 cups sugar snap peas, trimmed

1 cup frozen shelled edamame, thawed

1 bunch radishes, trimmed and thinly sliced

1 tablespoon extra-virgin olive oil

2 tablespoons minced shallots

¼ teaspoon fine sea salt

2 teaspoons finely grated lemon zest

1 teaspoon Earth Balance butter

¾ teaspoon umeboshi vinegar

Juice of ¼ lemon

¼ teaspoon freshly ground black pepper

Cook the snap peas, edamame, and radishes in boiling salted water for 1 minute. Drain and rinse under cold water immediately to stop the cooking process.

Heat the oil in a large skillet over medium heat. Add the shallots, and sauté for 2 to 3 minutes or until soft. Add the drained snap peas, edamame, radishes, and salt and cook for 1 minute or until heated through.

Remove from heat, and stir in the zest, butter, vinegar, lemon juice, and pepper. Serve warm.

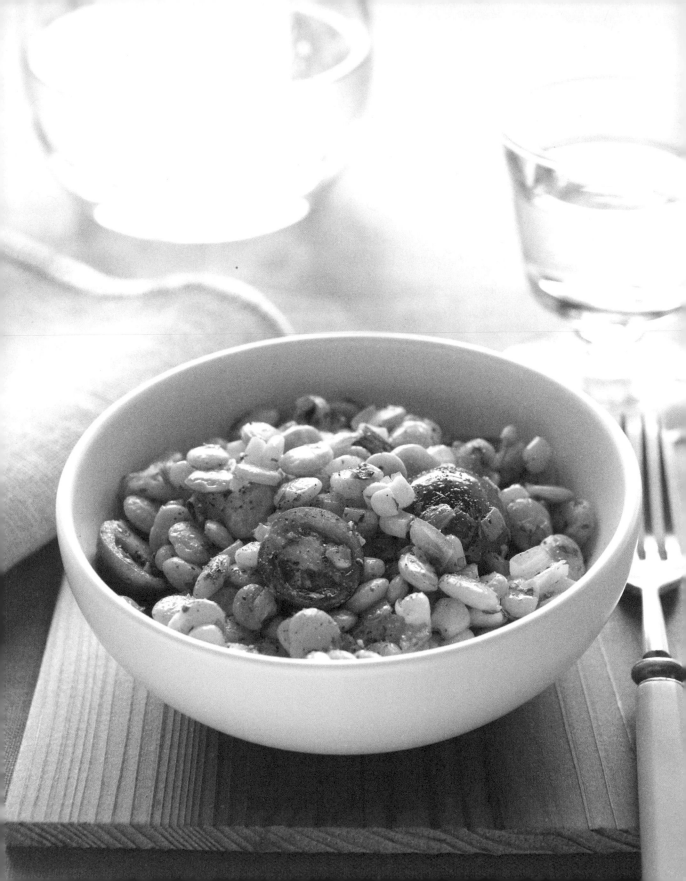

Summertime Succotash

This dish is pretty, fresh, and delicious. Try it with the Hot Rice with Cold Lemon, Basil, and Tomato (page 151) or Kim's Red Radish Tabbouleh (page 226). It's also great with white jasmine rice topped with toasted sunflower seeds. Complete the meal with some steamed bok choy or watercress.

SERVES 6

1 tablespoon Earth Balance butter

1 teaspoon olive oil

1 cup diced red onion

1 garlic clove, minced

1 (10-ounce) package frozen baby lima beans, thawed (see Note)

1 cup fresh or frozen corn

1 cup cherry tomatoes, halved

2 tablespoons chopped fresh parsley

2 tablespoons chopped fresh basil

1 tablespoon white or red balsamic vinegar (White is best, but who has white? I use red.)

Heat the butter and oil together in a large skillet over medium-high heat. Add the onion, and sauté for 5 to 7 minutes or until the onion begins to brown. Add the garlic, and cook 1 minute longer.

Stir in the lima beans, and sauté for 5 minutes. Add the corn and tomatoes, and sauté 1 minute longer or until just heated through. You don't want the tomatoes to collapse and release their juices. Remove from the heat, and stir in the parsley, basil, and vinegar. Serve warm or chilled.

Note: If you can get your hands on fresh lima beans for this, by all means use them! You will need about 2 cups of shelled beans, or about 2 pounds in the pod. Soaking them in water before using makes the end product less gas-producing. Blanch the fresh beans in a large pot of salted boiling water for 2 to 3 minutes or until tender but not soft.

Hearty Pinto Bean Stew

Remember eating beans 'n' franks? This dish reminds me of that. Great for kids, husbands, and boyfriends, these beans deliver tons of flavor. Add a tofu dog and serve with a salad for a family-style meal, or serve with Hot Rice with Cold Lemon, Basil, and Tomato (page 151) and collard greens to go the more sophisticated route.

SERVES 2

1 cup pinto beans, soaked overnight in water to cover

2 cups tomato soup (Imagine makes a good one)

2 teaspoons shoyu

1 teaspoon olive oil

½ onion, cut into chunks

1–2 garlic cloves, finely chopped

2 teaspoons chopped fresh basil or ½ teaspoon dried

Dash of dried oregano

Dash of red-pepper flakes

Fine sea salt to taste

Combine the tomato soup, 1 cup of water, shoyu, and oil in a large soup pot. Place over medium heat, and bring to a boil. Drain the soaked beans and add them to the stock. When the liquid returns to a boil, reduce the heat to medium-low, cover, and simmer for 30 minutes.

After 30 minutes of simmering, add the onion, garlic, basil, oregano, and red-pepper flakes. If the stew seems too thick, add more tomato soup or water. Place cover slightly askew over pot, and simmer 30 to 40 minutes longer or until the beans are very tender. Season to taste with salt.

Lentil Stew

This stew is hearty, healthy, and simple. It keeps well in the fridge for 3 or 4 days.

SERVES 6

½ teaspoon garlic powder

½ teaspoon paprika

½ teaspoon fine sea salt

¼ teaspoon ground cumin

¼ teaspoon dried oregano

½ teaspoon dried basil

2 tablespoons olive oil

2 garlic cloves, finely chopped

2 large onions, cut into chunks

2 celery stalks, diced

1 carrot, sliced

1 potato, cut into chunks

¼ cup shoyu

5 cups vegetable broth

3 tomatoes, cored and cut into chunks

1½ cups brown lentils

2 slices of your favorite bread, cubed

Extra-virgin olive oil

Combine the garlic powder, paprika, salt, cumin, oregano, and basil in a small bowl. Heat the oil in a large soup pot (you'll be adding a lot of liquid later, so make sure it's big enough) over medium-high heat, and add the garlic, onion, celery, carrot, and potato. Stir in half the seasoning mixture and the shoyu. Cook, stirring frequently, for 7 minutes or until the onions are tender.

Add 5 cups of water, the broth, tomatoes, and lentils. Bring to a boil over high heat, then reduce the heat and simmer with the lid askew for 30 minutes. Add the remaining seasoning mixture, and cook for 20 minutes longer or until the lentils are soft. Meanwhile, pan-roast the cubed bread in a dry skillet until nice and toasted. Ladle stew into the bowls, and garnish with croutons and a drizzle of olive oil.

SOUPS, SALADS, AND VEGETABLE DISHES

Be sure to eat plenty of vegetables every day—preferably with every meal. It doesn't have to be fancy; a serving of simple steamed greens like collards, watercress, or bok choy, or whichever vegetables you usually serve with your meals is just fine. A salad is another easy way to get vegetables into your meal, and as far as add-ins go, the sky's the limit. Whatever I have in the fridge qualifies: carrot shavings, avocado, cucumber, celery, sprouts, toasted sunflower seeds, even raisins.

For dressings, you have some great choices. I love Annie's Goddess Dressing or Shiitake & Sesame Vinaigrette. They're both vegan and incredibly tasty. Or mix up a double batch of My Basic Vinaigrette so you'll always have some on hand for a quick salad. I vary the ingredients every time I make it, using more or less citrus or adding flaxseed oil—I've even used truffle-infused olive oil in my more decadent moments.

Other veggie ideas:

- Steamed artichokes are an elegant, delicious option in the spring. My mother served them all the time when I was growing up. We dipped the leaves in butter and mayonnaise, and it was such a treat to eat the heart. As an adult, I've traded in the butter for Earth Balance and the mayo for Vegenaise, and I think they taste even better. Incredibly easy to make, you can simply walk away while the artichokes steam or use the time to cook the rest of your meal.

- Simple steamed broccoli dipped in Vegenaise is so good.

- Sweet potatoes: Bake one like a potato, slice it in half, and either serve plain or with a filling: Earth Balance with salt and pepper is great, as is vegan sour cream.

My Basic Vinaigrette

MAKES ABOUT ¼ CUP, ENOUGH TO DRESS A BIG SALAD FOR TWO PEOPLE

2 teaspoons olive oil

Scant ½ teaspoon umeboshi plum vinegar

Scant ½ teaspoon shoyu

Juice of ½ orange

Scant ½ teaspoon fresh lemon juice

Place the oil, vinegar, shoyu, and juices in a bowl or cup. Stir vigorously with a fork to mix. Pour onto the salad, and toss. If you feel it needs more salt after tasting the salad, add a drop more vinegar or shoyu.

Watercress, Beet, and Heirloom Tomato Salad

This salad was inspired by my friend Marta Alicia Barrientos, from El Salvador. As she would say, "It's nutreetious and deleecious!"

- 2 medium beets
- 1 bunch watercress, tough stems removed
- 1 tomato, preferably an heirloom variety, cut into bite-size pieces
- 1 tablespoon olive oil
- Juice of 1 lemon
- Fine sea salt
- Freshly ground black pepper

Preheat the oven to 425°F. Wrap the beets in foil, and roast for 40 to 60 minutes or until you can pierce them easily with a skewer. Allow the beets to cool a bit, then slip off the skins and slice the beets into quarters from root to stem. (If your beets are small, just halve them.)

Combine the beets, watercress, and tomato in a salad bowl. Mix the olive oil and lemon juice together, and pour over the salad; mix well. Add a couple pinches of salt and a little pepper to taste. Toss again, and serve.

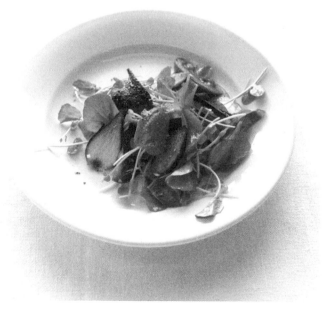

Alicia's Sexy Inspired Salad

I'm the salad maker of my household, and my inventions have morphed over the years. This is my current favorite. It's especially good because of the truffle oil, which, though a bit expensive, is used so sparingly it lasts forever and is really worth the cost. I like this salad best made right after arriving home with all our fresh produce from the farmers' market, but it's also a wonderful way to use up the odds and ends in the fridge. Try adding English peas, snap peas, or sprouts and serve with black bean stew and rice.

SERVES 2

Salad

Fresh salad greens such as red leaf, butter lettuce, or romaine

1 small handful of arugula

½ avocado, peeled and diced

½–1 heirloom tomato (optional, but nice)

¼–½ medium cucumber, chopped into bite-size pieces (peel only if the cucumber is not organic)

4 dandelion greens (optional, but good for you)

½ carrot, shaved with a vegetable peeler

3–4 chopped fresh basil sprigs

4–5 chopped fresh cilantro sprigs

1 teaspoon hemp seeds (optional)

1–2 tablespoons toasted sunflower seeds, lightly seasoned with shoyu (see Note)

Any other vegetables you like

Dressing

2½ tablespoons truffle-infused olive oil or extra-virgin olive oil

1½ tablespoons balsamic vinegar

Juice of ½ lemon

Juice of ½ orange

½ teaspoon grated vegan Parmesan cheese (Galaxy Foods makes a nice one that comes in a shaker like regular grated Parmesan)

Get a big salad bowl that makes you happy with lots of room to toss and play. Wash, tear, and throw in the lettuce. Add the arugula, avocado, tomato, and cucumber. Top with the dandelion greens, carrot shavings, and herbs. Sprinkle with the hemp and sunflower seeds.

Pour the dressing ingredients directly onto the salad and toss. (If you want to mix them first, go for it.)

> Note: Toasted seeds—sunflower, pumpkin, sesame—are a great addition to soups, salads, grains, and just about anything else. They are glorious little treasures that will make your tongue so happy. Christopher eats them right out of the jar as a snack.

Caesar Salad

This is the greatest Caesar salad, ever, on the planet. Period. All the components—croutons, dressing, greens—can be prepared and stored separately in th fridge for up to a week, so you can toss together a fresh Caesar for one or two whenever the urge strikes.

SERVES 6 TO 8

Croutons

½ teaspoon dried rosemary

½ teaspoon garlic powder

½ teaspoon fine sea salt

3–4 slices whole wheat sourdough bread, sliced into cubes (about 1½ cups)

Olive oil

Dressing

2 tablespoons blanched or roasted almonds

3 garlic cloves, minced

3 tablespoons Dijon mustard

2 tablespoons shoyu

1 tablespoon tahini

3 tablespoons fresh lemon juice

2 tablespoons extra-virgin olive oil

1 large head romaine lettuce, torn into bite-size pieces

½ sheet nori, cut with scissors into 2" x 4" strips

Preheat the oven to 325°F. Stir together the rosemary, garlic powder, and salt in a small bowl. Place the bread cubes in a large bowl, and drizzle with the oil. Toss well to distribute the oil. Sprinkle the herb mixture over the bread cubes, and toss again. Spread in a single layer on a baking sheet, and bake for 10 to 15 minutes or until the croutons are dry and lightly toasted. Cool completely.

Meanwhile, combine the almonds, garlic, mustard, shoyu, tahini, lemon juice, oil, and ¼ cup of water in a food processor or blender; process until smooth and well blended.

To serve, toss the lettuce and croutons together in a serving bowl. Add the dressing, and toss to coat. Sprinkle the nori over the salad, and serve right away.

Sicilian Collard Greens with Pine Nuts and Raisins

Beyond being incredibly yummy, this dish is also a sneaky way to introduce people to the glory of collard greens. For Superheroes who crave it regularly, you should substitute the balsamic vinegar for shoyu and the pine nuts for pumpkin seeds most of the time.

SERVES 2 OR 3

1 bunch collard greens

2 tablespoons pine nuts

3 garlic cloves, peeled and chopped

1 tablespoon olive oil

3 tablespoons raisins

2 tablespoons balsamic vinegar

Use a sharp knife to cut out the central rib and stem from each collard leaf. Rinse the leaves in a sink of cool water, lifting them into a colander to drain a bit (you want some water to remain on the leaves).

Toast the pine nuts over medium heat in a dry skillet for about 5 minutes or until golden. Shake the pan often to keep the pine nuts from burning. Transfer to a plate, and set aside.

Place the garlic and oil in a large skillet, and sauté over medium heat for 1 minute or until the garlic is fragrant. Add the damp collards and stir, then cover the pan and cook for 2 minutes longer. Add the raisins and pine nuts, and stir. Cover and cook for 2 minutes. Stir in the balsamic vinegar, cover, and continue to cook for 1 to 2 minutes longer.

Note: The stems of the collard greens are full of minerals, so if you want to use them, chop them into 1" pieces and cook for a couple of minutes before adding the collard greens.

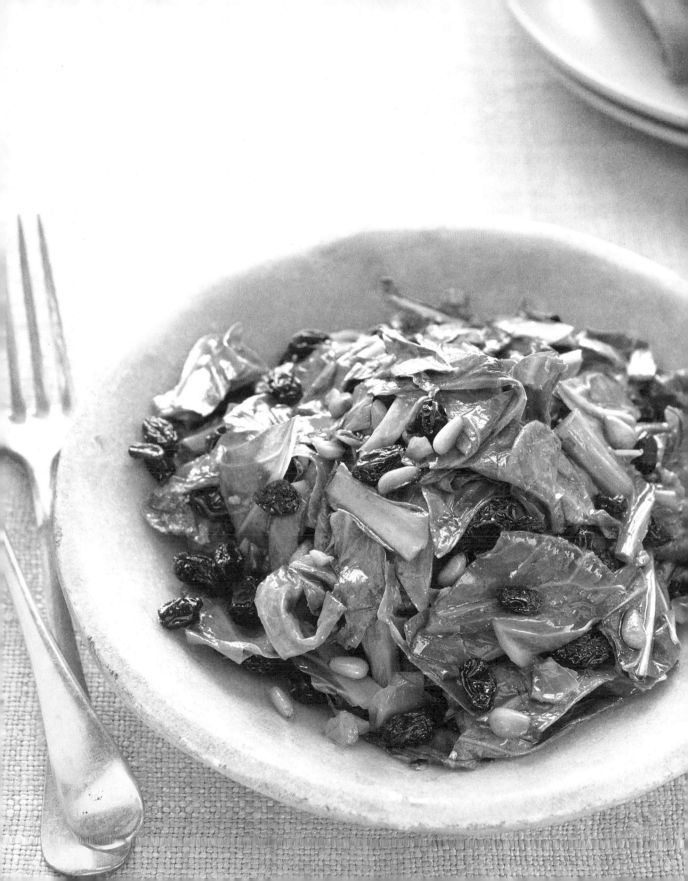

Warm Potato, Soybean, and Cucumber Salad

This recipe is from *Christina Cooks* by Christina Pirello. To me, it feels like something that would be served at a fancy luncheon for French ladies!

SERVES 4 OR 5

Salad

- 1 pound new or fingerling potatoes, unpeeled and cut into 1" cubes
- 1 cup frozen shelled edamame
- 1 red onion, halved and thinly sliced
- 1 small cucumber, halved lengthwise and cut into very thin half-moon slices (peel only if the cucumber is not organic)

Dressing

- ¼ cup umeboshi vinegar
- 1 tablespoon finely minced fresh ginger
- 1 garlic clove, finely chopped
- 1 tablespoon stone-ground mustard
- 4 tablespoons extra-virgin olive oil
- 2 teaspoons brown rice syrup
- 1 teaspoon white miso

Bring a pot of salted water to a boil, and cook the potatoes for 12 minutes or until just tender. With a slotted spoon or a skimmer, remove the potatoes from the pot, and transfer them to a mixing bowl. In the same water, cook the edamame for about 4 minutes or until just barely tender. Add the onion to the pot, and cook with the edamame for 30 seconds longer. Drain and add to the potatoes along with the cucumber. Combine gently.

Whisk together the dressing ingredients in a small bowl until well combined. Pour over the warm salad, and stir to coat. Serve warm.

DESSERTS

Who says you can't have your cake and eat it, too? All of the desserts in this section are 100 percent delicious, 100 percent vegan, and won't have you bouncing off the ceiling or leave you with a sickly sugar hangover the next day like conventional sweets can. However, they are not necessarily less caloric than their white-flour, refined-sugar siblings, so if you are primarily looking to drop a few pounds, don't go overboard in this section. Enjoy a beautiful piece of fruit after your meal and save the peanut butter cups for a once-in-a-while reward. The good news here is that because they won't cause those horrible blood sugar spikes that leave you crashed and craving more, more, more, it's easier to keep consumption of these yummies under control.

Ice pops are so simple that it's easy to forget them! Buy an ice pop mold and pour in a mixture of coconut, strawberry, and apple juices. That's my favorite, but any juice that you or your kids like will make a great ice pop. Freeze and enjoy on hot summer days.

Find a nondairy ice cream that you love. Start with scoops of ice cream and top them with whatever makes you happiest. Experiment to your heart's content. And don't forget the walnuts, or even try topping with ground-up graham crackers! If you want to start with a banana and make it a split, go for it!

Believe it or not, you can find vegan chocolate sauce (by Wax Orchard) and even faux marshmallow fluff (Ricemellow Creme Fluff). There's even soy whipped cream in a can (by Soyatoo)! If you can't get your hands on the chocolate sauce, just melt some dairy-free chocolate chips in a double boiler—or in a stainless steel bowl over boiling water—then drizzle over your ice cream.

Flour: Don't be discouraged from a recipe because you can't find the specific type of flour called for. Experiment and use whatever you have around the house. Spelt flour, whole wheat flour, unbleached all-purpose flour, barley flour, and brown rice flour can generally be substituted for one another.

Keep in mind, however, that if a recipe calls for pastry flour, you can only substitute it for another type of pastry flour. Bread flours are too dense and heavy for pastry recipes.

Chocolate-Apricot Coins

I took cooking classes with Laura Taylor and Karen Bryson-Pearson here in L.A. Both groovy, healthy ladies, they taught me these easy little sweets.

MAKES ABOUT 20

2 cups grain-sweetened, nondairy chocolate or carob chips

¼ cup maple syrup

2 tablespoons safflower oil

20 dried Turkish apricots, pounded into ¼" flat rounds

Place the chocolate chips, syrup, and oil in the top of a double boiler and place over a pot of simmering water. If you don't have a double boiler, place a stainless steel bowl over boiling water and melt the ingredients in it. Turn off the heat, cover, and let sit until the chocolate melts, 5 to 10 minutes.

While the chocolate melts, use a rolling pin or wine bottle to pound the apricots to an even ¼" thickness. Dip the apricots in the melted chocolate and place on a sheet of wax or parchment paper. Chill in the refrigerator until hardened.

Variation:
Quick Chocolate Ganache Strawberries

To make a fondue-like ganache, melt one cup of grain-sweetened, nondairy chocolate or carob chips with ½ cup soy milk (soy or soy/rice milk blend) over low heat. Whisk well to create a smooth texture. Dip the strawberries in the sauce. To make a candy-like coating for the strawberries, melt 1 cup of grain-sweetened chips with about ¼ cup nondairy milk. Set the dipped berries on parchment paper and chill.

Coffee Fudge Brownies

This dessert is *ridiculously* rich and *insanely* delicious. This brownie is your new boyfriend! It was inspired by my 14-year-old friend Gina Filippone, from Victoria, British Columbia. She baked a version of them one day while I was visiting, and they were so delicious I couldn't stop eating them. I've changed the original ingredients to make them healthier, and—can you believe it?—the healthy ingredients make them even better!

MAKES 12 BROWNIES

¾ cup whole wheat pastry flour

¾ cup brown rice flour

½ cup unsweetened cocoa powder

1 teaspoon baking powder

1½ teaspoons baking soda

1 teaspoon salt

1½ cups maple sugar

¾ cup soy/rice milk blend (or any nondairy milk)

¾ cup brewed decaf coffee

½ cup canola oil

½ cup walnuts, toasted and chopped (see Note)

Glaze

1½ cups grain-sweetened, nondairy chocolate or carob chips

½ cup Earth Balance butter

Preheat the oven to 325°F. Oil an 8" or 9" square baking pan.

Sift together the flours, cocoa powder, baking powder, baking soda, and salt in a large bowl. Stir in the sugar. In a separate bowl, stir together the milk, coffee, and oil. Add the wet ingredients to the dry ingredients, and stir to mix well. Stir in the walnuts.

Pour the batter into the prepared pan, and bake for 25 to 30 minutes or until a toothpick inserted in the center of the pan comes out clean. Place the pan on a wire rack to cool completely.

Once the brownies have cooled, prepare the glaze. Melt the chocolate chips and butter together in a double boiler until well combined and completely smooth. If you don't have a double boiler, place a stainless steel bowl over boiling water and melt the ingredients in it. Pour the warm glaze over the entire pan of brownies, smoothing it out over the surface. Chill in the fridge until the glaze has set, about 1 hour. Cut into squares and serve.

Note: To toast walnuts, spread nuts on a baking sheet, and place in a 350°F oven for 8 to 10 minutes or until nuts are lightly browned and fragrant. Stir nuts once or twice as they toast. Transfer the toasted nuts to a bowl to cool.

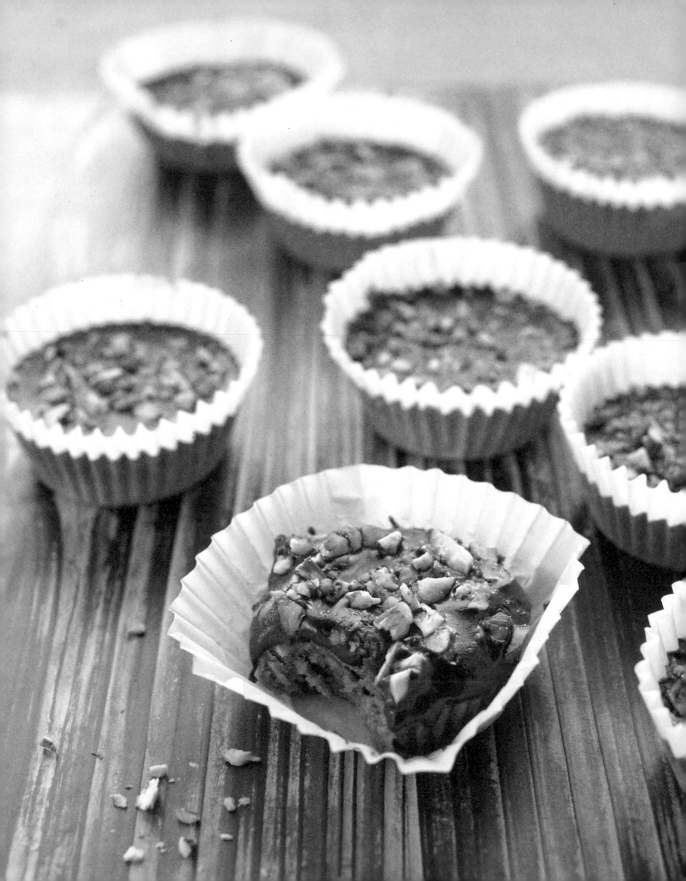

Chocolate Peanut Butter Cups

Back in the day, I was obsessed with Reese's Peanut Butter Cups. Now I make this healthier version and they are way better. In fact, I think they are the most ridiculously delicious things in the entire world. Look for graham crackers that are naturally sweetened or low in sugar (Health Valley makes a good one), and store the leftover crackers or crumbs in an airtight container for future use.

MAKES 12

10 graham cracker squares
(5 whole crackers)

½ cup Earth Balance butter

¾ cup crunchy peanut butter
(preferably unsweetened and
unsalted)

¼ cup maple sugar or other granulated
sweetener

1 cup grain-sweetened, nondairy
chocolate or carob chips

¼ cup soy, rice, or nut milk

¼ cup chopped pecans, almonds, or
peanuts

Line a 12-cup muffin tin with paper liners. (If You Care makes unbleached liners made from recycled paper.) Set aside.

Break the graham crackers into large chunks and place in a food processor or blender. Pulse on and off until they are ground to fine crumbs. Measure out ¾ cup of crumbs (reserve the rest for another use) and set aside. Melt the butter in a small saucepan over medium heat. Stir in the peanut butter, graham cracker crumbs, and maple sugar and mix well. Remove the mixture from the heat. Evenly divide the mixture, approximately 2 tablespoons per cup, among the muffin cups.

Combine the chocolate and milk in another pan. Stir over medium heat until the chocolate has melted. Spoon the chocolate evenly over the peanut butter mixture. Top with chopped nuts. Place in the refrigerator to set for at least 2 hours before serving.

Crispy Peanut Butter Treats with Chocolate Chips

These little yummies will blow your mind. Everyone—and I mean everyone—in your life will love these. You can serve them at parties, for after-school snacks, or as a regular dessert. They are also great for travel; I pack a big batch in my suitcase on most trips. Perfect for when I'm running late, have skipped a meal, or just want a dessert that won't bring me down, these treats are awesome.

MAKES 9 TO 12 SQUARES

1 box brown rice crisps cereal

1¾ cups brown rice syrup

Fine sea salt

¾ cup peanut butter or almond butter (preferably unsweetened and unsalted)

½ cup grain-sweetened, nondairy chocolate or carob chips

Pour the rice cereal into a large bowl. Heat the syrup with a pinch of salt in a saucepan over low heat. When the rice syrup liquefies, add the peanut butter and stir until well combined. Pour over the rice cereal. Mix well with a wooden spoon.

Once thoroughly mixed and cooled to room temperature, stir in the chocolate chips. Make sure the mixture is cool, or you will end up with melted chocolate instead of chocolate chips in your treats.

Turn the mixture out into an 8" × 8" or 9" × 13" baking dish. Wet your wooden spoon lightly and press the mixture evenly into the pan. Let cool for 1 hour—if you can—before cutting into squares or bars.

Variation:
Almond Raisin Bars

Substitute ¾ cup almond butter for the peanut butter and ½ cup dark or golden raisins for the chocolate chips (or use both chips *and* raisins . . . go crazy!).

Note: Without the chocolate chips, this dessert is totally fine for Superheroes.

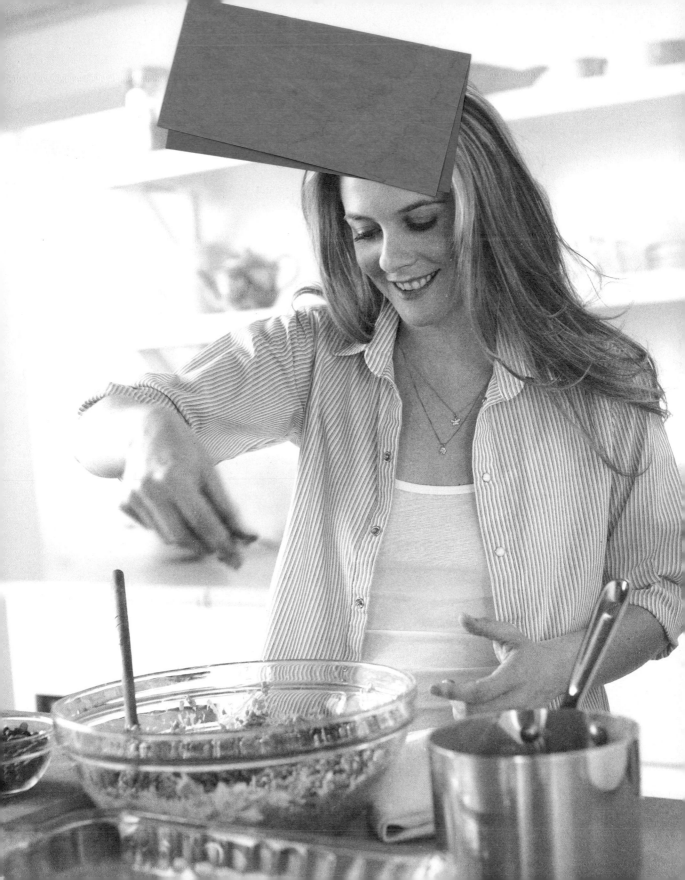

Oatmeal, Walnut, and Dried Plum Cookies

My friend Kristina Brindley is a wonderful vegan caterer who does home delivery. Her vittles are so delicious, I order from her almost every week. I think it's safe to say she is quite possibly the greatest dessert-maker to ever walk the earth—her desserts are insane! I'm not usually a big fan of oatmeal cookies, but I'm obsessed with these. (My mom, an oatmeal cookie connoisseur, just can't get enough.)

For more information on Kristina's delivery service, check out www.thekindlife.com.

MAKES 10 TO 12 COOKIES

1 cup quick-cooking rolled oats

¾ cup unbleached all-purpose flour

⅓ cup maple sugar

2 teaspoons baking powder

1 teaspoon baking soda

¼ teaspoon fine sea salt

⅓ cup maple syrup

½ cup safflower oil

1 teaspoon vanilla extract

½ teaspoon molasses

¼ cup chopped dried plums (or other dried fruit)

¼ cup finely chopped walnuts

Preheat the oven to 350°F. Line a baking sheet with parchment paper.

Combine the oats, flour, sugar, baking powder, baking soda, and salt in a large bowl. In a separate bowl, combine the syrup, oil, vanilla extract, and molasses. Add the wet ingredients to the dry ingredients, and stir to combine. Fold in the dried plums and nuts.

Using your hands, roll tablespoon-size scoops of dough into balls. Place the balls onto the prepared baking sheet, and press down slightly on the balls to flatten the tops. Bake for 8 to 12 minutes or until lightly browned. Transfer cookies to a baking rack to cool completely.

For variety, replace the all-purpose flour with whole wheat pastry flour, barley flour, spelt flour, or a gluten-free baking mix (choose one that does *not* include baking soda and baking powder). You can also substitute chocolate chips for the dried fruit and any kind of nuts for the walnuts.

Chocolate-Dipped Shortbread Cookies

I have a little *thing* for shortbread cookies. Luckily for me, these have simple ingredients and—except for the fact they're dipped in chocolate—could be a semiregular Superhero treat. They taste a bit like sugar cookies!

MAKES ABOUT 1 DOZEN

Cookies

1 cup whole wheat pastry flour

1 cup unbleached white flour

1 cup brown rice flour

1 teaspoon baking powder

½ cup safflower oil

⅔ cup maple syrup

2 teaspoons vanilla extract

1 teaspoon fine sea salt

Chocolate Coating

2 cups grain-sweetened, nondairy chocolate or carob chips

¼ cup maple syrup

2 tablespoons safflower oil

Preheat the oven to 350°F. Combine the flours and baking powder in a large mixing bowl. In a separate bowl, whisk together the oil, syrup, vanilla extract, and salt. Add the wet ingredients to the dry ingredients, and stir to form a smooth dough. If the mixture is too crumbly, add a bit of water, 1 teaspoon at a time, and up to 1 tablespoon more oil until the dough *just* holds together.

Roll the dough out to ½" thickness between 2 sheets of parchment or wax paper. Use cookie cutters or a knife to cut the dough into desired shapes. Arrange the cookies on the prepared baking sheet, and bake for 15 to 20 minutes or until lightly browned. Transfer the cookies to a baking rack to cool completely.

While the cookies are cooling, combine the chocolate chips, syrup, and oil in the top of a double boiler and place over simmering water. If you don't have a double boiler, place a stainless steel bowl over boiling water and melt the ingredients in it. Turn off the heat, cover, and let stand for 5 to 10 minutes or until the chocolate melts. Stir until smooth.

Dip each cookie halfway into the chocolate sauce, and place on a sheet of wax or parchment paper. Chill in the refrigerator until hardened.

Lemon–Poppy Seed Poundcake

I love me some poppy seeds, and this dessert totally delivers. It's pretty and is a perfect treat for guests or to serve with afternoon tea. I've given you two different glaze options here: One is sweet, glossy, and elegant while the other is fruity and colorful. They're both so delicious, I couldn't decide between them!

SERVES 8 TO 10

1 cup whole wheat pastry flour

1 cup all-purpose flour

⅓ cup maple sugar

2 teaspoons egg replacer (I like Ener-G)

2 teaspoons baking powder

1 teaspoon baking soda

¼ teaspoon sea salt

½ cup soy, rice, or nut milk

¼ cup fresh lemon juice

½ cup safflower oil

½ cup maple syrup

1 teaspoon lemon extract

2 tablespoons poppy seeds

Lemon Maple Glaze

½ cup maple syrup

½ cup lemon juice

2 teaspoons kuzu, diluted in a little bit of cold water

Berry Glaze

1 bag frozen berries, thawed

Maple syrup to taste

Vanilla extract to taste

Preheat the oven to 350°F. Oil the pans (you can use 3 mini loaf pans, a muffin tin, or 4 mini Bundt pans).

Combine the flours, sugar, egg replacer, baking powder, baking soda, and salt. In a separate bowl, combine the milk with the lemon juice and set aside for a few minutes; it will look curdled. Whisk in the oil, syrup, and lemon extract. Add the wet ingredients to the dry ingredients, and stir just until combined. Fold in the poppy seeds.

Pour the batter into the prepared pans, and bake for 15 to 25 minutes (mini loafs and muffins take about 15 to 18 minutes; loaf and Bundt pans take 20 to 25 minutes) or until a toothpick inserted in the center comes out clean. Cool the cake completely in the pans on a baking rack.

If using the Lemon Maple Glaze, combine the syrup and lemon juice in a saucepan over medium heat. Stir in the diluted kuzu, and continue stirring until the glaze comes to a boil. Simmer for 1 minute. Drizzle over the cake, and serve.

If using the Berry Glaze, whiz the berries in a blender with the syrup and vanilla extract to taste. Drizzle over the cake, and serve.

Peanut Butter Pie

This is CRAZY sweet and decadent. The chocolate ganache at the center of the pie makes this recipe a healthier version of Death By Chocolate. If you're a hazelnut nut, try using hazelnut butter instead of peanut butter. It's a little more expensive, but very elegant and delicious

SERVES 8 TO 10

1 vegan chocolate cookie crust (Arrowhead Mills makes one)

1 (10-ounce) bag grain-sweetened, nondairy chocolate chips

½ cup soy or hemp milk (do not use rice or nut milk)

1¼ cups peanut butter, divided

1 (12.3-ounce) box silken tofu (firm)

¼ cup maple syrup

1–2 teaspoons vanilla extract to taste

Preheat the oven to 375°F.

Bake the cookie crust for 4 to 5 minutes just to make it a bit crispy. Cool completely.

Melt the chocolate chips in the top of a double boiler set over simmering water. If you don't have a double boiler, place a stainless steel bowl over boiling water and melt the ingredients in it. Whisk in the milk until combined and smooth. With a measuring cup, scoop out about ¼ cup of the chocolate mixture, then pour the remainder into the cookie crust. Place the cookie crust in the refrigerator to cool completely.

While the filling chills, combine 1 cup peanut butter, the tofu, syrup, and vanilla extract in a food processor or blender; process until very smooth, scraping down the sides of the bowl as needed. Pour the peanut butter mixture on top of the chilled chocolate filling in the cookie crust, smoothing it out over the pie as you pour, and return the filled cookie crust to the refrigerator to chill for 1 hour or until firm.

To serve, return the reserved chocolate filling to the double boiler, or stainless steel bowl, and stir in the remaining ¼ cup peanut butter. Stir until the chocolate and peanut butter are very well combined and very warm. If the mixture seems too thick to drizzle, add some soy milk until it is runny enough to pour. Drizzle the mixture very generously over the chilled pie, or use a small spatula to spread it smoothly over the whole pie like icing. Refrigerate for 15 to 20 minutes before serving.

My Favorite Cupcakes

I love cupcakes . . . is there anyone out there who doesn't? These are light, springy, and delicious with a decadent fudgy frosting. These are best eaten right after they're made.

MAKES 12

Cupcakes

⅔ cup hemp or soy milk

1 teaspoon apple cider vinegar

⅔ cup agave nectar

⅓ cup safflower oil

2 teaspoons vanilla extract

1 cup all-purpose flour

⅓ cup whole wheat pastry flour

1 teaspoon baking powder

½ teaspoon baking soda

Pinch of fine sea salt

Fudge Frosting

½ cup (4 ounces) Earth Balance butter

½ cup agave nectar

2 teaspoons vanilla extract

⅓ cup unsweetened cocoa powder

½ cup soy milk powder

Note: Soy milk powder is sold in large amounts, so if you have a bunch left, you can add water to make it into soy milk. If you don't have soy milk powder, the frosting will be fine—just a little runnier.

Preheat the oven to 325°F. Line a 12-cup muffin tin with paper liners. (I use unbleached, recycled cupcake liners by a company called If You Care, available at Whole Foods.)

Combine the milk and vinegar in a medium bowl, and set aside for at least 5 minutes or until it bubbles a little. If it doesn't bubble, keep stirring the mixture until it does. Add the agave nectar, oil, and vanilla and stir.

In a separate bowl, combine the flours, baking powder, baking soda, and salt. Add the wet ingredients to the dry, mixing until no lumps remain.

Pour the batter into the prepared muffin tin, and bake for 18 to 22 minutes or until a toothpick inserted in the center of one cupcake comes out clean and the tops are slightly springy when pressed. Cool the cupcakes in the pan for 10 to 15 minutes, then cool completely on a baking rack before frosting.

To make the Fudge Frosting, use a mixer to cream the butter together with the agave nectar in a mixing bowl until very smooth. Add the vanilla extract and about half the cocoa powder, mix on low speed to combine, then add the remaining cocoa powder. Add in the soy milk powder, and beat at medium-high speed until fluffy. If it is runny, refrigerate the frosting until it sets up a little.

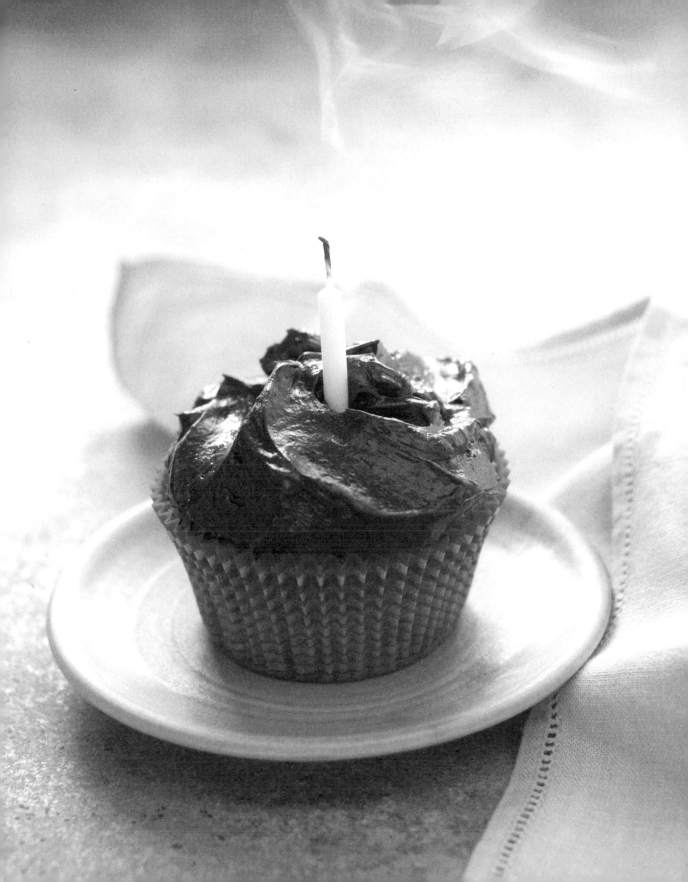

Mixed Berry Cheesecake

The last time I made this was when we had some friends over for movie night. We started with the Waffle, Sausage, and Cheese Panini (page 153) with a side of Sicilian Collard Greens with Pine Nuts and Raisins (page 176) and finished off the meal with this cheesecake—and then we watched *The Hunchback of Notre Dame* starring Charles Laughton. What an amazing movie!

SERVES 8

¾ cup Earth Balance butter

2 cups graham cracker crumbs (see Note)

1 (12-ounce) package silken tofu

1 cup nondairy cream cheese

1 tablespoon safflower oil

¼ cup maple syrup plus an additional 1 to 2 teaspoons if using a fresh fruit topping

¼ cup soy milk

2 teaspoons arrowroot

1 teaspoon vanilla extract

½ teaspoon lemon or orange extract (optional)

Fresh mixed berries for topping (or frozen mixed berries, thawed)

Preheat the oven to 350°F. Oil an 8" or 9" springform pan.

Melt the butter in a small saucepan. Turn off the heat, and stir in the graham cracker crumbs. Press the crumb mixture into the bottom and slightly up the sides of the prepared pan, and bake for 5 minutes. Let cool on a baking rack.

Combine the tofu, cream cheese, oil, ¼ cup syrup, milk, arrowroot, vanilla extract, and citrus extract (if using) in a blender or food processor and process until smooth. Pour the mixture into the graham cracker crust, and smooth the top with a spatula.

Bake the cheesecake for 45 minutes to 1 hour. Let the cheesecake cool to room temperature. If using fresh berries, toss them with 1 to 2 teaspoons syrup to create a slightly glazed effect. Top the cheesecake with the berries, and chill until you're ready to serve.

Note: To make graham cracker crumbs, place graham cracker squares in a sealed plastic bag and smash with a rolling pin, or grind graham cracker squares in a food processor. You'll need 12 to 13 graham cracker squares to make 2 cups graham cracker crumbs.

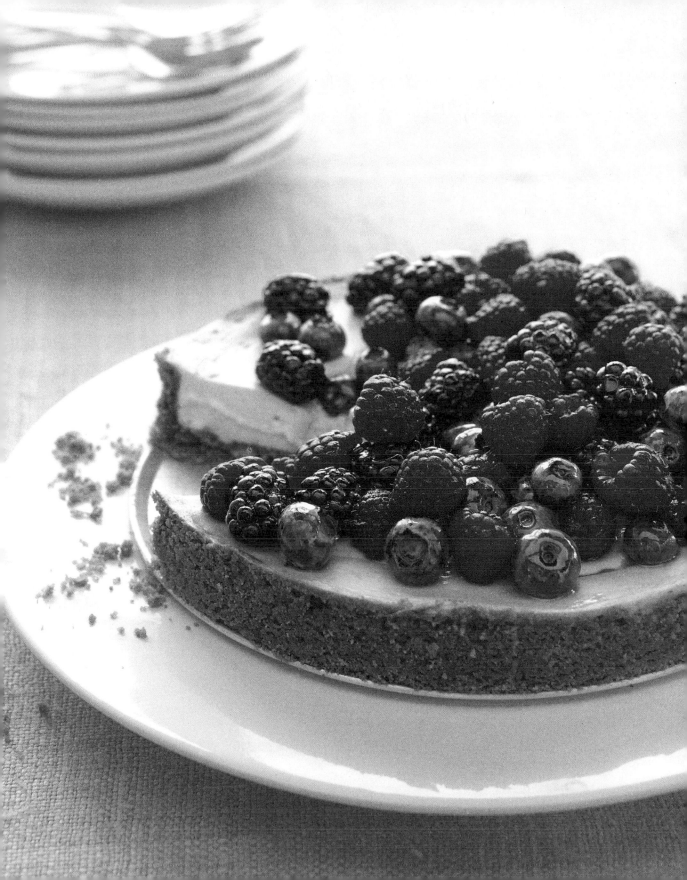

Peach Crumble

This dessert has a wonderful crumbly granola crust that will blow your socks off. In fact, I love the crust so much I've given this recipe almost as much crust as filling! You'll see why when you taste it. Of course, it's best made with fresh peaches, but you can also use frozen when you crave this crumble out of season. For a crunchier topping, use less maple and brown rice syrup.

I would consider this a regular Superhero dessert if it weren't for the flour. Any baked flour product can make you feel a little gunked up and get in the way of your Superpowers, so go easy. A couple of times a week is fine.

SERVES 4 TO 6

2½–3 cups sliced fresh or thawed frozen organic peaches

1 cup organic blueberries

1¾ cups apple juice

2 tablespoons kuzu

1 teaspoon fresh lemon juice

2 teaspoons vanilla extract

Pinch of fine sea salt

Topping

3 cups rolled oats

2 cups barley flour, spelt flour, brown rice flour, or sweet rice flour

¼ teaspoon fine sea salt

¼ teaspoon ground cinnamon

¾ cup safflower oil

¾ cup brown rice syrup

¼ cup maple syrup

1 cup chopped pecans or walnuts

Preheat the oven to 350°F.

Combine the peaches and blueberries in a 9" square baking pan.

Reserve ¼ cup of the apple juice in a small bowl, and heat the remaining 1½ cups in a small saucepan. Place the kuzu in a small bowl, and add in the reserved apple juice. Let the kuzu mixture sit for about 10 seconds so that the kuzu can dissolve into the liquid. Stir with a fork, and immediately whisk the kuzu mixture and the lemon juice into the hot apple juice, stirring continually to prevent lumps from forming. Bring to a boil, then reduce the heat and simmer for 2 minutes. Turn off the heat, and add the vanilla extract and the salt. Pour over the peaches and blueberries in the pan.

To make the topping, dry-roast the oats, flour, salt, and cinnamon in a skillet over medium-low heat for about 5 minutes. Heat the oil and syrups together in a separate pan, then pour over the flour mixture and mix well. Stir in the nuts.

Crumble the topping over the fruit, then cover the pan with foil and bake for 30 minutes. Remove the foil, and bake 15 to 25 minutes longer or until the topping is golden and the fruit filling bubbles a little. (Try to handle the foil with care so you can reuse it another time.) Cool crumble for about 30 minutes before serving.

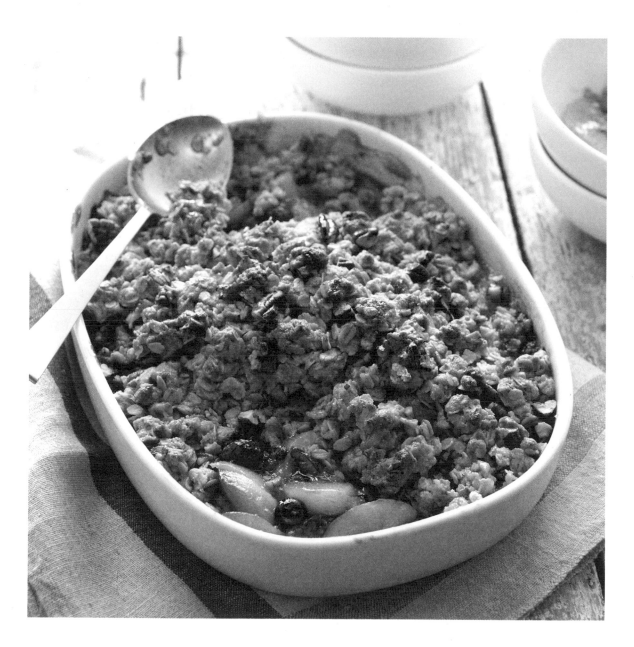

BREAKFAST

Becoming vegan may not mean a whole lot of big changes at breakfast time if you're basically a grab-and-go kind of morning eater, especially during the week. Cereal with fruit and milk, a piece of toast, or a bagel with tofu cream cheese are all easygoing options that will get you out of the house in 5 minutes or less.

- Go crazy with whole grain toast, your favorite nut butter, and fruit-sweetened jam. Dalfour makes an amazing strawberry jam.
- Find a whole grain, fruit juice–sweetened cereal and eat it with soy milk, rice milk, or my favorite: a soy/rice blend made by Eden.
- Thinking about making your own nut milk? Soak ½ cup almonds in water overnight. Discard the soaking water and transfer the almonds to a blender. Add 4 cups water, a dash of vanilla extract, and blend until smooth. Voilà!

When you do have a bit more time to cook, check out some of these cool breakfast options.

Quick Date-Apple-Cinnamon Oatmeal

I used to eat the presweetened, instant oatmeal that came in a packet until I joined the cast of a play about Orthodox Judaism in which I portrayed a lesbian who has a cocaine overdose on stage . . . anyhoo, another actress in the show, Lesa Carlson, taught me how to make this oatmeal! I love using dates from the farmers' market.

MAKES 1 SERVING

1 cup organic rolled oats

2 tablespoons maple syrup

2 tablespoons chopped walnuts

⅓ crisp apple, cut in cubes

About 5 dates, pitted and chopped

Fine sea salt to taste

3 shakes of ground cinnamon

Scant 1 teaspoon flaxseed oil

Bring a kettle of water to a boil.

Combine the oats, syrup, nuts, apple, and dates in a bowl. Add a pinch or two of salt, then pour on enough hot water to just cover the oats; don't add too much or it will be watery. Cover the bowl with a plate or pot lid, and let the oatmeal stand until the oats have absorbed the water. Stir, and add a little more water if the oats look too dry. Let the oatmeal cool a little, and then drizzle with the flaxseed oil. Enjoy.

Whole Wheat Biscuits

These biscuits are sublime at breakfast, but can also be used as a snack or served at a lovely tea. Try them with Earth Balance butter and jam. They're so good.

MAKES 10 BISCUITS

2 cups whole wheat pastry flour

1 tablespoon baking powder

½ teaspoon fine sea salt

½ cup safflower oil

Approximately ½ cup plain nondairy milk (more or less as needed)

Preheat the oven to 450°F.

Combine the flour, baking powder, and salt in a large bowl. Slowly pour in the oil, mixing with a fork until the mixture is combined. It will be quite crumbly. Add the milk a little at a time, stirring with a fork. You want to use just enough milk to bring the mixture together.

Gather the dough into a ball, and place it on a lightly floured surface. Knead the dough about 25 times, then smooth the dough into a ball and pat it into a ½"-thick round disk. Use a 2½" biscuit cutter or the rim of a glass or jar to cut out biscuits, gathering the scraps and rerolling them to make a few additional biscuits. Place the biscuits on an ungreased baking sheet. If you like the sides crispier, place them about 1" apart. For softer sides, have the biscuits touching.

Bake on the center rack for 10 to 12 minutes or until the bottoms are golden. Serve hot or warm.

Traditional English Breakfast

Having British parents, I grew up on breakfasts of toast covered with cheese, tomatoes, or baked beans. Those days aren't entirely over; whenever we visit my parents, Christopher and my mother make this awesome vegan version of the traditional English breakfast. We also served it at our postwedding brunch!

If you like your greens sautéed, it will make the dish a little heavier but totally delectable. Spinach tastes great with garlic and lemon juice. Add vegan bacon, sausage, and hash browns to make it a royal feast!

SERVES 2

1 tomato

Fine sea salt and freshly ground black pepper to taste

Earth Balance butter

8 button mushrooms, halved

½ bunch kale or spinach

1 can vegetarian Heinz baked beans (the most authentic but they contain sugar) or a healthier brand

4 slices French baguette (I like sourdough)

2 slices vegan Cheddar cheese (optional)

Preheat your broiler.

Cut the tomato in half. Sprinkle the cut surfaces with a pinch of salt and a pinch of pepper, then top with a small amount of butter. Arrange the tomato halves on a baking sheet, cut sides up, and slide under the broiler for 3 to 6 minutes or until bubbly. Remove the tomato halves from the broiler, but leave the broiler on.

Melt 1 tablespoon butter in a skillet over medium heat. Add the mushrooms, and sauté for 4 to 5 minutes or until cooked through but still firm. Sprinkle with salt and pepper.

Heat water in a steamer to boiling, then steam the greens just until tender, 4 minutes for kale and 2 minutes for spinach. While the greens cook, heat the beans in a saucepan.

Arrange the bread slices on a baking sheet, and place the baking sheet under the broiler for 1 minute. Flip the bread slices, top 2 with a slice of cheese, and return to the broiler until the bread is golden and the cheese melts. Butter the other 2 pieces of toast, if you like. You should be sort of dancing between all of these steps, as you want to keep everything warm and have it all ready at the same time.

Place a piece of cheese toast and plain toast on each plate, and ladle some of the beans onto the plain toast. Add some mushrooms, kale or spinach, and a tomato half to each plate. Eat it all together. Delicious.

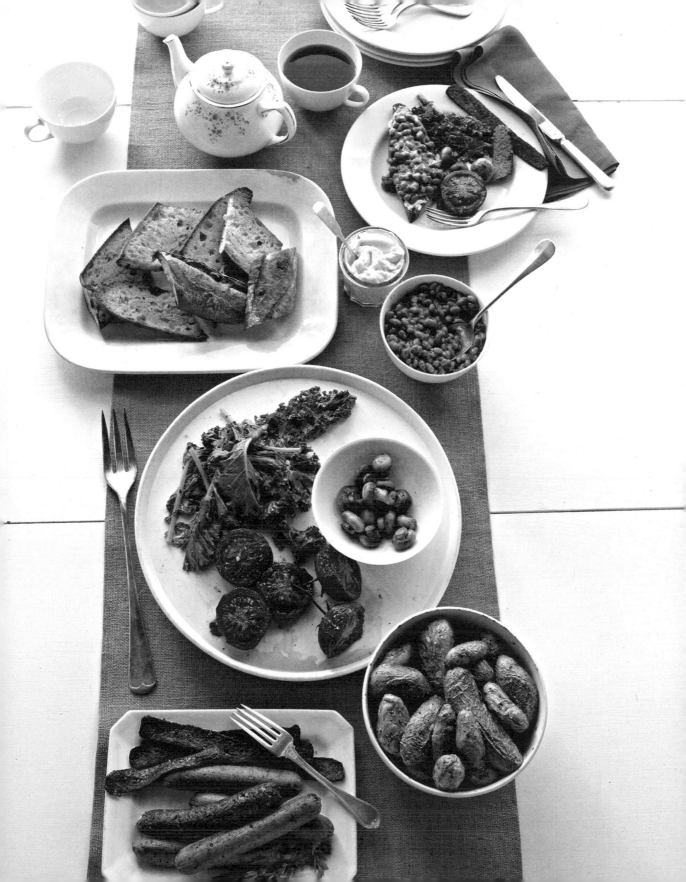

Crocodile Crunch

This chunky, funky festival of fruit is colorful and nutritious. It's especially fun for kids because it includes a bright green sauce made with spirulina, which has a tendency to get all over teeth, lips, and little hands. I was first introduced to a version of this recipe by Laura and Woody Harrelson; there was a time when they made it every day for breakfast, no matter where they were in the world. Feel free to use whatever seasonal, local fruit you love.

SERVES 2

2–3 cups of bite-size pieces of fresh fruit, such as kiwifruit, strawberries, bananas, avocados, apples, pears, or mango

2 teaspoons spirulina

1½ tablespoons any nondairy milk (I use soy or hemp because they're creamier)

2 teaspoons almond butter (for this recipe, I like to use raw)

1½ tablespoons maple syrup

2 tablespoons fresh orange juice

2 tablespoons shaved fresh or dried coconut

½ cup kamut flake cereal

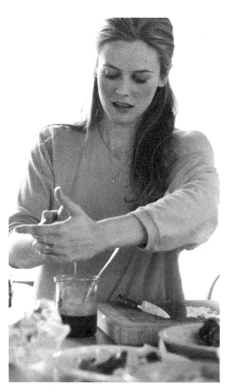

Divide the fruit into 2 serving bowls.

Use a fork to stir together the spirulina and soy milk in a small glass. Add the almond butter, and mix again. Stir in the syrup and orange juice, and give it a final stir. The sauce should be smooth and neither too thick nor too runny.

Pour the sauce over the fruit, and sprinkle with the coconut and cereal. Serve immediately.

Mom's Granola

I think this is the greatest granola that ever lived. As a little kid, I often woke up to the smell of my mother's granola baking in the oven. I loved it so much I could never wait for it to cool, so I'd eat it right off the pan! With a little healthy tweaking, this version's just as good—great with any kind of nondairy milk, as a snack, or on top of a dessert. It will also last for weeks or even months stored in a glass container. Thank you, Mom!

MAKES 2 QUARTS

6 cups quick-cooking oats

½ cup maple sugar

¾ cup wheat germ

½ cup shredded coconut

½ cup sunflower seeds

1 cup raisins

½ to 1 cup of walnuts (optional)

½ cup safflower oil

⅓ cup maple syrup (sweetest version) or brown rice syrup (slightly milder)

1½ teaspoons vanilla extract

Preheat the oven to 350°F.

Spread the oats on a rimmed baking pan, and bake for 10 minutes. Transfer the oats to a large mixing bowl, and add the sugar, wheat germ, coconut, sunflower seeds, and raisins, or walnuts if using. Stir to mix well, then add the oil, syrup, and vanilla extract. Mix until everything is moistened.

Spread half of the mixture on each of 2 rimmed baking sheets (or bake in 2 batches), and bake for 10 minutes. Stir after 5 minutes to brown evenly.

Let the baked granola cool on the pans, then transfer it to a bowl and stir until crumbly. Store in an airtight container.

Pumpkin Bread

While on vacation in Maui, Christopher and I discovered a magical place called Laulima Farms. At their stand, they sold smoothies, salads, and fresh coffee harvested from their own coffee bean crop. Their blender was powered by a bicycle, so I had to pedal for a few minutes to get my smoothie. How fun is that? We went every morning to get our treats, and this bread was my favorite. Because the Laulima Farms people have the magic touch, I think it was a tad yummier there, but what doesn't taste better in Maui?

SERVES 8 TO 10

5 cups cooked pumpkin (fresh is best, but canned will do; see Note)

2 cups maple sugar

2 "eggs": either 2 tablespoons flaxseeds pureed with 6 tablespoons water or 2 eggs' worth of egg replacer

1 cup almond milk or other nut milk

¾ cup safflower oil

1 teaspoon vanilla extract

4 cups spelt flour

3 teaspoons baking soda

3 teaspoons baking powder

1 tablespoon ground cinnamon

1 teaspoon ground nutmeg

¾ cup grain-sweetened, nondairy chocolate or carob chips

1 cup whole macadamia nuts (save a little bit of chocolate and nuts to sprinkle on top at end, if you want)

Preheat oven to 350°F. Oil two 9" × 5" glass loaf pans.

Combine the pumpkin puree, sugar, "eggs," milk, oil, and vanilla extract in a mixing bowl. In a separate bowl, combine the flour, baking soda, baking powder, cinnamon, nutmeg, and most of the chocolate chips and nuts if reserving some to sprinkle on top. Add the wet ingredients to the dry ingredients until just combined.

Fill the prepared pans with the batter. Top with the reserved chocolate chips and nuts. Bake for 45 minutes to 1 hour or until the top springs back when pressed with a finger.

Let the loaves cool in the pans for a few minutes, then turn out onto a baking rack to cool completely.

Note: To use fresh pumpkin, cut the pumpkin in half and scoop out the seeds. Place the pumpkin, cut sides down, in a baking dish with ¼" water inside. Bake at 400°F for 45 to 60 minutes or until very soft. Cool, cut, and puree the pumpkin until smooth. You might need to add a little bit of water if the pumpkin is on the dry side and has a hard time moving in the blender.

SNACKS, DRINKS, AND PARTY FOOD

On pages 84–85, I offered some suggestions of convenient snack foods to stock up on for those times when the temptation to be naughty is especially strong. When I have a bit more time, though, I like to skip the packaged snack foods—however healthy and natural—and cook up one of these extra-delish snacks. Most of them can also double for a casual get-together or buffet-style meals. Another recipe that makes a great snack or party food is Radicchio Pizza with Truffle Oil (page 144), and of course you can never go wrong with chips, salsa, and guacamole.

The drinks make a lovely addition to an afternoon tea or luncheon. Make them by the pitcher to have on hand for unexpected guests or for postworkout rehydration instead of buying pricey (and eco-unfriendly) sports drinks.

If it's just me, the fridge, and the munchies, I might opt for one of these easy pick-me-ups:

- My favorite late night snack is toast spread with Earth Balance butter, topped with sliced tomatoes, a little sprinkle of fine sea salt, and some chopped fresh basil. Crazy delicious.

- Another quick and easy snack I love is an open-faced sandwich made with anything I can find in the fridge.

- Next time you serve hummus, go beyond carrots and celery for dipping; try endive, steamed pea pods, or green beans. They will make your hummus platter fresh and different.

- Make a cheese and cracker platter using Follow Your Heart vegan cheese with a variety of whole grain crackers.

Artichoke, Mushroom, and Leek Crostini with Pesto

These are so good, it's ridiculous! Sophisticated, fancy, and a complete and utter yum-fest, these crostini will blow you away. Even though the combination of toppings tastes best, each tastes great by itself. Serve them at your next party.

SERVES 2

3 tablespoons olive oil

2 teaspoons balsamic vinegar

2 tablespoons mirin

2 teaspoons shoyu

Salt

3–4 garlic cloves, thinly sliced

2 cups thinly sliced leek

2 cups sliced button mushrooms

Artichoke Spread

1 can whole, water-packed artichoke hearts, drained

1 tablespoon olive oil

½–1 teaspoon umeboshi vinegar

Pesto

1 cup fresh basil leaves

¾ cup raw pine nuts

¼ cup lemon juice

1–2 tablespoons umeboshi vinegar

¼ cup olive oil

4–6 thick slices whole grain baguette

Finely chopped flat-leaf parsley

Preheat the oven to 400°F. Line a baking sheet with parchment.

Combine the oil, vinegar, mirin, shoyu, and 2 pinches of salt in a skillet over medium heat. Add the garlic, leek, and mushrooms. Cover the pan and when you hear sizzling, gently shake the skillet, holding the lid in place. Reduce the heat to low and braise until the leek is quite tender and deeply browned, 5 to 10 minutes. Remove the lid and allow any remaining liquid to cook off. Remove from heat and stir gently to combine.

Blend the artichoke hearts, olive oil, and umeboshi vinegar in a food processor until smooth. Remove from the food processor and set aside.

Blend the basil, pine nuts, lemon juice, umeboshi vinegar, and oil in the food processor until smooth. Adjust seasonings to taste.

Brush the bread lightly with oil on both sides. Arrange the bread on a baking sheet and sprinkle lightly with salt. Bake until the bread is lightly browned and crispy at the edges.

Spread the artichoke mixture on the bread, mound the leek mixture generously on top, and finish with a dollop of pesto and a sprinkle of parsley. Serve.

Artichoke Dip

Another of my mother's staples, this quick and easy recipe has been a party classic since the dawn of time. Now that I've un-dairied it, it will rule forever!

MAKES ABOUT 3 CUPS

2 (8.5-ounce) cans quartered artichoke hearts in water, drained

1 cup Vegenaise

1 cup grated soy Parmesan

1 garlic clove, finely chopped (optional)

Paprika

Crackers or endive leaves for dipping

Preheat the oven to 350°F.

Use a wooden spoon to mash up the artichokes in a mixing bowl. Add the Vegenaise, cheese, and garlic (if using) and combine well.

Scrape the dip into a baking dish, and bake for 30 minutes or until heated through and browned on top. Sprinkle with paprika, and serve with crackers or endive leaves.

Raw Balls

When I was deep into the raw food movement, I spent a lot of time with my friend Juliano, a raw food chef here in L.A. My raw balls are inspired by his raw balls, and they work equally well as a snack or dessert. Eat them straight out of the freezer.

MAKES 10 TO 12 BALLS

½ cup walnuts

½ cup pitted dates

Scant ½ cup raw carob powder

Scant ½ cup maple syrup

½ cup almond butter

½ teaspoon vanilla extract

¼ teaspoon fine sea salt

½ cup whole almonds

2 cups shredded unsweetened coconut

Place the walnuts in a food processor and process until coarsely ground. Add the dates, and pulse until well combined with the nuts. Add the carob powder, syrup, almond butter, vanilla extract, and salt. Process until the mixture is thick and smooth. Add the almonds, and pulse a few times until combined; you want them to remain in crunchy chunks.

Form the mixture into golf-ball-size balls with your hands. Roll the balls in coconut. Place in a sealed container in the freezer until hardened.

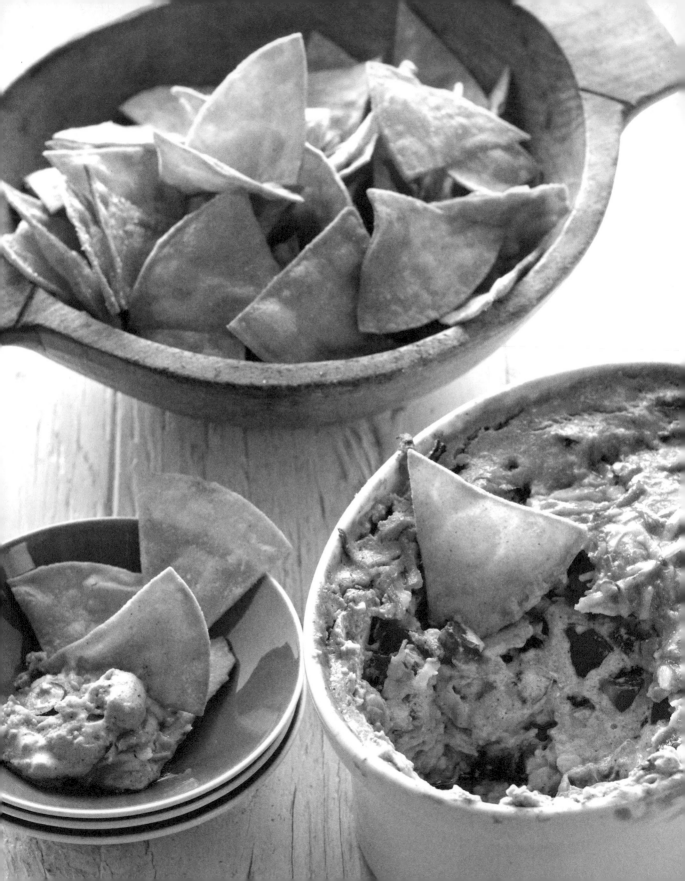

Cheesy, Oozy Guacamole Bean Dip

This dip is quick, easy, and delicious—the perfect thing to bring to a party. Make it in a glass dish to display all the pretty layers. Great for meat-eating friends.

SERVES 8

1 (16-ounce) can refried beans

3 large avocados

3 tablespoons fresh lime juice

2 (8-ounce) containers nondairy sour cream

1 packet taco seasoning (see Note)

½ cup diced mild green chiles, drained

½ cup sliced black olives, or more if you like

5 tomatoes, chopped

2 cups shredded vegan Cheddar cheese

Preheat the oven to 350°F.

Spread a layer of refried beans in the bottom of an 8" × 8" quart glass baking dish. Pit and peel the avocados, and place in a bowl. Mash the avocados together with the lime juice, and spread on top of the refried beans. Stir together the sour cream and taco seasoning, and spread over the avocado.

Sprinkle the chiles over the sour cream, and top with a layer of black olives. Add the tomatoes, and sprinkle with the cheese. Heat the dip for 15 to 30 minutes or until heated through and the cheese is a bit melted.

Serve warm or at room temperature.

> Note: We use Bearitos organic taco seasoning, but it does contain a touch of cane sugar. If you're avoiding all white sugar, make your own by combining chili powder, ground cumin, onion powder, hot paprika or cayenne, and salt.

Variation:

For chips, there are some pretty healthy baked organic tortilla chips on the market, but you can also make your own by cutting up Ezekiel sprouted grain tortillas and baking them in the oven until crisp or dry-roasting them in a frying pan.

Egg Salad Sandwiches

When I was a kid, my mom invited friends over for tea all the time. I would eat tons of chocolate-covered biscuits, sponge cake, finger sandwiches—and drink lots and lots of tea. Can you imagine all the sugar and caffeine running through my little body? These days, our tea parties are just as elegant and dainty, without the next-day payback. Make your own party spread with 2 or 3 kinds of little sandwiches (try thin cucumber slices and vegan mayo or Yves "ham" and vegan Cheddar). Remove the crusts, cut the sandwiches into little triangles, and bring on the tea and cookies!

SERVES 4

2 (12-ounce) cakes firm tofu

2 small onions, diced

2 celery stalks, diced

2 tablespoons shoyu

1 tablespoon safflower oil

1 teaspoon turmeric

½ teaspoon fine sea salt

1 teaspoon Vegenaise, or more to taste

4–8 thin slices whole wheat bread

Paprika (optional)

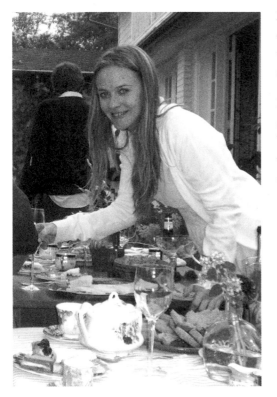

Mash the tofu in a mixing bowl until chunky but not completely smooth. Add the onions, celery, shoyu, oil, turmeric, and salt and mix well. Stir in the Vegenaise and refrigerate until ready to use.

Divide the egg salad among 4 slices of bread. You can serve them open-faced or top with a second slice of bread, as you prefer. If serving open-faced, sprinkle with a bit of paprika. For tea sandwiches, slice off the crusts, cut diagonally into 4 small triangles, and serve.

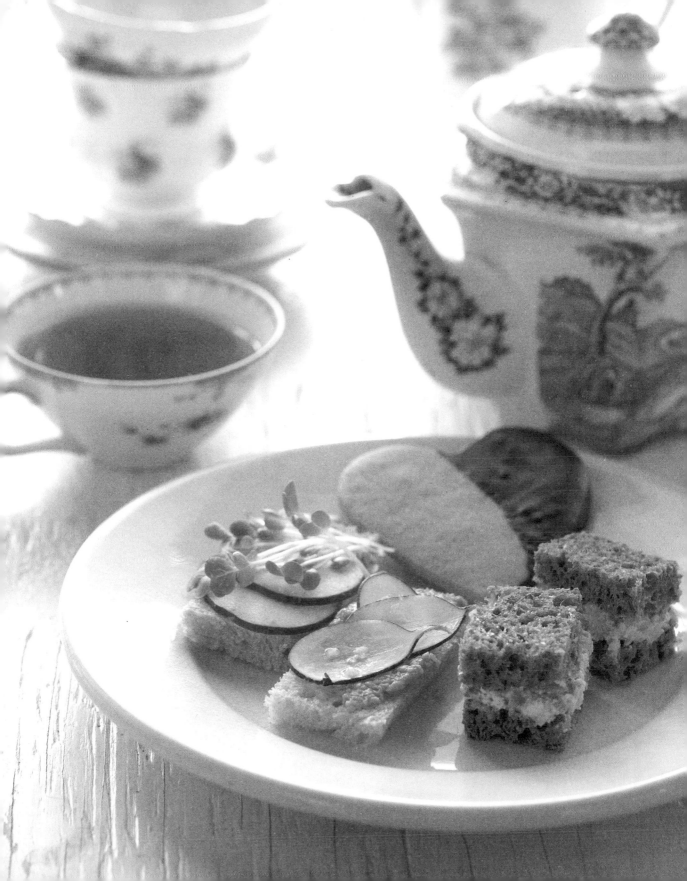

Warm Spicy Wine

There's nothing like mulled wine when it's cold outside. It's a wonderful winter treat and especially good for holiday parties. I like this drink as much as I like saying its Nordic name: Glögg (the ö sounds like the oo in "book"). Come on . . . say it with an accent! I share my love of Glögg with my friend Mark Bridges, who designed the costumes for *There Will Be Blood* and *Boogie Nights* and is one of the most talented people I know. Mark, who is German, calls it Glühwein ("Gloo-Vine"), which is just as much fun to say. He always brings a big pot of it to my parties.

SERVES 6 TO 8

1 bottle sulfate-free organic red wine (Trader Joe makes a good one)

1 cup Madeira

1 cup freshly squeezed orange juice (optional)

¼–½ cup maple syrup

5 whole white cardamom pods, cracked (optional)

2 whole cloves

1 (4") cinnamon stick

2 slices fresh or dried orange with peel (optional)

Combine all the ingredients in a large stainless steel saucepan, and heat slowly over low heat without boiling. Strain, and serve immediately. For a stronger flavor, turn off the heat, cover, and let the spices steep for several hours or overnight. Strain, and reheat gently .

Fruit Smoothies à la Alicia

I love smoothies and am always playing with different flavors and combinations. I'm not generally a big fan of the taste of stevia, but I actually really like it in smoothies!

SERVES 1

½ cup almond milk or other nut milk

½ cup soy milk or rice milk

¾ banana, preferably frozen

1 cup frozen strawberries

2 drops stevia or 1 teaspoon maple syrup or to taste

¼ teaspoon vanilla extract (optional)

1 whole cinnamon stick (optional)

Combine everything in a blender and whiz until smooth!

- Toss in a whole cinnamon stick and blend it along with the fruits for a nice little crunch.

- Raisins, dates, and nuts make great additions to a smoothie.

- In the summer, make smoothies as a cooling dessert.

- Leftover smoothies can be poured into ice pop molds. Kids (and big kids like me and Christopher) go nuts for them.

- When your favorite fruit is in season, buy up a bunch and freeze it for smoothies and other desserts later in the year.

Hot Chocolate

This recipe has a sophisticated taste with deep, rich flavors. You'll find it's not too sweet.

SERVES 1

1 cup soy/rice milk blend

1 teaspoon unsweetened cocoa powder

1 tablespoon grain-sweetened, nondairy chocolate or carob chips

¼ teaspoon vanilla extract

1 teaspoon maple syrup

Optional toppings: vegan marshmallows, nondairy whipped topping, or chocolate shavings

Whisk the milk, cocoa powder, chocolate chips, vanilla extract, and syrup together in a small saucepan. Place over medium heat, and cook until the chocolate chips are melted, whisking occasionally. Serve naked or with your choice of topping!

Peach and Mint Iced Tea

Smack dab in the middle of summer, when peaches are at their peak, this tea is elegant and refreshing.

SERVES 8

4–6 kukicha or green tea teabags

4 ripe peaches, pitted and cut in ¼" pieces

1 small bunch fresh mint

Maple syrup to taste (optional)

Bring water to a boil in a kettle, and place the teabags in a heatproof pitcher. Add 8 cups of boiling water to the pitcher, and steep for 10 minutes. Remove and discard the teabags, and allow the tea to cool to room temperature.

When cooled, add the peaches and the mint to the tea. Sweeten with maple syrup to taste, if desired, and chill until ready to serve.

Pomegranate and Lime Iced Tea

Ooooh, make a nice big batch of this on a hot summer afternoon and keep it in the fridge for a couple of days! It's beautiful, refreshing, and healthy.

SERVES 8

6–8 kukicha or green tea teabags

2 cups unsweetened pomegranate juice

¼ cup maple syrup

3 limes, thinly sliced

Bring water to a boil in a kettle, and place the teabags in a heatproof pitcher. Add 8 cups of boiling water to the pitcher, and steep for 10 minutes. Remove and discard the teabags, and allow the tea to cool to room temperature.

Stir in the pomegranate juice and maple syrup. Add the limes, and chill until ready to serve.

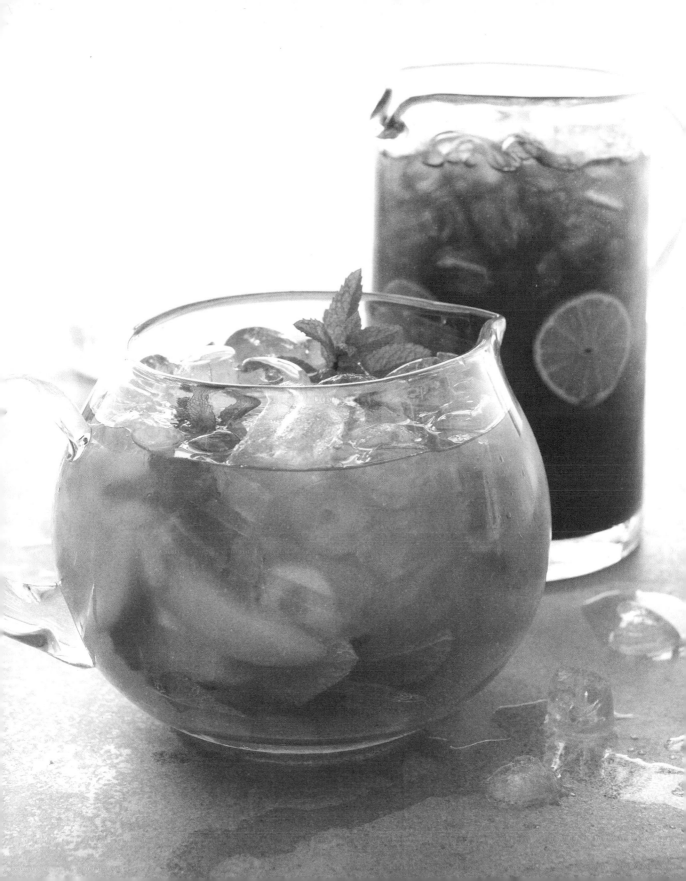

15

Superhero Recipes

With this group of recipes, you can experience the Kind Foods in all their glory.
Most are quite simple, a few are more elaborate, but every one is designed to develop
and nurture your Superhero powers. I think you'll be amazed by how good you will
feel on a diet of real, clean, wholesome food.

Here are some tips for Superhero cooking:

- In order to stick to the Superhero plan to the greatest degree possible, it's
  important to plan ahead. You may need to soak beans or cook some grains the
  night before, so have a rough vision of what you're going to eat in the coming
  day. Things go much more smoothly when you have a plan.

- Always cook more than you need. Leftover grains, beans, soups, and desserts
  keep well for a couple of days; and having the building blocks of a quick meal
  ready to roll in the fridge is vital to maintaining a Superhero lifestyle from one
  day to the next.

- Try to get the bulk of each day's cooking done in one session so other meals can
  be put together really quickly from the leftovers.

- The Superhero plan will introduce you to quite a few new foods like daikon,
  burdock, millet. They were once all new to me, too, but now they've become a
  regular part of my diet and I love them. Don't be intimidated by a recipe that
  calls for seemingly exotic ingredients; you'll soon realize that Superhero
  cooking is actually very simple and easy.

GRAIN ENTRÉES

Just like in the Vegan diet, the cornerstone of the Superhero plan is whole grains, and the component you should start with when you are planning a meal. For me, more often than not that grain is rice, though I also love quinoa, millet, barley, and couscous. I always make enough rice for a few meals at a time because it makes life so much easier; I can turn the leftover rice into breakfast porridge, fried rice for lunch, or add it to salads and burritos at dinner. It's also great to combine rice with other grains. Try rice with barley, whole wheat berries (3 parts rice to 1 part other), or sweet brown rice (1:1).

When you're keeping it simple on the grain front, think about serving them embellished with one of these flavor-enhancing garnishes:

- Chop enough scallions, chives, arugula, parsley, or cilantro to last for 2 to 3 days and store in old jam jars in the fridge. Any of these will give grain extra flavor, color, and overall sparkle. I prefer to chop them fresh each time, but when life gets crazy, this shortcut really helps.

- Roast sunflower or pumpkin seeds and sprinkle with shoyu (below). Make enough for 2 weeks and keep them in a jar. Use them as a condiment at the table since you can put them on anything!

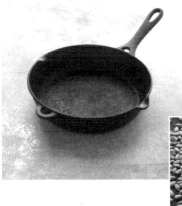

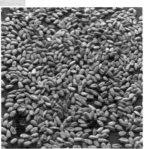

To make toasted seeds: Rinse the seeds and drain immediately in a fine sieve. Transfer to a hot pan over medium heat, and stir constantly as they dry and become golden brown and a little puffed up. They may begin to pop, and some popping is okay, but if the seeds begin to pop right out of the pan, reduce the heat. Remove from the pan when done and sprinkle with a few drops of shoyu, stirring to combine. Keep small batches (about 1 cup) of toasted seeds in a jar in the fridge for up to 2 weeks. Toasted seeds make even the simplest meals delicious.

Clean, Mean Burritos

If my husband had to name his favorite thing to eat, it would definitely be burritos. I'm not as into burritos, but I love these because they're so healthy and fresh. Use any cooked or raw vegetables you like in the filling; burritos are a great way to use up leftover roasted veggies or any kind of salad. You can also dice up a packaged, prebaked tofu and use in place of the beans. So good!

SERVES 1

1 whole grain tortilla (Ezekiel is my favorite)

½ cup cooked rice

½ cup cooked beans (such as kidney, black, or pinto)

Chopped onion, cucumber, avocado, sliced radishes, sprouts, pressed salad (pages 255–256), and/or shredded lettuce (½ cup in all)

2 tablespoons chopped fresh cilantro

Tofu Cream (page 225)

Warm the tortilla in a dry skillet until pliable, or wrap it in a dampened dish towel and heat in a 300°F oven for 5 or 6 minutes.

Place the rice in the center of the warmed tortilla, and mound the beans on top of the rice. Add the vegetables, sprinkle with cilantro, and top with the Tofu Cream (make sure not to overload the tortilla, or it will be hard to fold properly).

Fold the two sides of the tortilla in over the filling, then flip up the bottom edge and roll as tightly as possible. Enjoy!

Tostadas (Kinda)

With a healthy portion of both grains and beans, this is a colorful, complete meal and yet *another* great way to use leftovers. I know that "tostada" means toasted, but I prefer my tortilla to remain warm and only lightly dry-roasted in this dish. That's the "kinda" part. If you want to toast your tortilla more, go for it. I find that tostadas are a great vehicle for Tofu Cream (page 225), which is an awesome, versatile condiment. If there are non-Superheros at the table, they may want to add vegan cheese, tomatoes, or hot sauce, but these are delicious either way.

SERVES 2

2 teaspoons olive oil

¼ cup half-moon onion slices

2 pinches of fine sea salt

1 carrot, julienned

1 celery stalk, thinly sliced

¼ cup corn kernels, fresh or thawed frozen

2 whole wheat tortillas

1 cup cooked brown rice

1 cup cooked beans (such as pinto, black, kidney, or azuki)

½ cup alfalfa sprouts

1 small cucumber, chopped (peel only if the cucumber is not organic)

½ avocado, peeled and cubed or sliced

A few large dollops of Tofu Cream (page 225) per serving

1 radish, thinly sliced (optional)

1 teaspoon arugula, chopped (optional)

1–2 teaspoons chopped fresh cilantro or 1 teaspoon chopped fresh parsley

1 teaspoon toasted sunflower seeds (page 215) or Gomashio (page 232)

Heat the olive oil in a small skillet over medium heat. Add the onion and a pinch of sea salt and sauté for 2 to 3 minutes. Add the carrot, celery, and corn with another pinch of salt and stir until just tender for 5 to 6 minutes. If the vegetables start to stick or become too brown before they are tender, add 1 to 2 tablespoons water.

Heat the tortillas in a dry skillet over high heat. Layer each tortilla in this order: rice, beans, sautéed veggies, sprouts, cucumber, Tofu Cream, and avocado.

It's always nice to have some sort of garnish, so sprinkle with radish and arugula as desired. If you like cilantro, you should definitely add a bunch. If not, try a little chopped parsley. Top it all off with sunflower seeds or gomashio.

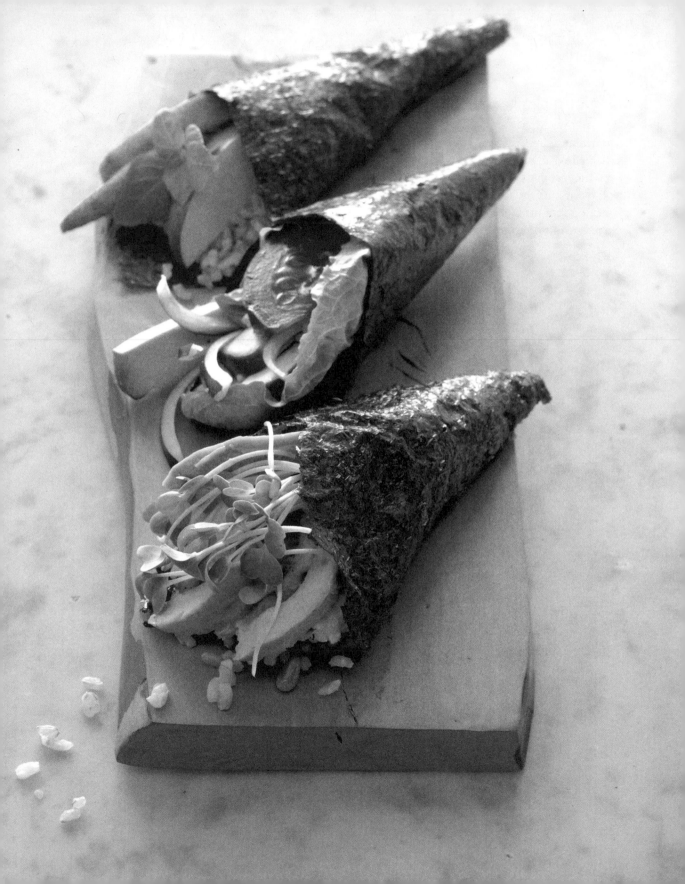

Toasted Nori Burritos

My friend Renée taught me to make these nori rolls when we were driving to a concert called "Reggae on the River" in Northern California. In the car, she had brought along romaine lettuce, basil, cilantro, avocado, apple, and hummus; and we wrapped them all up in the nori and ate them as we traveled. It was a delicious, refreshing, crunchy snack that kept us going for 2 days! Below is a variation on that nori burrito, but know that you can make one out of almost anything.

SERVES 2

1 umeboshi plum

1 cup cooked brown rice (leftover is great)

2 sheets toasted nori

2 romaine lettuce leaves

1 avocado, sliced

1 apple, sliced

4 fresh basil leaves

Leaves from 6 cilantro sprigs

Leftover cooked kale or salad greens

Tear the umeboshi plum into little pieces and discard the pit. Place half the rice on each sheet of nori and top with the remaining ingredients. Roll the nori into a cone shape around the filling; if it's rolled tightly, you can seal the edges by wetting your finger to dampen the edges of the nori.

Note: Serve a half sheet of nori at dinner to use as a wrapper for any leftovers or food that might need refreshing. Nori makes everything taste great!

Thin Mushroom "Pizzas"

Pretty, fancy, and totally delicious, these things are freaking amazing. Even you Flirts will love them.

SERVES 8

12 dried shiitake mushrooms

1 cup dried porcini mushrooms

1 tablespoon olive oil plus more for drizzling over the tortillas

1 onion, halved and cut in half-moon slices

3 garlic cloves

2 pinches of fine sea salt

2 cups fresh button mushrooms, sliced

A few drops of shoyu to taste

8 whole wheat tortillas (Ezekiel brand is my favorite for this)

1 cup Tofu Cream (page 225)

8 to 10 black olives, sliced

Chopped fresh basil for garnish

Preheat the broiler.

Soak the shiitake and porcini mushrooms in water to cover for 30 minutes in a small bowl. Remove the mushrooms from the water. Cut out and discard the tough shiitake stems.

Heat the oil in a skillet over medium heat. Add the onion, garlic, and a pinch of salt and cook for 2 to 3 minutes, or until the onion and garlic begin to soften. Add the shiitake and porcini mushrooms and cook for 5 to 7 minutes, or until the mushrooms are tender. Add the button mushrooms with a pinch of salt and the shoyu. Cook for 2 minutes and set aside.

Drizzle the tortillas lightly with olive oil and toast under the broiler until almost crisp, being careful not to burn. Spread a thin but generous layer of Tofu Cream on each tortilla and top with the cooked mushrooms and olives. Drizzle with a little more olive oil and broil again until the tortillas are just crisp. Garnish with chopped basil before serving.

Rice Waffle with Vegetable Mélange

Mina Dobic is an amazing woman who used a macrobiotic diet to combat her cancer. Her book, *My Beautiful Life*, is truly inspiring reading for anyone. Mina is responsible for guiding me to full Superhero status, and she inspired this recipe.

This dish reminds me of a Chinese mu shu dish—so yummy—and it's a complete meal, with grains, protein, and veggies all in one. If you don't have a waffle iron, you can cook the batter like pancakes in a skillet.

SERVES 2 TO 4

Waffles

2 cups cooked brown rice

1 cup whole wheat pastry flour

1 tablespoon mellow miso mixed with 3 tablespoons water

Vegetable Mélange

2 teaspoons dark sesame oil

1 cup half-moon onion slices

1 cup seitan, thinly sliced

1 cup carrots, sliced

1 teaspoon shoyu

2 cups broccoli florets

Sliced black olives (optional)

Stir together the rice, flour, miso, and 1 cup of water in a large mixing bowl. Heat a waffle iron, and coat lightly with oil. Pour in about ½ cup of batter, depending on the size of your waffle iron, and cook until browned. Transfer the cooked waffle to a plate to keep warm, and repeat with the remaining batter.

Heat the oil in a skillet over medium-high heat. Add the onion, and sauté for 2 minutes. Add the seitan to the skillet, and sauté for 1 minute longer. Arrange the carrots on top of the seitan and onions, and add 3 tablespoons of water to the pan. Cover the pan and simmer for 7 minutes, adding more water if the pan gets too dry. Add the shoyu and broccoli to the pan, and simmer 3 minutes longer. Stir to combine the ingredients and remove the pan from the heat.

Arrange a waffle on each serving plate, and top each waffle with a heap of sautéed veggies and seitan. Sprinkle with olives, if using, and serve warm.

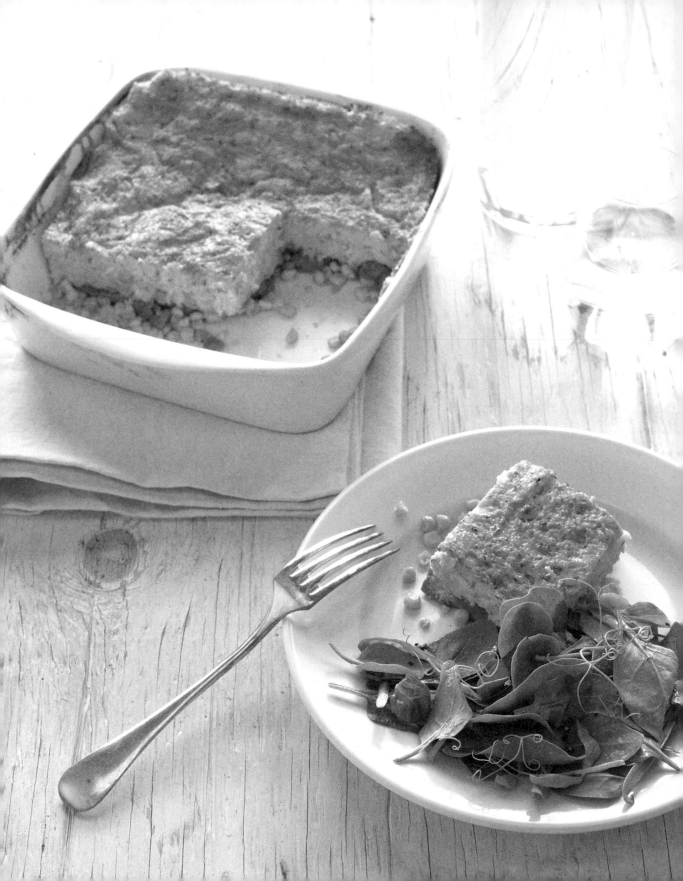

Polenta Casserole with Seitan

This dish is elegant, delicious, and satisfying—great for brunch. Because it incorporates a grain, vegetables, and seitan, it's a complete meal. A nice side of greens would make it absolutely perfect.

SERVES 6

1½ cups polenta or cornmeal or 1 cup millet

1 medium-size head cauliflower, cut in large pieces

1 cup peas, fresh or frozen and thawed

2 pinches fine sea salt

1 (8-ounce) package seitan, sliced

Kernels from 2 ears of corn or 1 cup thawed frozen kernels

6 asparagus spears, cut into 1" pieces

1½ teaspoons roasted sesame tahini

⅓ cup soy milk

1½ tablespoons shoyu plus more for sprinkling on top

2 teaspoons umeboshi vinegar

¼ cup chopped fresh parsley

Fresh basil leaves for garnish

Place the polenta or millet in a large heavy pot. Add the cauliflower, peas (if using fresh), salt, and 5 cups of water (add just 3 cups if using the millet). Bring to a boil, reduce the heat, cover, and simmer the polenta for 30 minutes (cook for 25 minutes if using the millet). Polenta must be stirred frequently as it cooks to prevent it from sticking or becoming lumpy, but you don't need to stir millet.

Preheat the oven to 350°F. Lightly oil an 8" × 8" casserole dish.

While the cauliflower mixture cooks, arrange the sliced seitan in the casserole dish. Layer the corn kernels on top, and then add the asparagus.

Remove the polenta mixture from the heat. Add the tahini, milk, shoyu, and umeboshi vinegar and mash with a potato masher or fork until the mixture resembles mashed potatoes. Add the chopped parsley and peas (if using frozen) and mix well. Spoon the mashed mixture into the casserole dish over the vegetables and smooth the top. Poke a few small holes in the surface, and sprinkle with a little extra shoyu (this makes the top crispy).

Bake for 30 to 40 minutes. Let the casserole cool for 15 minutes before cutting into squares. Garnish with the basil, and serve.

Quinoa with Basil and Pine Nuts

Quinoa is a funky, crazy little grain that's really high in protein, but I love its unique and wonderful flavor. You'll see when you make this dish; it's perfect for a light lunch served with some steamed greens or as the complement to a hearty bean dish. To give the quinoa a richer, nuttier flavor, pan-roast the rinsed quinoa until it's golden before boiling.

SERVES 2

1 cup quinoa

Pinch of fine sea salt

½ cup pine nuts or cashews

1 tablespoon olive oil

1 generous handful fresh basil leaves, chopped

Place the quinoa in a strainer and rinse well. Combine the quinoa with 2 cups of water and the salt in a saucepan and bring to a boil. Reduce the heat, cover, and simmer for 20 minutes.

While the quinoa cooks, heat the pine nuts in a small dry skillet over medium heat. Toast until the nuts are just starting to turn golden, about 6 to 7 minutes, shaking the pan frequently to prevent burning. Transfer to a serving bowl to cool.

Add the quinoa to the serving bowl with the pine nuts and fluff with a fork. Add the olive oil and basil, stir to combine, and serve.

Dolma with Tofu Cream

I love this dish because it's light yet satisfying. The cabbage leaves, yummy filling, and Tofu Cream complement each other *perfectly*.

SERVES 6

2 cups brown rice

1 small head green cabbage for wraps or 1 jar grape leaves, drained

1 cup diced seitan

1½ cups diced onions

½ cup diced carrots

1 cup finely chopped fresh parsley

2 garlic cloves

¼ cup olive oil

1 tablespoon umeboshi plum paste

3 tablespoons dark miso

¾ teaspoon shiso powder

½ cup fresh lemon juice

¾ cup Tofu Cream (opposite)

Combine the rice and 3½ cups water in a saucepan. Bring to a boil, reduce the heat to low, cover, and cook for 45 to 55 minutes, or until the rice is tender. Set aside to cool.

Bring a large saucepan of water to boil over high heat. Separate 12 or so leaves from the cabbage head and add to the boiling water. Cook until soft, about 2 minutes. Drain in a colander.

In a mixing bowl, combine the cooked rice, seitan, onions, carrots, parsley, garlic, oil, and umeboshi plum paste. Dissolve the miso and shiso powder in a small amount of water and add to the vegetable mixture, mixing well.

Take a green cabbage leaf, fill it with approximately ½ cup of the filling, and roll up burrito-fashion to enclose. Repeat with the remaining cabbage leaves and filling, making about 12 rolls in all. Arrange the cabbage rolls in layers in a medium-size pot. Pour the lemon juice and ½ cup of water over the rolls, cover, and bring to a boil over high heat. Reduce the flame to low, and simmer (over a flame deflector if you have one) for 30 minutes. If all the liquid hasn't evaporated, keep the pot over low heat, covered, until all of the water is gone. Serve the cabbage rolls hot or at room temperature with a dollop of tofu cream on top.

Tofu Cream

SERVES 8

1 (14-ounce) package firm tofu	3½–4 tablespoons Vegenaise
1½ tablespoons umeboshi plum paste	6 tablespoons fresh lemon juice

Rinse the tofu and place on a plate with a second plate on top. Place a heavy weight (like a kettle full of water) on top of the plate. Set aside for 10 minutes to press out the excess liquid.

Transfer the pressed tofu to the basket of a steamer set over a pot of boiling water. Cover the pot, and steam the tofu for 3 to 5 minutes. Let cool.

Place the steamed tofu, umeboshi plum paste, Vegenaise, and lemon juice in a food processor and puree until smooth, pulsing the processor on and off and using a spatula to scrape down the sides often. Transfer to a tightly sealed container, and chill for an hour before serving. The Tofu Cream will keep for 2 or 3 days in the refrigerator.

Kim's Red Radish Tabbouleh

Kimberly Stakal is a cool vegan chef who lives in Chicago. While helping me test some of these recipes, she came up with this tabbouleh dish. It's fresh, light, and a great way to eat bulgur wheat. Rock on, Kimberly!

SERVES 2

¼ teaspoon fine sea salt

1 cup bulgur wheat

3 tablespoons fresh lemon juice

2 tablespoons olive oil

½ cup finely chopped fresh parsley

2 scallions, white and green parts minced

½ cup thinly sliced radishes

Bring 1½ cups of water and the salt to a boil in a saucepan. Place the bulgur and boiling salted water in a heatproof bowl. Stir once, then cover the bowl with a plate and set aside until the grain has absorbed all the water, about 20 to 30 minutes.

Stir in the lemon juice, oil, parsley, scallions, and radishes and mix well. Add more lemon juice and salt to taste.

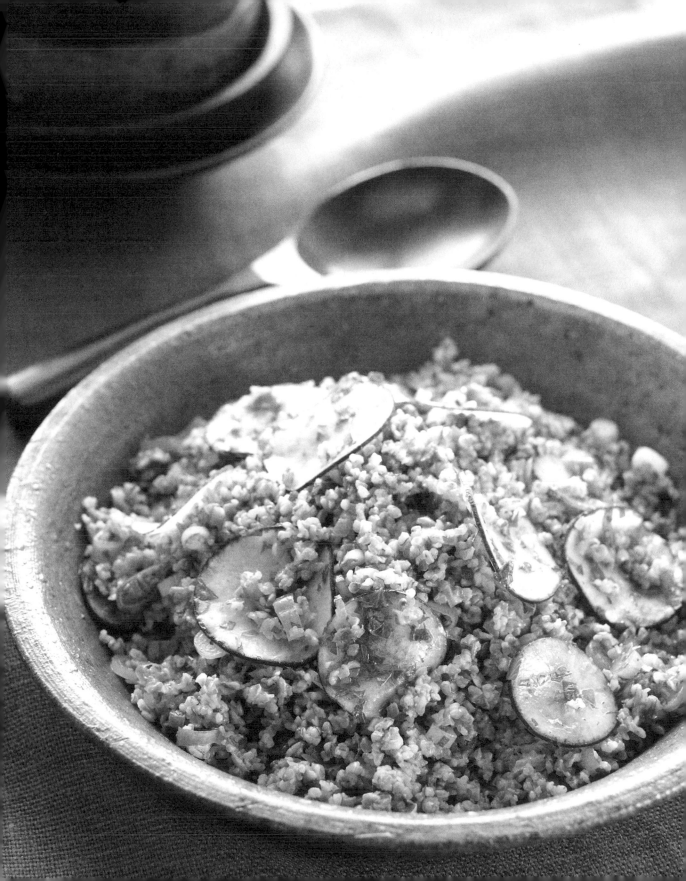

Risotto with Oyster Mushrooms, Leeks, and Peas

I found a version of this dish at every French restaurant I visited while shooting a film in Lithuania. When I got back home, I re-created my own healthier version that's now one of my favorite things to serve for a light lunch. White rice is less Superhero than brown rice, so if you want to eat this kind of dish more than once or twice a week, substitute brown rice for the Arborio.

SERVES 4 OR 5

3 tablespoons olive oil

¾–1 cup oyster mushrooms or 1 cup button mushrooms, sliced

2 pinches of fine sea salt

½ cup thinly sliced leeks

½ cup fresh or thawed frozen peas

1–2 garlic cloves, minced

¾–1 cup onion, chopped

1 cup Arborio rice

½ cup mirin or white wine

Bring 5 cups of water just to a boil in a saucepan. Remove from the heat and cover to keep warm.

Meanwhile, heat 1 tablespoon of the oil in a skillet. Add the mushrooms and a pinch of salt and stir until the mushrooms soften (this will happen quickly for oyster mushrooms, longer for other varieties). Add the leeks and a pinch of salt and sauté for 1 minute, or until the leeks soften. Add some water to the pan, 1 tablespoon at a time, if the vegetables become dry or start to stick to the pan.

If you are using fresh peas, blanch them for 1 minute in a small pot of boiling water, and then add them to the sautéed vegetables. If using thawed frozen peas, just mix them straight into the sautéed vegetables. Remove from the heat and set aside.

Heat the remaining 2 tablespoons oil in a medium skillet over medium heat. Add the garlic and onion and, when the onion begins to sizzle, add a dash of salt. Sauté until the onions soften, about 1 to 2 minutes. Stir in the rice and toast the grains until they are opaque, about 2 to 3 minutes. Stir in the wine and cook until it has evaporated. Reduce the heat to medium-low and begin adding the warm water by ladlefuls, stirring it into the risotto, and adding more liquid only when the previous addition has been absorbed. After the rice has cooked for 20 minutes, season to taste with salt. The total cooking time should be 25 to 30 minutes. The risotto will be creamy, but the rice should retain some firmness.

Add the sautéed vegetable mixture to the risotto and stir together until hot. Serve warm.

Fried Udon Noodles

Udon noodles generally turn up in a big bowl of broth, but I like the texture of these soft noodles when they've been fried briefly. You can mix them up with anything else you want: broccoli, 'shrooms, tofu . . . whatever makes you salivate. Get creative and clean out your fridge!

SERVES 2

1 (8-ounce) package udon noodles

2 tablespoons olive oil

2 cups sliced green cabbage

1 cup half-moon onion slices

2 teaspoons finely chopped garlic

¾ teaspoon fine sea salt

¾ teaspoon freshly ground black pepper

1½ tablespoons sweet paprika

Chopped fresh parsley for garnish

Bring a large pot of water to a boil. Add the udon noodles and cook just until al dente; drain and keep warm.

Meanwhile, heat 1 tablespoon oil in a large skillet over medium heat. Add the cabbage and cook, stirring occasionally, until very tender, about 15 minutes. Add a tablespoon or so of water to the pan if the cabbage begins to stick or burn.

Heat the remaining 1 tablespoon oil over medium-high heat in a separate pan. Add the onions, garlic, salt, pepper, and paprika and cook until the onions are translucent, again adding a touch of water if the onions start to stick. Add the onions to the skillet with the cabbage and stir to combine. Add the drained noodles and toss together until heated through. Sprinkle with parsley and serve hot.

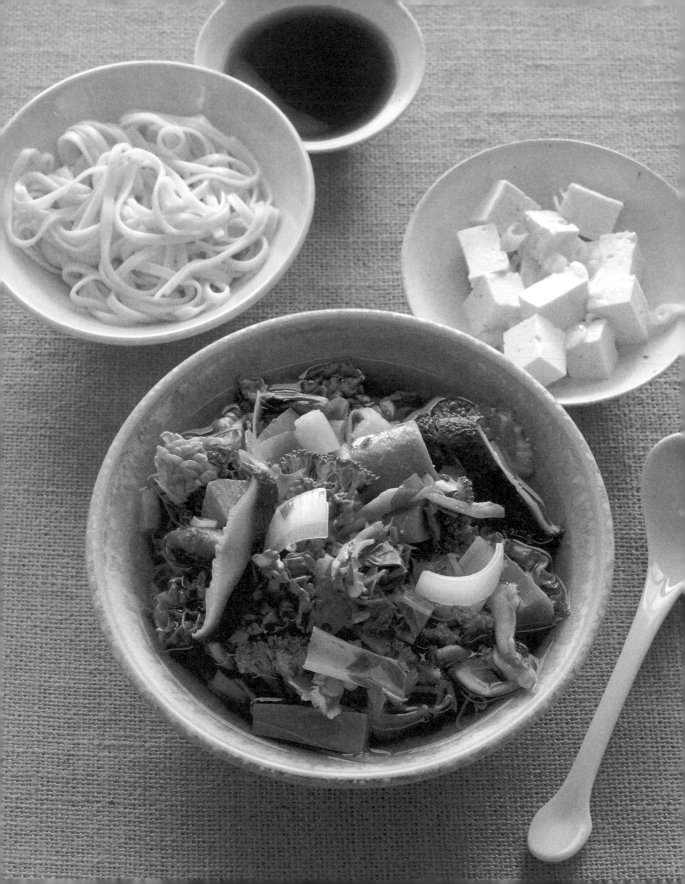

Nabeyaki Udon

This is a traditional Japanese dish that is generally cooked in an earthenware or iron pot. This dish is so full of noodles and vegetables that it's pretty much a complete meal as is, but if you want more protein, add some tofu cubes to the simmering broth or serve a protein on the side. Either way, this dish is light, fresh, and satisfying. The shiitake mushroom soaking water gives the broth a deep flavor.

SERVES 2

1 dried shiitake mushroom

1 tablespoon maitake mushrooms

Sauce

2–4 teaspoons shoyu

3–4 tablespoons water or soaking water from shiitake mushroom

5–8 drops ginger juice (grate a 1" piece of ginger and squeeze out the juice with your fingers)

½ teaspoon fresh lemon juice or rice vinegar

1 carrot, cut into bite-size pieces

1 stalk broccoli, cut into bite-size pieces

1 leek, white and green parts, cleaned and cut into large bite-size pieces

2 bok choy leaves, cut into bite-size pieces, or 1 baby bok choy

1 handful bean sprouts

2–3 napa cabbage leaves or collards, roughly chopped

4–6 dandelion greens, roughly chopped

1 (8-ounce) package udon noodles

1" piece kombu

Place the shiitake and maitake mushrooms in a small bowl with water to cover. Soak for 30 minutes or until softened. Bring a large pot of water to a boil for the noodles. Stir together the sauce ingredients in a small bowl and set aside.

Arrange all the vegetables on a plate near your stove. Remove the mushrooms from their soaking liquid, reserving the liquid. Slice and add to the plate with the vegetables.

Cook the noodles in the boiling water until just al dente; drain and set aside.

In a nabe or ceramic pot that is safe for use on the stovetop (if you don't have one, you can use a regular pot), bring 2 to 3 cups water and the mushroom soaking liquid to a boil. Add the kombu and mushrooms and lower the heat so the water is simmering. Begin adding the vegetables one at a time, starting with the carrots and other vegetables that take longer to cook. Most of the vegetables shouldn't take longer than 2 minutes to cook. You want them fresh and light, not mushy or overcooked.

Bring the nabe pot to the table. Give each person 3 bowls: 1 for their noodles, 1 for their nabe vegetables, and 1 small bowl for their dipping sauce. Everyone takes from the big nabe pot, dipping their vegetables and noodles in the dipping sauce as desired. The whole meal is pretty and fun and healing.

Make sure to drink the vegetable broth at the end. It has a very subtle flavor and all the goodness of the vegetables that cooked in it.

Variations:

You can lay fried mochi on top of the vegetables and garnish with toasted nori pieces and scallions! If you feel particularly ambitious, serve topped with a few pieces of Vegetable Tempura (page 274).

Gomashio

I guarantee you will love gomashio; it's a delicious condiment that tastes amazing on top of any grain or vegetable dish. It's also incredibly good for you. Since it's made from calcium-rich sesame seeds and magnesium-rich sea salt, it's great for the bones and is good for the overall nervous system. Gomashio aids in digestion and adds extra vitamins and minerals to your meal. Black sesame seeds are higher in minerals than tan sesame seeds, but I love them both so I switch off from batch to batch. Just keep the ratio 1 part salt to 18 parts seeds.

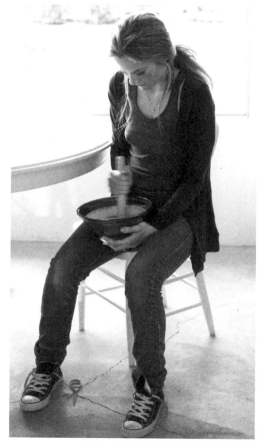

You will need a suribachi—a grooved Japanese mortar and pestle—to make gomashio. They're really cheap and useful for lots of things, so definitely get one! Unfortunately, an electric coffee grinder won't grind the salt and seeds together as well.

Gomashio will last about 2 weeks in an airtight container. Limit your consumption to about 1 to 3 teaspoons of gomashio a day, or you'll get too much salt in your diet.

Heat 1 teaspoon of fine sea salt in a small dry skillet over medium heat. Heat until the salt is really dry, stirring often, about 2 or 3 minutes. Be careful not to let it burn. Pour the roasted salt into a suribachi, and grind to a fine powder. Rinse 6 tablespoons of sesame seeds in a fine mesh strainer. Place the seeds in the same dry skillet, and toast over medium heat until the seeds have a nutty aroma, puff up a little, and crush easily between your fingers.

Add the sesame seeds to the suribachi with the sea salt, and grind until the seeds are 80 percent crushed. Transfer the gomashio to a glass jar with a tight lid, and store in the refrigerator for up to 2 weeks.

Basic Rice

Sometimes a simple bowl of plain rice is just the perfect thing, especially if I've been eating lots of complicated, fun food. When it's fresh out of the pot, I like hot rice sprinkled with Gomashio, sunflower seeds toasted with shoyu (page 215), or fresh chopped cilantro, parsley, or chives for a bright color and flavor. Come to think of it, all that stuff is great on leftover rice, too! With some veggies on the side, I'm all set.

SERVES 2

1 cup short- or medium-grain brown rice, soaked in water overnight if possible

Pinch of fine sea salt

Wash the rice by placing it in a pot. Cover with water and swish it around with your hands. Pour off the water, replace with fresh water, and allow the rice to soak for 1 hour or up to overnight. Drain the rice through a strainer. (Sometimes I skip these steps.) Return the rice to the pot and add 2 cups of water and the salt. Bring to a boil over high heat, then cover. Place the pot on a flame deflector if you have one, and turn the heat down as low as it will go.

Simmer the rice for 50 minutes, then turn off the heat and let the rice sit for a few minutes longer with the lid still on. Serve warm.

Fried Rice

Fried rice is one of those endlessly adaptable recipes that will come out slightly different each time, depending on the type of vegetables and rice you use. It works well with long-grain or medium-grain brown rice—you can even use sweet brown rice, which makes it nice and sticky. Here is a combination I like using short-grain brown rice. It's quick, easy, tastes great, and is great for you.

SERVES 1 OR 2

1–2 tablespoons dark sesame oil

1 teaspoon finely chopped garlic

2 pinches of fine sea salt

¼ cup thinly sliced lotus root rounds

¼ cup thinly sliced daikon rounds

¼ cup thinly sliced carrot

1 cup cooked short-grain brown rice

Shoyu to taste

Brown rice vinegar to taste

½ cup chopped bok choy or small broccoli florets

¼ cup finely chopped scallions, white and green parts

Heat the oil in a wok or large skillet over medium-high heat. Add the garlic and a pinch of salt and cook, stirring constantly, for 10 seconds. Add the lotus and daikon and another pinch of salt and stir-fry for 2 minutes. Add the carrots and cook for 2 minutes longer. If the vegetables begin to stick, add a little water, a tablespoon at a time, to the wok.

Add the rice to the wok and sprinkle with 3 tablespoons of water. Season the rice with shoyu and vinegar, add the bok choy, and stir-fry for 2 to 4 minutes, or until the rice is hot and all the liquid has been absorbed. Stir in the scallions just before serving. Serve hot.

Rice Pilaf with Caramelized Onions

This recipe by Christina Pirello comes from her book *Christina Cooks*. There are so many delicious flavors and textures in this dish that it becomes much more than the sum of its parts. It's good enough to serve at a dinner party.

SERVES 4 TO 6

2 tablespoons plus 2 teaspoons extra-virgin olive oil

½ red onion, cut into thin half-moon slices

3 pinches of fine sea salt

Mirin or white wine

4–5 slices fresh ginger, cut into fine matchstick pieces

1 small carrot, finely diced

1 small parsnip, finely diced

½ cup pecans, lightly oven-roasted and coarsely chopped

3 tablespoons pumpkin seeds, lightly pan-toasted

2 cups cooked short-grain brown rice

Brown rice vinegar

2–3 scallions, white and green parts thinly sliced on the diagonal, for garnish

Place 2 tablespoons oil and the onion in a medium skillet over medium heat. When the onion begins to sizzle, add a generous pinch of salt and sauté for 3 to 4 minutes. Add a generous sprinkle of mirin and reduce the heat to low. Cook, stirring frequently, for about 15 minutes, or until the onion begins to caramelize (this may take as long as 20 minutes).

While the onion cooks, place the remaining 2 teaspoons oil, the ginger, carrot, parsnip, and a generous pinch of salt in a large skillet over medium heat. When the vegetables begin to sizzle, add a pinch of salt and sauté until just tender, about 10 minutes. Turn off the heat and stir in the pecans and pumpkin seeds just to coat with oil. Add the rice and a generous splash of vinegar and stir to combine. Transfer to a serving bowl and top with the caramelized onions. Sprinkle with the scallions and serve.

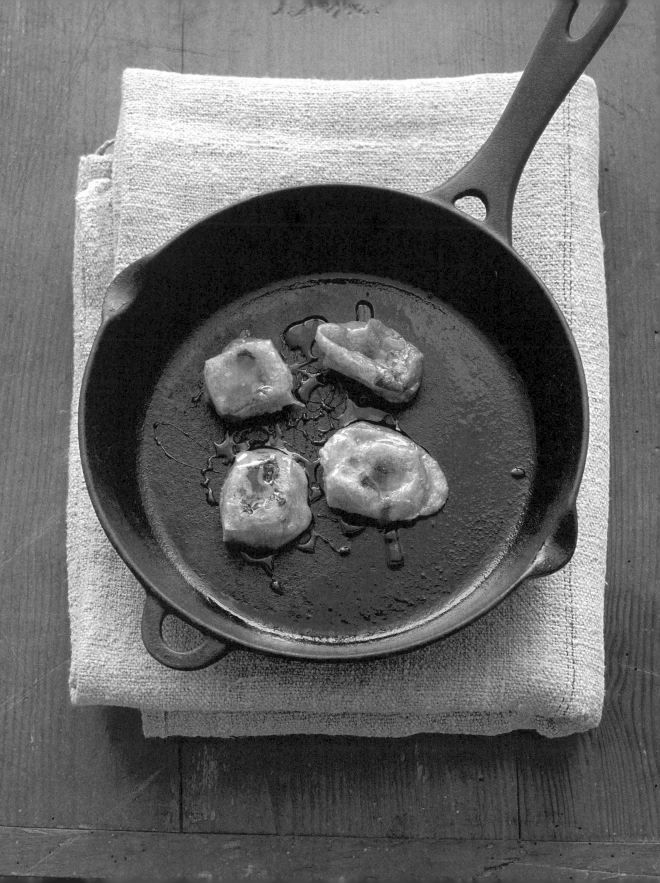

Pan-Fried Mochi

Mochi is made from sweet rice, and it's sticky and gooey and freakin' delicious. Often served at breakfast (see Mochi Waffles, page 286), mochi can also be the grain component of any meal. My two favorite ways of using mochi are as croutons (see Note) for garnishing soups or as a snack on its own. Either way, to me it tastes best pan-fried with either sweet or savory flavorings. You could also make this with flavored mochi if you like; mugwort is one I use sometimes.

SERVES 2

Sweet Version

1–2 teaspoons sesame or olive oil

2 to 4 pieces unflavored mochi, each 1" x 2"

Shoyu

Brown rice syrup (about 1 tablespoon per serving)

Heat the oil in a cast-iron or stainless steel frying pan over medium heat. Place the mochi pieces into the pan, making sure they don't touch. Cover, reduce the heat to low (or place the pan on a flame deflector if you have one), and cook for exactly 4 minutes. Flip the mochi, add about 2 drops of shoyu to each piece, cover, and let cook for another 4 minutes. The mochi should begin to get gooey, puff up a little, and morph into funny shapes.

Transfer the mochi to serving plates and drizzle with rice syrup. Yum.

Savory Version

2 to 4 pieces unflavored mochi, each 1" x 2"

¼ sheet nori per serving

Grated daikon (about 1 tablespoon per serving)

Follow the same cooking instructions as above, but skip the brown rice syrup. Instead, place the cooked mochi onto a little sheet of nori, top with grated daikon, and wrap up to make a mochi burrito.

Note: To make croutons for soup, cut the mochi into smaller pieces and cook as above without any of the additional flavorings or ingredients.

Ginger Pasta with Zucchini

While shooting Kenneth Branagh's *Love's Labour's Lost*, I stayed in a hotel in London; in the room below me was another actress in the movie, Stefania Rocca. A beautiful and spunky Italian, she always had a huge group of friends visiting her, cooking pasta, drinking wine, and having a good time. Over the weeks that we worked and lived as neighbors, Stefania taught me a lot about cooking—she was into health food and really knew her pasta. This dish was born of that education, and it reminds me of that time. It's simple, earthy, and nourishing. Grazie, bella!

Superheroes shouldn't eat pasta every day, but 2 or 3 times a week is just fine.

SERVES 2

8 ounces whole wheat penne

2 pinches of fine sea salt

¼ block firm tofu, cut into bite-size cubes

1 tablespoon olive oil

½ onion, chopped

½ zucchini, halved lengthwise and thinly sliced

Shoyu to taste

1–2 teaspoons ginger juice (grate a 2" piece of ginger and squeeze out the juice with your fingers)

Bring a large pot of water with a generous pinch of salt to a boil. Cook the pasta according to package directions until al dente; drain and set aside.

Mash the tofu with a fork in a small bowl and set aside.

Heat the oil in a skillet. Add the onion and a pinch of sea salt and sauté until the onion is translucent, about 3 to 4 minutes. Add 1 or 2 tablespoons of water to the pan if the onions begin to stick. Add the zucchini and sauté for 2 to 3 minutes, or until it softens, then add the mashed tofu and shoyu to the skillet. Sauté 2 minutes longer, then stir in the ginger juice and cooked pasta. Toss all the ingredients together over medium heat until the pasta is heated through and all the liquid has been absorbed.

Variation:

Use steamed kabocha squash, stir-fried red onion, corn, mushrooms, and umeboshi plum paste in place of the tofu, onion, zucchini, and ginger. It's great when the squash becomes soft enough to coat the pasta!

PROTEIN DISHES

I try to eat a good variety of beans, and my regulars are azukis, chickpeas, lentils, black soybeans, kidney, and pinto. Variety is important because each bean contains different nutrients that the body needs. I also eat tempeh or tofu, but only a couple times a week each.

Although I've included some fancy bean dishes in this book, beans cooked simply are really good sometimes—like kidney beans with a little shoyu and parsley or maybe with some sautéed leeks mixed in. Mmm . . .

Basic Bean Cooking

Rinse and sort through beans, discarding any debris. Soak the beans in water to cover generously for 6 to 8 hours (overnight is easiest).

To cook, strain and rinse the soaked beans.

Place the beans in a pot with fresh water to cover generously. Add a 1" square kombu per cup of beans.

Bring to a boil over medium-high heat, then lower the heat to a simmer and cook for 3 to 5 minutes. This will allow gases to release from the beans. If any foam is produced, skim it off with a spoon.

Cover the pot and cook the beans over low heat (or over a flame deflector if you have one) until tender, usually about 45 minutes to 1 hour.

Season with shoyu (½ to 1 teaspoon per cup of beans) and let simmer at least 5 more minutes.

Cooking times will vary depending on the recipe and what type of bean you are using. You may need to add more water to the cooking beans if the water level in the pot gets low.

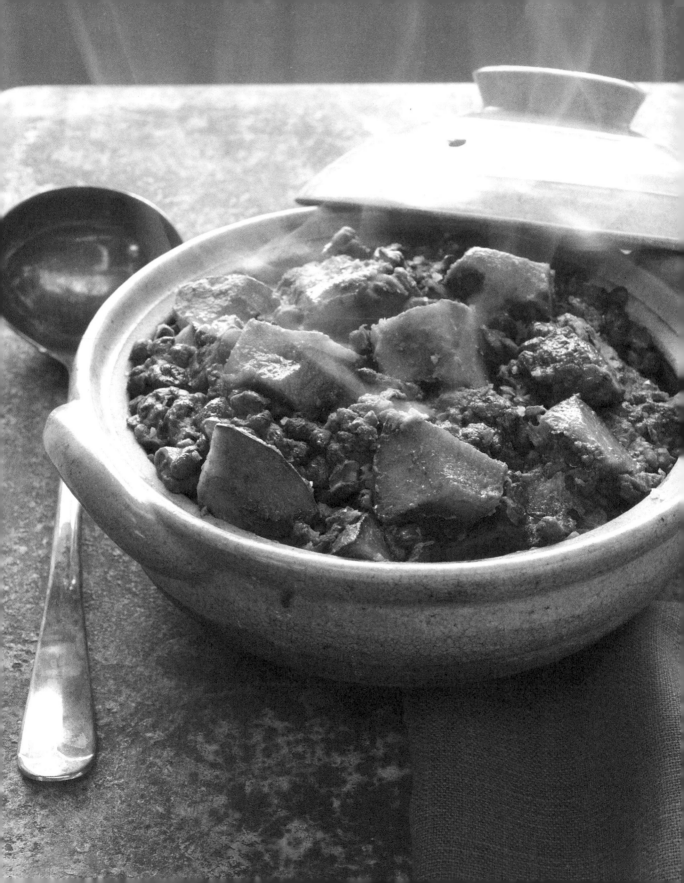

Azuki Beans with Kabocha Squash

This is a very traditional macrobiotic recipe, which may sound a little ho-hum, but it's actually incredibly good. Originally cultivated in Japan and revered for their healing properties, azuki beans are said to strengthen the kidneys' functions. This dish is high in potassium and iron, so serve it at least once a week if you can and you will feel its power. If you prefer the squash with a softer, stewier texture, add it to the beans 10 or 15 minutes earlier.

SERVES 4

4"–6" piece of kombu

1 cup dried azuki beans

2 cups kabocha squash cut into large chunks (peel only if the squash is not organic)

1 teaspoon shoyu

Chopped fresh cilantro or parsley for garnish

Combine the kombu and the beans in a bowl and cover with water by an inch or two. Soak overnight. The next day, drain the kombu and beans and discard the soaking water. Slice the kombu into 1" × 1" squares and place them in a heavy pot with a heavy lid, preferably enameled cast iron. Add the beans and enough fresh water to just cover the beans. Bring to a boil.

As the beans boil, strain off any foam that rises to the top. Let the beans boil, uncovered, for about 5 minutes, as this allows gases to release. Cover the pot, reduce the heat to low (and place on a flame deflector, if you have one), and simmer for about 40 minutes. Check the beans every 10 minutes or so, adding water to the pot when the water level appears to dip below the bean level. After 40 minutes, arrange the squash on top of the beans and add more water to keep the beans covered. Cook for another 20 minutes, or until the beans seem soft and tender. Add the shoyu to the beans, and cook 10 more minutes. Serve garnished with the cilantro or parsley.

Variations:

You can use any kind of winter squash (buttercup, butternut, Hokkaido pumpkin, delicata, and so on) or even carrots in place of the kabocha squash in this dish.

You can also make a soup from azuki beans and sweet vegetables. Follow the same directions, but use more water and a variety of sweet vegetables (such as onions, carrots, squash, and corn). Season with shoyu, and garnish with scallions. This is also deeply nourishing and revitalizing.

Black-Eyed Pea Croquettes with Dijon Glaze

Jessica Porter wrote *The Hip Chick's Guide to Macrobiotics*, which contains this recipe by her friend Lisa Silverman. Now I don't know Lisa, but I love her because anyone who can come up with this recipe, all on her own, is a *genius*! These croquettes are ridiculously easy and will please the whole family. The outsides of the croquettes get crispy in the hot oil, but the insides stay moist so they're crunchy and satisfying—perfect for Flirts and people who think they don't like beans! Although barley malt is best for the glaze, if you can't get your hands on it, use rice syrup.

MAKES 12 MEDIUM-SIZE CROQUETTES, SERVES 4

2 cups black-eyed peas, soaked overnight in water to cover

2 tablespoons chopped fresh parsley or cilantro

½ teaspoon fine sea salt

1 tablespoon shoyu

1 teaspoon ground cumin

2 cups safflower oil for frying

Dipping Sauce

½ cup barley malt syrup or rice syrup

1 tablespoon Dijon mustard

Drain the soaked beans and transfer to a food processor. Add the parsley or cilantro, salt, shoyu, and cumin. Blend until the beans are chopped to fine shreds, but don't blend them to a pulp. The mixture will be slightly wet but should hold together. Form the bean mixture into something between football- and UFO-shaped croquettes in the palms of your hands.

Heat 1" of oil in a cast-iron skillet to about 350°F. To test the oil, drop in a tiny amount of croquette mixture. If it bubbles furiously and rises to the top, the oil is ready. Do not let the oil get so hot that it smokes. You may need to make little adjustments to the heat under the oil throughout the cooking process to avoid burning the croquettes.

Place 4 croquettes in the oil and fry for about 4 minutes on each side. Use a slotted spoon to transfer the fried croquettes to a plate lined with paper towels or a paper grocery bag to drain.

To make the dipping sauce, stir together the barley malt syrup and mustard in a small saucepan. Warm the sauce over low heat until it bubbles.

Serve the croquettes while still hot. Drizzle with the dipping sauce or serve it alongside the croquettes in individual dipping bowls.

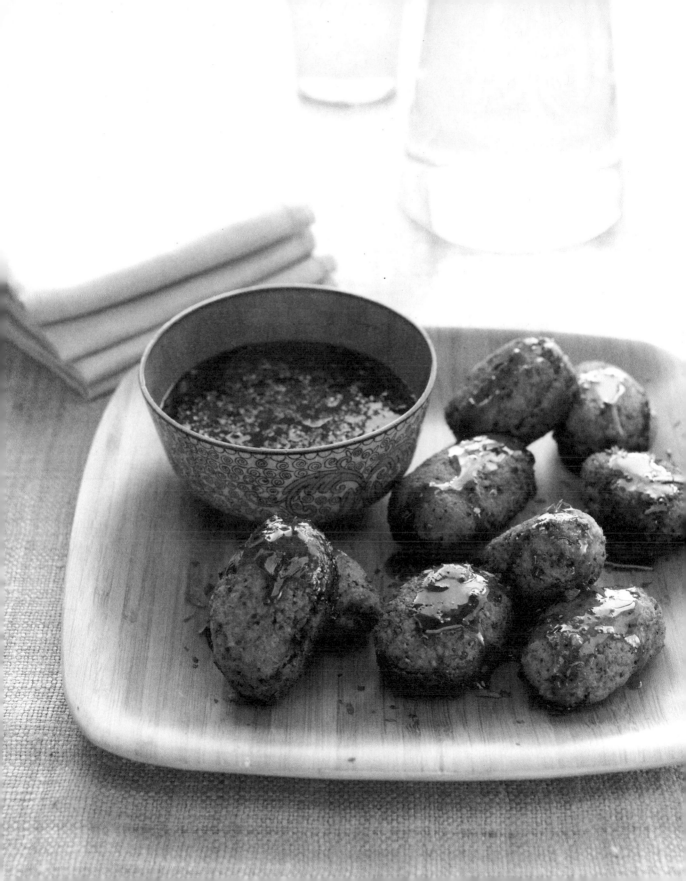

Hijiki-Tofu Croquettes

I know these may sound weird, but trust me, they are really delicious. I love the cookbook *Christina Cooks,* and this recipe is an adaptation from it. I can't think of a better way to serve seaweed to skeptics. And they're not just for Superheroes—they work equally well as party fare or snack food for everyone.

SERVES 5

Croquettes

½ (14-ounce) block extra-firm tofu, crumbled

¼ cup dried hijiki, rinsed well and soaked in water to cover until softened

Soy sauce

Mirin

1 carrot, diced

¼ cup diced burdock

¼ cup shelled hemp seeds

Pinch of fine sea salt

¼ cup whole wheat pastry flour, if needed

Safflower oil for frying

Sauce

1 tablespoon ginger juice (grate a 2" piece of ginger and squeeze out the juice with your fingers)

Generous pinch of red-pepper flakes

3 tablespoons soy sauce

1 teaspoon mirin

1 teaspoon fresh lemon juice

5 romaine lettuce leaves

1 cucumber, cut into very thin diagonal slices (peel only if the cucumber is not organic)

To make the croquettes, place the tofu in a mixing bowl and mash with a fork to create a coarse paste.

Drain the soaked hijiki and chop into small pieces. Place the hijiki in a small saucepan with enough water to just cover. Season lightly with soy sauce and mirin, cover, and bring to a boil over medium heat. Add the carrot and burdock to the pan, reduce the heat to low, and cook until all the liquid has been absorbed, about 30 to 35 minutes. Add the hemp seeds and a pinch of salt and stir together to create a stiff dough, adding the pastry flour if needed. Using your hands, shape the dough into football-shaped croquettes about 1" in diameter.

Heat 2 to 3 inches of the oil in a deep pot over medium heat. When the oil is hot, increase the heat to high, and gently drop 3 or 4 croquettes into the oil. Cook until golden and crisp on the outside, about 3 minutes. Use a slotted spoon to transfer the fried croquettes to a plate lined with parchment paper or paper grocery bag (which hopefully you don't have because you only use canvas bags!) to drain. Cook the remaining croquettes in batches.

To make the sauce, whisk all the ingredients together in a small bowl. Adjust the seasonings to your taste.

To serve, arrange the lettuce leaves on individual salad plates. Distribute the cucumber slices evenly among the plates. Divide the croquettes among the plates, and drizzle with the sauce.

Fruity French Lentils

This is a great summer dish and perfect for lunch, but it's also very versatile; you can use apricots, figs, persimmons, or other fruits in place of the raspberries. Made with fall fruits like pears or dried cranberries, this would be a lovely part of a holiday meal. It's light with a surprising combination of ingredients that complement each other beautifully.

SERVES 2

1 cup green lentils

Pinch of fine sea salt

½ cup fresh raspberries or fruit of your choice

⅛ cup chopped fresh basil

⅛ cup chopped fresh parsley

½ cup chopped walnuts

½ cup fresh orange juice

1 teaspoon strawberry jam

Sort through and rinse the lentils; drain and place them in a saucepan with 2 cups of water. Bring to a boil, add a pinch of salt, and simmer until tender, about 30 minutes. Drain any remaining cooking liquid and rinse under cold water to cool.

Combine the fruit, basil, parsley, and walnuts in a mixing bowl. Stir the lentils into the fruit mixture, and mix again.

Stir together the orange juice and jam in a small bowl. Pour over the lentil mixture, and mix well. Chill for 30 minutes before serving.

Tuna Salad Sandwich (Kinda)

By "kinda" I mean this sandwich doesn't *exactly* replicate tuna, but then it's not *trying* to . . . it's an independent sandwich with a life of its own! The tempeh offers a richness and deliciousness that is unique. The salad mixture is great on a piece of toast, in a sandwich, or as part of a composed salad plate, and I encourage all Flirts or Vegans to try it.

SERVES 4

1 (8-ounce) package tempeh

1 red onion, minced

¼ cup umeboshi vinegar

1 celery stalk, chopped

½ carrot, chopped ·

½ cup fresh or frozen and thawed corn kernels

⅓ cup fresh or frozen and thawed peas

½ small cucumber, chopped (peel only if the cucumber is not organic)

¼ cup chopped kosher dill pickles

1 tablespoon Vegenaise

½ tablespoon Dijon or stone-ground mustard

1 tablespoon fresh lemon juice

2 tablespoons chopped fresh dill or to taste

1 tablespoon drained capers

2 tablespoons chopped fresh parsley

Bring water to a boil in a pot fitted with a steamer basket. Cut the tempeh in half, and place in the steamer basket. Steam for 20 minutes. Set aside to cool.

Bring a small saucepan of water to a boil. Add the onion, and boil for 10 to 15 seconds. If you dig raw onion, you can skip this step. Use a strainer or slotted spoon to transfer the onion to a mixing bowl. Keep the water boiling in the pot on the stove.

Add the vinegar to the onions, stir well, and set aside to marinate for 30 minutes.

While the onion marinates, blanch the celery, carrots, corn, and peas in the reserved boiling water for 10 seconds each, scooping them into a mixing bowl as each vegetable is done. Set aside to cool.

Drain the marinated onions through a sieve, and rinse quickly under running water. Squeeze the excess liquid from the onions, and add to the bowl with the vegetables. Cut the cooled tempeh into small cubes, and add to the bowl along with the cucumber, pickles, Vegenaise, mustard, lemon juice, and dill, if using. Stir well to combine. Serve topped with capers and parsley.

Tofu Salad

Try this salad as an open-faced sandwich on toast or enjoy it just straight from the bowl. Tofu is really cooling, so this dish is wonderful in the summer, but feel free to make it all year round.

SERVES 1 OR 2

¼ cup fresh or frozen and thawed peas

⅓ (14-ounce) package firm tofu

¼ cup finely chopped celery

3 olives, chopped

1 tablespoon rinsed capers

2–3 slices kosher dill pickles, chopped

2 tablespoons finely chopped scallion or chives

1 tablespoon finely chopped parsley

1 tablespoon Vegenaise

1 tablespoon umeboshi vinegar or 2 teaspoons umeboshi plum paste

1 tablespoon fresh lemon juice

Whole wheat pitas (optional)

Green leaf lettuce leaves

1 red radish, thinly sliced

Bring a saucepan of water to a boil. Add the peas, and blanch for 3 minutes or until the peas are bright green. Drain and set aside.

Wrap the tofu in cheesecloth or a clean dish towel and place on a plate. Place a second plate on top of the tofu, and place a weight on top of it for 10 minutes to press out the liquid. Bring water to a boil in a steamer or a pot fitted with a steamer basket. Unwrap the tofu and place it in the steamer basket. Cover the pot and steam the tofu over boiling water for 5 minutes. Carefully remove the tofu and transfer to a bowl. Mash with a fork to make it crumbly. Add the peas, celery, olives, capers, pickles, scallion or chives, parsley, Vegenaise, vinegar, and lemon juice. Taste the mixture. If it is too bland, add more umeboshi vinegar, a little at a time, to taste.

Spoon the tofu salad into warmed pitas with the lettuce leaves and sliced radishes, or serve on the lettuce leaves and garnish with the radishes.

SOUPS AND SALADS

Soup is an important part of the Superhero diet, so I try to have it at least once a day, and often more. Luckily, making soup (especially miso) is easy and even relaxing. Here are a few tips for making great soup:

- Use what you have: I love to clean out my fridge as I cook and put everything to good use. I find the things that need eating, the things that need donating to the dogs, and the things that have lost that loving feeling as they start to become compost all by themselves. More often than not, the things that still have some vitality end up in my soups (often in some version of my Magical Healing Soup, page 251).

- Top it off well: Croutons are a great addition to soups. Make one of the garlic bread recipes on page 147, and then cut the bread into cubes to make croutons! Or you can skip the garlic and go for plain. Mochi also makes great croutons. Cut the mochi into little cubes, and fry (with or without oil) or bake in the oven until they puff up.

- For miso soup: All miso soups have about 1" to 1½" of wakame seaweed per cup of liquid. I generally just cut mine dry with scissors over the soup. And all miso soups should contain no more than 1 teaspoon of miso paste per cup of liquid.

- One super important note: Never boil miso! Boiling kills its powerful enzymes, so add the miso at the end of the cooking time and simmer for just 2 to 3 minutes.

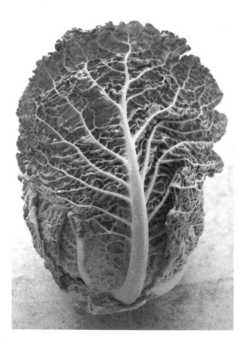

Dandelion, Bok Choy Miso Soup

It's hard to believe that you can throw together a soup this healing and nourishing in just about 10 minutes, but it's true. Serve it any time of day, including breakfast! This recipe includes two different flavors of miso—it's not necessary that you use both, but I think it tastes better. If you only buy one miso, make it barley since it's the most medicinal. Once you've mastered this soup, play with a combination of vegetables, but always include the wakame and miso. Try combining daikon with celery, or leek with chopped dandelion greens, and scallion. You can also top the soup with nori and plain croutons.

SERVES 2 OR 3

¼–½ cup onion, cut into large dice

1 whole scallion, roots and all, sliced thinly on the diagonal (see Note)

2" piece dried wakame, cut into small pieces with scissors

1 teaspoon sesame oil

2" x 4" piece brown rice mochi, quartered

Shoyu

¼ cup diced rutabaga

¼ cup diced green cabbage

2 large bok choy leaves, white and green parts chopped separately

1½ teaspoons barley miso

1½ teaspoons mellow white miso

5–7 dandelion leaves, leafy parts only, cut into bite-size pieces

1 sheet nori

Bring 2½ cups of water to a boil in a medium pot. Lower the heat, and add the onion, scallion, and wakame. Simmer while you prepare the mochi.

In a skillet, heat the oil over medium-low heat. Add the mochi to the pan, cover, and cook for 3 to 4 minutes, checking to make sure the mochi doesn't burn. Flip the mochi, drizzling each side with a couple drops of shoyu. Cover the pan, and cook for 3 to 4 minutes longer. The mochi is done when it expands and begins to look puffy.

While the mochi cooks, continue adding vegetables to the soup. Start with the rutabaga. When it has simmered for 5 minutes, add the cabbage and white part of the bok choy. Simmer for 1 minute. Place the miso in a small cup, stir in a few tablespoons of the soup broth, and then add it to the soup. Simmer the soup for 2 minutes, making sure not to boil the miso. Stir in the dandelion greens and the green part of the bok choy just until wilted and still bright green. Remove the pot from the heat.

To serve, ladle the soup into small bowls. Rip the nori into bite-size pieces, and sprinkle on each serving. Top with a fried mochi square.

Note: The hairy root end of the scallion is full of good energy and extra good for you.

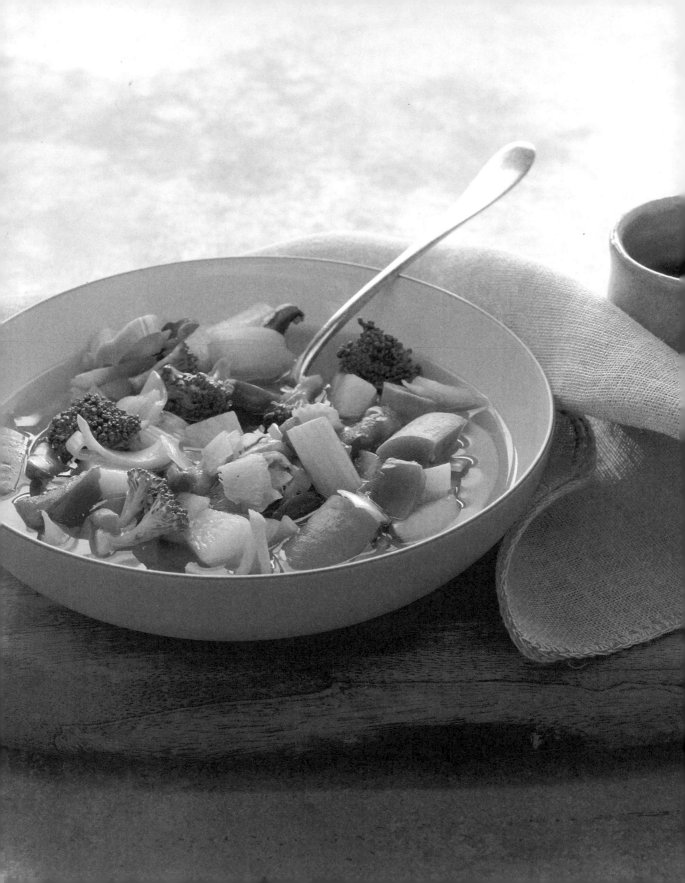

Alicia's Magical Healing Soup

Welcome to your new chicken soup. I make this when I'm just not feeling right and, for real, it heals me. And it's different every time; some days certain things appeal to me and other days they just don't sound right at all, so making this soup is all about listening to your intuition. I always begin by pulling everything out of the fridge that sounds remotely yummy to me, and then I sort of edit as I go along. This is a combo that ends up on my table a lot, but you can really use any vegetables you like. Consider adding lotus root, burdock root, dried shiitake mushrooms (presoaked), collards, kale, garlic, bok choy, cilantro—anything that sounds good to you. And although they're nightshades, I even use a little potato and tomato once in a blue moon if it feels right.

SERVES 2

½ medium carrot, cut into large chunks

¼ medium daikon, cut into large chunks

¼ red onion, cut into large chunks

2–3 celery stalks, chopped (I love the middle part sooo much that I usually eat it before it makes it into the soup!)

3–4 small broccoli florets

4 button mushrooms, sliced

2–3 trumpet mushrooms, sliced

½ medium leek, halved then cut into large chunks and swirled in a bowl of water to dislodge any grit

Ginger juice to taste (grate a 1" piece of ginger and squeeze out the juice with your fingers)

Shoyu to taste

1 whole scallion, roots and all, thinly sliced on the diagonal

¼ bunch watercress, tough stems discarded

Mochi, chopped or shredded (optional)

Toasted nori pieces (optional)

Bring 3 cups of water to a boil in a large pot. Add the carrot and daikon. Reduce the heat to a simmer. Add the red onion, and cook for 2 to 3 minutes. Add the celery, broccoli, mushrooms, and leek. Add the ginger juice and shoyu to the broth to taste. Simmer until the vegetables are cooked through but still slightly firm, about 5 minutes. Add the scallion, and turn off the heat. (If you prefer the scallions raw, add them just before serving.) To serve, ladle the soup into bowls. Top each serving with some watercress, mochi, and nori.

Note: You can make this soup into a miso soup by adding about 2 to 3 teaspoons of miso paste at the end. Dilute the miso with a little soup broth, and add it to the soup at the end of cooking, allowing it to simmer for about 2 to 3 minutes.

Hearty Kinpira Stew

This soup is delicious and sooo good for you. Because it's warming and strengthening, I have it almost twice a week in winter, but it's appropriate any time of the year. Kinpira stew is earthy and makes me feel strong.

SERVES 4 TO 6

Sesame oil

1 cup burdock, sliced into thin matchstick pieces

Pinch of fine sea salt

1 cup carrot, sliced into thin matchstick pieces

1 cup lotus root, sliced into thin rounds

1 cup thinly sliced kabocha squash (peel only if the squash is not organic)

1 cup onion, diced

1 tablespoon sweet white miso (see Note)

1 tablespoon barley miso

Brush the bottom of a soup pot lightly with oil. Place the pot over medium heat. When the oil is hot, add the burdock and a pinch of salt. Sauté for 5 minutes, stirring constantly. If the burdock starts to stick to the bottom of the pan, add a little more oil or a little water.

Layer the carrot, lotus root, and squash on top of the burdock. Cover the vegetables with water, and bring to a boil. Lower the heat and simmer, covered, for 30 to 40 minutes or until the vegetables are very soft. Add more water from time to time as needed if the water level becomes too low.

Add the onion to the pot, and simmer until very soft, about 10 to 15 minutes. Combine the misos in a small cup, and dilute them with a little of the soup broth (you may add more miso later to taste). Slowly add the diluted miso mixture to the pot, and stir gently. Simmer for 3 minutes more, taking care not to let the soup boil once the miso has been added. Serve immediately.

Note: If you have to choose one miso, the barley is more medicinal.

Creamy Sweet Kabocha Squash Soup

This soup is so simple it's ridiculous, and yet it's truly delicious and good for you. It soothes the digestion process and helps me to feel centered and calm. I like to make a pot of it and eat it for a few days.

SERVES 3 OR 4

4 cups kabocha squash, peeled and cut in 2" cubes

2 pinches of fine sea salt

Minced fresh parsley

Place the squash in a saucepan with 3½ cups of water. Bring to a boil, and add a small pinch of salt. Cover, lower the heat, and simmer for 15 minutes, until the squash is soft. Mash the squash with a potato masher, or blend with a handheld blender, right in the pot. Add another pinch of salt (or 1 teaspoon shoyu), and simmer for 7 to 10 minutes longer. Serve the soup hot with a sprinkle of parsley on top.

To make the sweetest version, here are some tips on finding the sweetest winter squash:

- For kabocha and buttercup: Make sure the squash is a dark green with one bright orange spot on it—that's where it sat and grew on the ground. The darker the green, the sweeter the squash.

- For butternut: A darker beige exterior is better, verging on orange.

- For all squash: Avoid squash that feels light in weight. That means it's dry inside—and less flavorful—so heavier is better.

- Some old-time, organic squash growers will actually cure their squash by letting it sit in a cool dark place for a while. Ask at the farmers' market to see if any of your local growers do that. Cured squash tends to be sweeter.

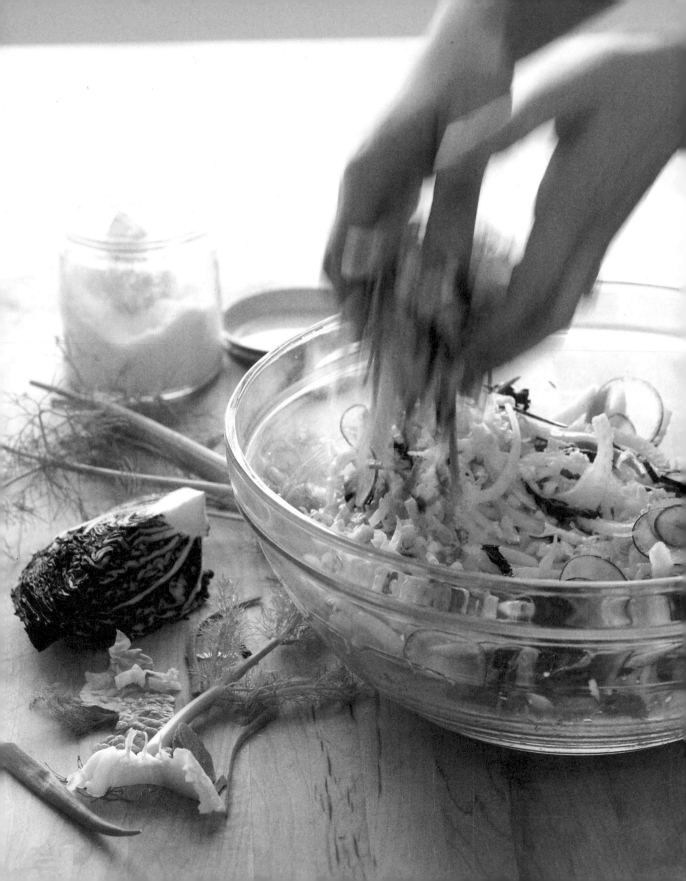

Radicchio, Radish, and Fennel Pressed Salad

Pressed salads are an interesting twist on fresh salads; by lightly salting and pressing the vegetables, they become more digestible while retaining all their live enzymes. In fact, the word *salad* comes from the Italian *herba salata*, which means "salted herb." Pressed salads are crunchy and refreshing. Have some pressed salad as a side dish a couple of times a week. They will keep in the fridge for up to 2 days, but after that, pressed salads will become too limp and wilted. So freshly pressed is best! You're going to be using your bare hands for pressed salads, so make sure you wash them with biodegradable soap instead of the heavy-duty chemical stuff.

This amazing combination of tastes will wake up any palate.

SERVES 6 TO 8

½ head napa cabbage, thinly sliced

¼ head radicchio, thinly sliced

5–6 red radishes, thinly sliced

1 fennel bulb, stalks and fronds removed, thinly sliced

1 carrot, thinly sliced

2–3 scallions, thinly sliced

2 teaspoons fine sea salt

Combine the cabbage, radicchio, radishes, fennel, carrot, and scallions in a large bowl. Mix the vegetables together with your hands, and then slowly add the salt a little at a time. Massage the salt into the vegetables using your hands. If, after a few minutes, the vegetables do not start to wilt or exude liquid, add a little bit more salt. Continue to massage the vegetables until they are wilted and liquid gathers at the bottom of the bowl. You should be able to "wring out" the salad, almost as you would a washcloth.

Next, mound all the vegetables together at the bottom of the bowl to form a little hill. Cover with a plate small enough to fit inside the bowl and place a weight on top (I like to use a full tea kettle or a big gallon glass bottle filled with water). Press the salad for 35 minutes to 1 hour. Pour off the excess liquid, and give the salad a good squeeze with your hands. Taste it, and if it tastes salty, give the salad a quick and gentle rinse under cold water, then squeeze it once again.

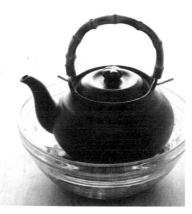

Cabbage, Radish, and Cucumber Pressed Salad

This salad is made by the exact same technique as the previous recipe but uses vinegar rather than salt to wilt the vegetables to give it a different flavor. Slice all the veggies as thinly as you possibly can.

SERVES 2 OR 3

5–6 leaves napa cabbage, thinly sliced

3 red radishes, thinly sliced

3 whole scallions, thinly sliced on the diagonal

½ cucumber, thinly sliced on the diagonal (peel only if the cucumber is not organic)

1 orange or apple, peeled and thinly sliced

1½ tablespoons umeboshi vinegar

1 tablespoon balsamic vinegar or brown rice vinegar (see Note)

1 tablespoon toasted sunflower seeds

Combine all the vegetables and fruit in a mixing bowl. Add the vinegars and massage the vegetables with your bare hands until they begin to wilt and release some liquid. This may take a few minutes. Don't be afraid to get into it; really squeeze the vegetables and have fun. The massaged vegetables should feel quite wet by the end. Form into a mound and place a small plate on the vegetables within the bowl and place a weight on top (a full tea kettle or big jar of apple juice) to press the vegetables. Press for 20 to 30 minutes. Pour off the excess fluid, and give the salad a good squeeze with your hands. Taste it; if it tastes salty, give the salad a quick and gentle rinse under cold water, then squeeze it once again. **Add the sunflower seeds and toss into the salad before serving.**

Note: If you make this often, make sure to use the brown rice vinegar most of the time as balsamic vinegar is more acidic. Whole Foods makes a good, clean balsamic vinegar with no added sugars.

SUPERHERO VEGETABLE DISHES

By now you surely know what an important role dark leafy greens play in the Superhero diet. Calorie-for-calorie, they are the most nutrient-dense foods on the planet, so please eat leafy greens with your meals as often as you can—at least once a day but 2 or 3 times a day is even better. They are true super-foods, and you will soon fall helplessly and hopelessly in love with them.

If greens don't turn your crank (yet), make a delectable sauce to eat with them. I like Ume-Sesame Dressing (page 259), Tahini Dressing (page 259), or the flaxseed and ume vinegar combo from the Baby Bok Choy Drizzled with Ume Vinaigrette recipe (page 265) on just about anything. Even a simple sprinkle of toasted sunflower seeds makes me happy! However, you will be surprised when—after a while—you really appreciate the taste of naked collards and kale. You'll see . . .

And feel free to think beyond the steamer or skillet. Grilled zucchini and onions on the barbecue are one of my favorite dishes in summer—they are so delicious. Cut the zucchini and onions into nice thick slices, add oil, sprinkle with salt and pepper, and grill. This is a great way to cook virtually any vegetable you love. And don't forget baked sweet potatoes!

Quick, Easy Snack

Steam or toast a piece of bread. Take 2 tablespoons good-quality, unpasteurized sauerkraut (Goldmine and Eden make good ones) and squeeze it to remove excess salt and fluid. (If it's too salty for your taste, you might want to rinse it and squeeze it again.) Slice or mash up ½ avocado. Spread the avocado on the toast, then top with the sauerkraut and a sprinkle of paprika.

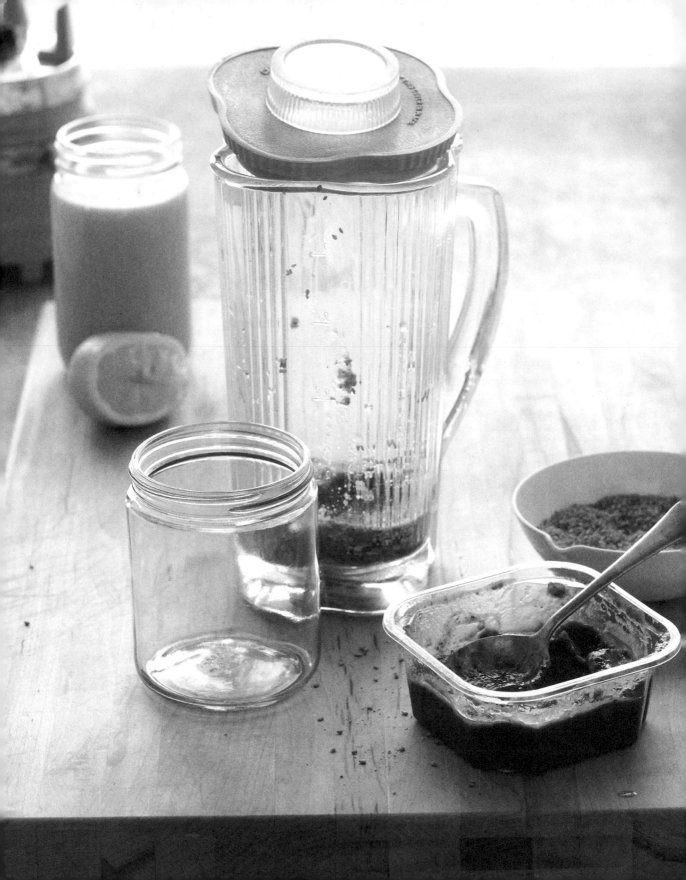

Tahini Dressing

One of my favorites things is a big plate of steamed vegetables—leeks and beets are the absolute best—drizzled with tahini dressing. It's also delicious over brown rice, noodles, pressed salads, as a flavorful garnish on soups, or as a spread for sandwiches.

I don't have tahini dressing every day—maybe once or twice a week.

MAKES ABOUT 1 CUP

½ cup tahini, raw or roasted

Juice from 1¼ lemons

1–2 teaspoons shoyu

Less than ¼ garlic clove, to taste

Dash cayenne (optional)

1 teaspoon umeboshi vinegar (optional)

Combine the tahini, lemon juice, shoyu, garlic, cayenne (if using), vinegar (if using), and ½ to ¾ cup of water in a blender. Puree until very well combined. Refrigerate in a tightly sealed jar. This will keep for about 4 days. You can add basil, cilantro, parsley, miso, and ume vinegar for variation, but if you add herbs, the dressing will only last for 2 days.

Ume-Sesame Dressing

This dressing is a more recent member of my repertoire, thanks to Mina Dobic. It's sooo freaking good. I love it the most on dinosaur kale. It keeps well in a jar in the fridge for 3 to 4 days.

MAKES ABOUT 1½ CUPS

½ cup sesame seeds

1 tablespoon umeboshi plum paste

Place the seeds in a strainer, and rinse under cool running water. Shake off as much moisture as possible, and then empty the seeds into a medium skillet. Toast the seeds over low to medium heat, stirring often, until all of the moisture has evaporated and the seeds puff up a little and give off a nutty scent.

Transfer the seeds to a blender. Add the umeboshi plum paste and ¾ cup of water. Blend until the seeds are very finely ground, then add the remaining ½ cup of water. The dressing should be nice and thick.

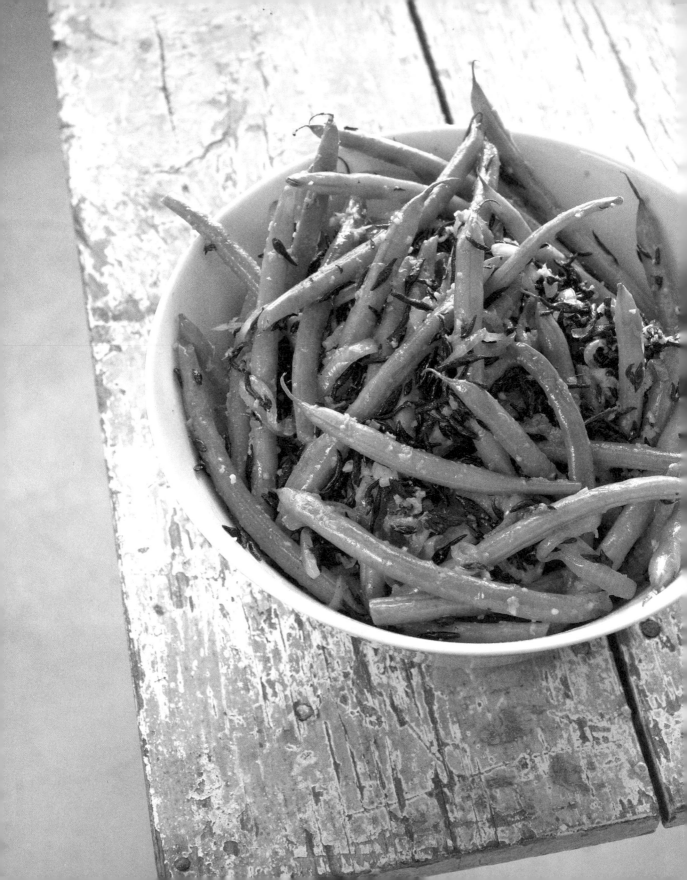

Gingered Green Beans with Hijiki

If hijiki and arame were siblings, hijiki would be the big brother and arame the shy sister. Hijiki is bigger, more mineral-rich, and has a stronger taste. It's also amazing for you. Alternate between brother and sister (¼- to ½-cup servings) week to week. As you get acquainted with this recipe, you can add more or less green beans.

SERVES 2 TO 4

½ cup dried hijiki

1 tablespoon shoyu

2 tablespoons olive oil

½ cup onion, halved and sliced

1 tablespoon finely chopped garlic

Pinch of fine sea salt

2 cups fresh green beans

Juice from 2 tablespoons grated ginger

Place the hijiki in a small bowl, and cover with hot water. Soak for about 30 minutes, then drain and rinse in a colander to rid the hijiki of any remaining grit.

Combine the hijiki with the shoyu and water to almost cover in a saucepan. Cook, uncovered, over medium heat until the water has nearly evaporated, about 30 to 40 minutes.

While the hijiki cooks, heat the oil in a skillet over medium-high heat. Add the onion, garlic, and salt and sauté for about 4 minutes, or until translucent. Cut the tips from the green beans, and add to the onions. Cover and cook until the green beans are tender-crisp, about 3 to 5 minutes. Add the hijiki and ginger juice. Mix well, and cook for 1 to 2 minutes longer to marry the flavors. Serve immediately.

Arame Turnovers

This yummy recipe comes from *Christina Cooks*. It's a great, sneaky way to get sea vegetables into little kids (and big ones, too). Because they're cooked in phyllo dough, they are elegant, delicious, and great for parties.

SERVES 2 TO 4

½ cup dried arame, rinsed well and set aside to soften (do not soak)

Shoyu

Mirin

2 shallots, thinly sliced

1 small carrot, cut into fine matchstick pieces

¼ cup fresh or frozen and thawed corn kernels

3 sheets phyllo dough, thawed

Extra-virgin olive oil

¼ cup toasted almonds, ground into a fine meal

Rinse the arame under running water, and set aside for a few moments to soften. Place the arame in a small saucepan with enough water to half-cover. Add generous dashes of shoyu and mirin, and bring to a boil over medium heat. Cover the pot, reduce the heat to low, and simmer for 15 minutes. Add the shallots, carrot, and corn to the pot in layers, cover, and simmer until all the cooking liquid has been absorbed into the dish, about 5 minutes.

Preheat the oven to 350°F and line a baking sheet with parchment paper.

Cut the phyllo dough sheets lengthwise into four equal strips. Lay 1 phyllo strip on a dry work surface, covering the remaining phyllo with a damp towel. Brush the phyllo strip with oil and sprinkle with some of the ground almonds. Lay another strip on top, brush with oil, and sprinkle with some of the ground almonds. Lay a third sheet on top. Spoon about 3 tablespoons of the arame mixture onto one corner. Fold the phyllo around the filling as you would fold a flag, forming a layered triangle. Place on the prepared baking sheet. Repeat with the remaining phyllo and filling to make 4 turnovers.

Brush each turnover lightly with oil, and bake for 15 to 20 minutes, or until the phyllo is crisp and golden brown. Serve warm.

Arame with Carrots and Onions

I know a lot of people are grossed out at the idea of seaweed, but I promise you this is a really delicious vegetable dish. Serve it in small portions—maybe ¼ to ½ cup—and I really think you'll like it. Arame is great for your hair, skin, nails, and bones. Try to have an arame dish at least once a week.

SERVES 4 TO 6

1 ounce dried arame (about one large handful)

1–2 teaspoons toasted sesame oil

½ cup onion, cut into half-moon slices

Fine sea salt

½ cup carrot, cut into fine matchstick pieces

Shoyu to taste

Chopped scallion for garnish

Soak the arame in water to cover for 5 minutes. Lift the arame out of the soaking water, leaving any grit behind. If the arame strands seem long, cut them into approximately 2" pieces.

Heat the oil in a skillet over medium-high heat. Add the onion and a tiny pinch of sea salt. Sauté for 1 to 2 minutes. Add the carrot to the skillet, and then scatter the arame on top. Without stirring, add enough water to the skillet to just cover the vegetables, leaving the arame just above the liquid. Add about 1 teaspoon shoyu or less. Bring to a boil, reduce the heat to low, and cover the skillet. Simmer for about 25 to 30 minutes. Sprinkle in a few more drops of shoyu. Cover and cook 4 to 5 minutes longer, then remove the cover and cook until almost all the liquid has evaporated. Stir the vegetables and arame to combine, and cook another minute or two, or until the liquid is entirely evaporated. Garnish with scallion, and serve.

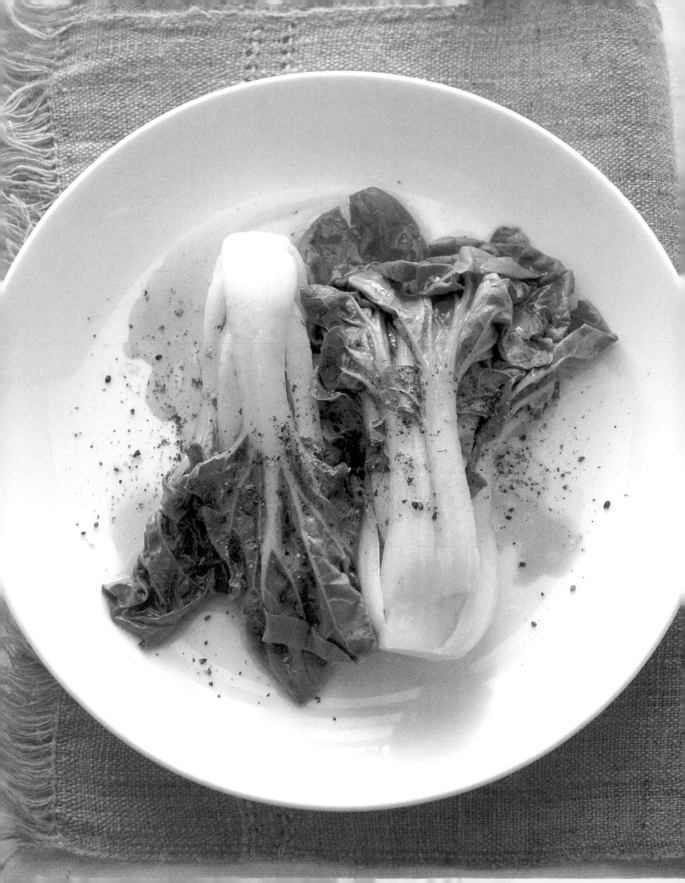

Baby Bok Choy Drizzled with Ume Vinaigrette

I've highlighted (and photographed) the bok choy version of this dish because it's so pretty, but this same recipe made with cabbage and leeks is just as delicious and worthy of equal attention. Christopher and I absolutely *lived* off cabbage and leeks for years. I beg you to try both versions. There's something about the combination of the flaxseed oil, the sour of the vinegar, the freshness of the green and the seeds. . . . *Oh my God.*

SERVES 2

1–2 small heads bok choy (left intact) or ½ large head bok choy (chopped into bite-size pieces)

1 tablespoon umeboshi vinegar

1 tablespoon flaxseed oil (if you can't get flaxseed oil, substitute extra-virgin olive oil, but the flaxseed oil is way yummier)

1 teaspoon Gomashio (page 232, optional)

Bring water to a boil in the bottom of a steamer or a pot fitted with a steamer basket. Add the bok choy and steam for 1 to 2 minutes until the vegetable is just starting to wilt. Transfer to a serving platter.

Mix the vinegar and oil together in a small bowl, and drizzle over the steamed bok choy. (You may not need it all.) Serve sprinkled with the gomashio.

Variation:

You can serve lightly steamed leeks and cabbage the same way. Be sure to steam the leek and cabbage separately, as it's nice to keep their flavors pristine and their cooking times may vary depending on the size and thickness of the vegetables. Top with toasted sunflower or pumpkin seeds seasoned with a few drops of shoyu (page 215).

Notes:

- People tend to throw greens in a steamer and just walk away, so it's alarmingly easy to overcook bok choy. I recommend you always err on the side of undercooking it, since it's so water-dense that it continues to cook a little after being removed from the steam. What you're aiming for is crunchiness without bitterness.

- After you get familiar with this recipe, you may decide you want to use less vinegar. Find the oil to vinegar ratio that works best for you.

Cuban-Style Roasted Sweet Potatoes

Ahh, the sweet potato! I make this recipe with yellow-fleshed sweet potatoes (not garnet yams, which have a totally different flavor). Though they are not related to white potatoes botanically, they have the same satisfying texture and they're sweet! When I eat a sweet potato, I feel like I'm getting away with something. Feel free to cut it in any shape you want for this recipe, but I prefer it in big pieces.

SERVES 4

3 large sweet potatoes, peeled and quartered (about 3 pounds)

4 tablespoons extra-virgin olive oil

Fine sea salt to taste

Freshly ground black pepper to taste

1 large garlic clove, minced

1 tablespoon fresh lime juice

1½ tablespoons chopped fresh parsley

Heat the oven to 400°F. Line a baking sheet with parchment paper, and set aside.

Place the sweet potatoes in a medium bowl, toss with 2 tablespoons of the oil, and season to taste with salt and pepper. Spread the potatoes on the prepared baking sheet, and roast until they can be pierced easily with a knife but still offer some resistance, about 30 minutes. Let cool for 15 minutes or so.

Transfer the potatoes to a large bowl, and toss with the garlic, lime juice, parsley, and remaining 2 tablespoons of oil. Adjust the seasoning to taste with salt and pepper. Serve warm or at room temperature.

Scarlet Roasted Vegetables

I call these scarlet vegetables because the beets bleed into the others, making everything red, messy, and yummy. This is a pretty dish, perfect for Thanksgiving or any time.

SERVES 4 TO 6

4–6 shallots, peeled and halved lengthwise

3 large beets, cut into 1" chunks

2 parsnips, quartered lengthwise

1 large fennel bulb, halved, cored, and thickly sliced

1–2 cups kabocha squash, cut into big chunks (peel only if the squash is not organic)

3–4 celery stalks, cut in 1" pieces

3–4 dried bay leaves

½ cup pecan halves

6–8 dried apricots, coarsely chopped

1–2 teaspoons shoyu

Grated zest of 2 lemons

2–3 tablespoons extra-virgin olive oil

Juice of 1 lemon

2 tablespoons chopped fresh parsley

Preheat the oven to 350°F. Lightly oil a large, shallow baking dish.

Combine all of the vegetables, bay leaves, pecans, apricots, shoyu, lemon zest, and oil in a mixing bowl. Mix the vegetables to coat them well.

Transfer the vegetables to a prepared baking dish, and spread out evenly. Cover with aluminum foil, and roast for 40 minutes, or until the vegetables are soft when pierced.

Remove the aluminum foil, and roast for 15 minutes longer to let the vegetables brown a little. Remove from oven, and toss with the lemon juice. Garnish with the parsley.

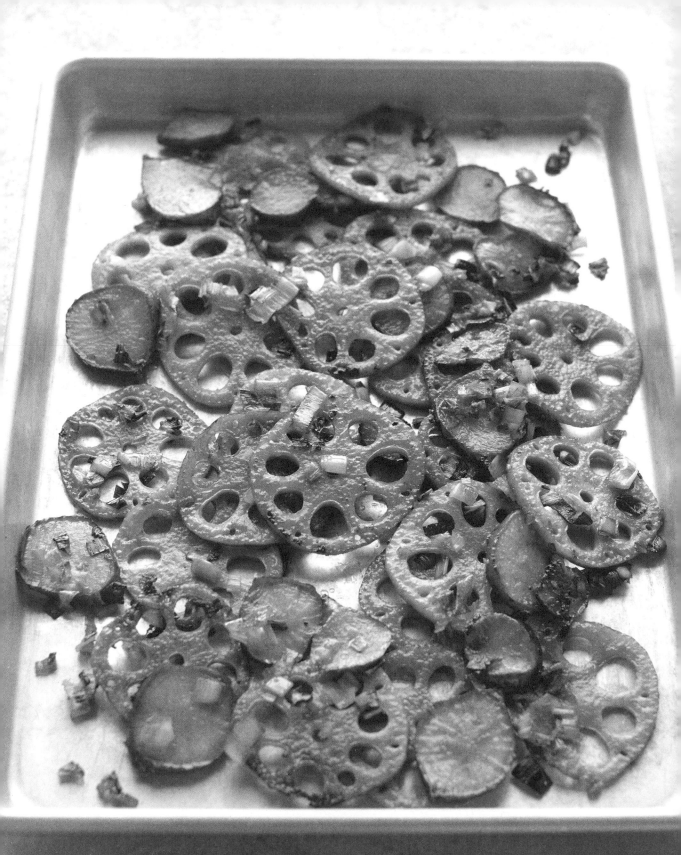

Maple-Roasted Lotus Root, Sunchokes, and Leeks

This recipe sounds exotic, but it tastes like candy to me . . . savory candy. You *must* try it.

SERVES 4 TO 6

- 4" piece of lotus root (about ½ of a medium root), sliced into thin rounds
- 3 sunchokes (also called Jerusalem artichokes), thinly sliced
- 2 small or ½ of a large, thick leek (white part only), sliced into thin half-moons
- 2 garlic cloves, pressed or minced
- 1 tablespoon olive oil
- 1 teaspoon shoyu or 3 pinches fine sea salt
- 1 tablespoon maple syrup

Preheat the oven to 375°F.

Place all the vegetables and garlic in a bowl. Add the oil, and toss to coat. Spread the veggies onto a baking sheet.

Roast the vegetables for 12 minutes, then sprinkle with the shoyu and syrup; stir to coat. Return the vegetables to the oven, and roast an additional 10 minutes. At this point, check to see if the vegetables are tender and becoming golden; if not, return to the oven for 5 to 10 minutes longer. Serve warm.

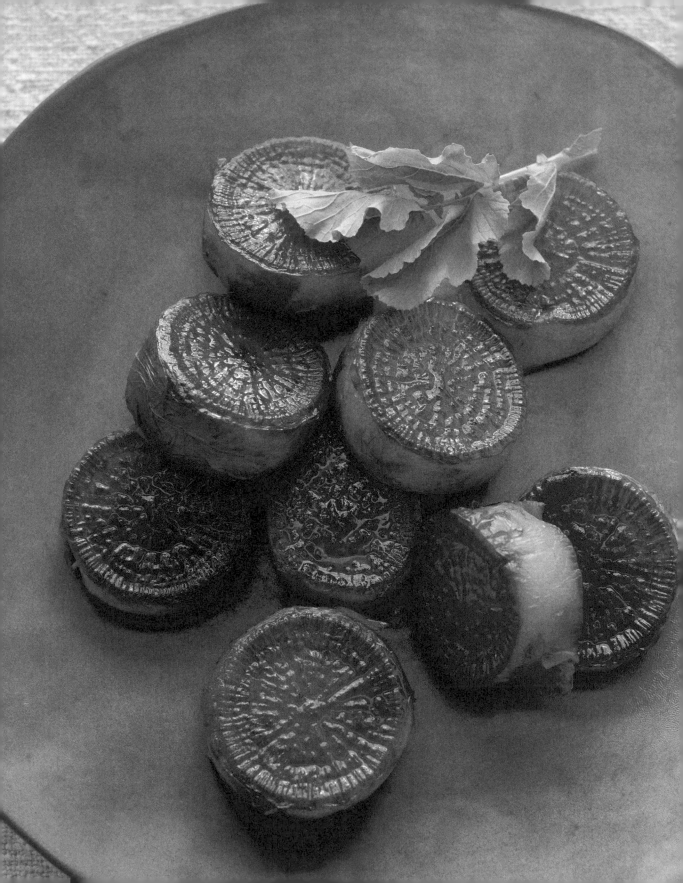

Braised Daikon in Mirin and Shoyu

This dish smells ridiculously good and should be eaten relatively soon after it is prepared. It was inspired by John Medeski—of the amazing musical trio Medeski, Martin, and Wood—a wine connoisseur and foodie.

SERVES 2 OR 3

1 large daikon (roughly 1 pound but size doesn't really matter)

2 tablespoons shoyu

¼ cup mirin

2"–3" strip kombu

Slice the daikon into ¾" rounds, and place them in a skillet in a single layer. Add water almost to cover the daikon. Add the shoyu, mirin, and kombu. Bring the liquid to a boil over high heat, then reduce the heat to very low, cover the pan, and simmer the daikon for 30 minutes, or until all liquid has been absorbed.

Christopher's Cauliflower Steaks

Christopher and I ordered this dish at a really fancy restaurant in New York. We both loved it so much that he started making his own version at home. It's so simple and so good.

SERVES 4

1 medium to large head cauliflower

1 large fennel bulb, stalks and fronds removed

2 tablespoons olive oil

Fine sea salt

Freshly ground black pepper

Preheat the oven to 375°F. Slice the cauliflower as you would cut a loaf of bread, making ½"- to ¾"-thick slices per person. Arrange the slices on a lightly oiled baking sheet. Slice the fennel bulb, and arrange on the same baking sheet or use a second sheet if necessary. Brush the cut surfaces of the cauliflower and fennel with the oil, and season lightly with salt and pepper.

Roast the vegetable steaks until they are light brown, about 15 minutes, then flip the slices, brush with more oil, and return to the oven until browned and tender, about 15 minutes.

Carrot and Burdock Kinpira

This traditional Japanese (and macrobiotic) dish should be eaten a couple times a week. Burdock strengthens and purifies the blood, while carrots are full of phytonutrients. Together they make a really strengthening dish that makes me feel grounded and energized . . . and it tastes really good.

SERVES 4

About 1 teaspoon sesame oil (toasted or plain)

1 cup burdock, cut into matchstick pieces

2 pinches fine sea salt

1 cup carrots, cut into matchstick pieces

Shoyu to taste

A few drops of ginger juice (grate a ½" piece of ginger and squeeze out the juice with your fingers)

2 tablespoons toasted sesame seeds

2 teaspoons chopped parsley for garnish

Heat a small amount of oil in a skillet over medium-high heat. Add the burdock, a pinch of salt, and cook, stirring continually, for 2 to 3 minutes. Add the carrots, another small pinch of salt, and cook, stirring continually, for 2 to 3 minutes longer.

Add enough water to just cover the bottom of the skillet to create steam. Cover the pan, and reduce heat to low. Simmer/steam for 7 minutes. Sprinkle ½ to 1 teaspoon of shoyu on the kinpira, cover, and let cook for 4 minutes longer. The kinpira should be almost dry. Remove from the heat, add the ginger juice, and toss. Add sesame seeds and parsley, toss again, and serve.

Notes: In fall and winter, make a longer kinpira, one that simmers for 20 to 30 minutes. This will make the vegetables sweeter, softer, and easier to digest. It will also be more strengthening and warming to the body. Follow the above directions, but add more water at the beginning and check the vegetables halfway through to make sure they're not drying out or burning. Add small amounts of water throughout the cooking if necessary.

To make matchsticks, slice the vegetable (carrot or burdock) thinly on the diagonal. After making 6 or 8 slices, lay them down, slightly overlapping one another like fallen dominoes. Chop along the fallen slices lengthwise in order to get the longest matchsticks possible. Repeat until you have as much as you need.

Nishime

Pronounced Ni-*shee*-may, this is another traditional macrobiotic dish and it's great for the stomach, spleen, and pancreas. The slow stewing of the vegetables in their own juices makes them fall-apart-in-your-mouth soft and sweet. The whole vibe of the dish is really calming and centering. I always feel good after eating nishime; it's my new comfort food. Superheroes should eat nishime 2 or 3 times a week. Carrot and burdock is another yummy combination, but note that it will take a little longer to cook.

Here are my favorite vegetables to use, in order of how much I love them in this dish. But have fun and play with what you like best: kabocha squash, daikon, celery, onion, sweet potato, rutabaga, green cabbage, carrot, burdock, and lotus root.

Layer the vegetables in the pot beginning with the vegetables that cook in the least time and ending with those that take the longest. Cut larger chunks of vegetables in colder months and smaller chunks in warmer months. Try to use as little water as possible. The perfect nishime will have little or no water left at the end of cooking. Try to use 3 to 5 vegetables at a time. Three (not including the kombu) are ideal.

SERVES 4

1" piece dried kombu seaweed

1 cup red onion, cut into chunks

1 cup celery, cut into 2" pieces

1 cup daikon, cut into 1" rounds

1 cup unpeeled kabocha squash, cut into medium chunks

Shoyu to taste

Place the kombu in the bottom of a medium pot or Dutch oven. Layer in the vegetables one at a time, starting with the red onion, celery, daikon, and lastly the squash. Add about 1 inch of water. (Using as little water as possible will create a sweeter dish.) Cover and bring to a boil, then reduce the heat to low and simmer for 20 minutes. The cooking liquid should be greatly reduced. Sprinkle with shoyu to taste, and cook 5 minutes longer, or until the vegetables are tender and the water has nearly all evaporated. Scoop the vegetables onto serving plates.

Note: If there is still a lot of water left in the pot when the vegetables are cooked and tender, lift the cooked vegetables out of the cooking water and place in a serving dish. Dissolve 1 tablespoon kuzu in 2 tablespoons cold water. Add the dissolved kuzu to the hot cooking liquid, and bring to a boil. Pour this "gravy" over the vegetables, and serve.

Vegetable Tempura

People tend to freak out about fried foods, but here's the deal:

- Deep-fried food that is cooked properly is not fatty. Most of the oil should drain off of properly cooked, crispy tempura.

- As long as you are using good-quality oil, deep-fried food is a healthy part of a healthy diet. It helps to keep the body warm and supports strong physical activity—great for kids and athletic grown-ups.

- Tempura or other deep-fried food once a week on a Superhero diet will not cause you to gain weight. If anything, it will make you feel satisfied and happy, which will help you stick to the diet. So enjoy a few pieces of tempura!

- Always serve tempura with a tablespoon of grated daikon and eat it as you go; this helps to counteract any excess oil you might be getting with the tempura.

These are my favorites, but choose whatever vegetables you like. It's best to make the batter in small batches, so if you plan to serve more people, make multiple batches of batter.

SERVES 2

Tempura Batter

1 cup whole wheat pastry flour or ½ cup each whole wheat pastry flour and rice flour

1–2 tablespoons kuzu or arrowroot

Pinch of fine sea salt

Dipping Sauce

1 teaspoon shoyu

3–5 drops ginger juice (grate 1" fresh ginger and use your fingers to squeeze out the juice)

Safflower oil, enough to fully cover vegetables while frying

2–4 (¼"-thick) slices onion

¼"-thick slices carrot, cut on the diagonal

2–4 (¼"-thick) slices unpeeled kabocha squash

2–4 small broccoli florets

2–4 (¼"-thick) slices burdock, cut on the diagonal

1 tablespoon finely grated daikon per person

*　　*

To make the batter, stir together the flour, kuzu, and salt in a mixing bowl. Stir in 1 cup of water, and mix just until combined. If the batter is very thick, stir in another tablespoon or so of water; if it is too loose and runny, add a touch more flour. Cover the bowl and refrigerate the batter for 30 minutes; don't let it stand too long, or it will become too thick.

To make the dipping sauce, combine the shoyu and ginger juice with ½ cup of water in a small saucepan. Bring to a boil, and simmer over medium heat for 3 to 4 minutes.

Pour 2 to 3 inches of oil into a deep skillet or small, deep pot. Heat the oil slowly until very hot and a drop of the batter sizzles on contact with the oil.

One at a time, dip a vegetable slice in the batter, allowing the excess to drip back into the bowl, and carefully lower it into the hot oil. Do not overcrowd the pan. Cook until the batter becomes crisp and is just starting to look pale golden in places, and the vegetable floats to the surface of the oil; don't let them brown. Use tongs to transfer the finished tempura to a plate lined with paper towels or clean dish towels.

Serve hot with the dipping sauce and grated daikon.

> Note: You can refrigerate the used oil and reuse it once or twice.

Squash 'n' Onions

As a die-hard squash lover, it was difficult to select my favorites from among all my squash recipes. But in the end, this dish won out. Simple and lovely, it's good for Flirts, vegans, family dinners, parties—you name it. To find the sweetest butternut squash, look for one that is a darker beige in color and heavier in weight.

SERVES 4

1 medium butternut squash (about 1 pound but weight doesn't really matter), preferably organic

2 medium onions

1 tablespoon olive oil

½ teaspoon dried oregano

¼ teaspoon fine sea salt (optional)

Wash and scrub the squash, but don't peel it unless it's not organic. Cut the squash into 2" pieces. Peel the onions, halve lengthwise, and slice crosswise in ½" slices.

Heat the oil in a 2-quart saucepan. Add the onions, and sauté until transparent, about 5 minutes. Add the squash and oregano. Sauté for another 2 or 3 minutes. Add ½ cup of water to the skillet and, if using, the salt. Cover the pan, reduce the heat to low, and simmer for 25 minutes.

Radish Umeboshi Pickles

Pickles are magic foods that aid in digestion, deliver good-quality enzymes to the body, and add a colorful, crunchy element to your meal. A few slices of pickles (about 1 tablespoon total) every day is perfect. Just eat them at the end of your meal, or feel free to cut them into tiny pieces to sprinkle on your grain or to just chomp on. If the pickles taste really salty, you can rinse or even soak them for a few minutes.

SERVES 12

6 red radishes, washed and thinly sliced

½ cup umeboshi vinegar

Place the radish slices in a glass jar. Pour the vinegar and 1 cup of water over the radishes in the jar until they are completely submerged. (If you need to make additional brine, combine 1 part vinegar to 2 parts water.) Cover the container with a cheesecloth, and secure with a rubber band. Pickles need air in order for fermentation to take place. Let stand at room temperature for at least 24 hours or up to 3 days. Rinse the pickles in fresh water before serving. After 3 days, let your pickles live in the refrigerator. They will be fine for about 10 days, but they will get saltier and stronger as they sit, so the older they are, the more rinsing and possibly soaking they will need before eating.

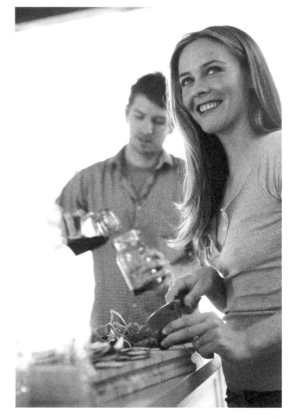

SUPERHERO DESSERTS

To keep your Superhero powers at their peak, it's best to have dessert no more than once every other day, but if you're newly off of sugar and it still feels strange and foreign to you, have as many Superhero desserts as you need to keep yourself comfortable.

If you need a quick dessert, have a piece of seasonal fruit or 1 tablespoon peanut butter with some strawberry jam. Apple slices dipped in almond butter and maple syrup are also incredibly yummy. Try almond or hazelnut (or any flavor you like) amasake. It's a thick, milkshake-y drink made from fermented sweet brown rice and is available at most health food stores.

The desserts in the Vegan section are okay for Superheroes every once in a while. For example, Crispy Peanut Butter Treats with Chocolate Chips (without the chocolate chips!) on page 184 are basically Superhero fare, as is the Peach Crumble on page 194.

If you think you're going to lose it and buy some desserts made with nasty foods, by all means, make one of the sexier vegan desserts. They're always a better choice than a store-brought dessert and will satisfy you completely.

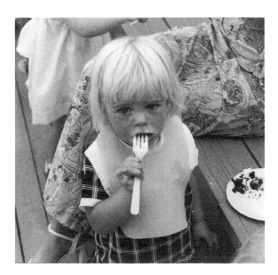

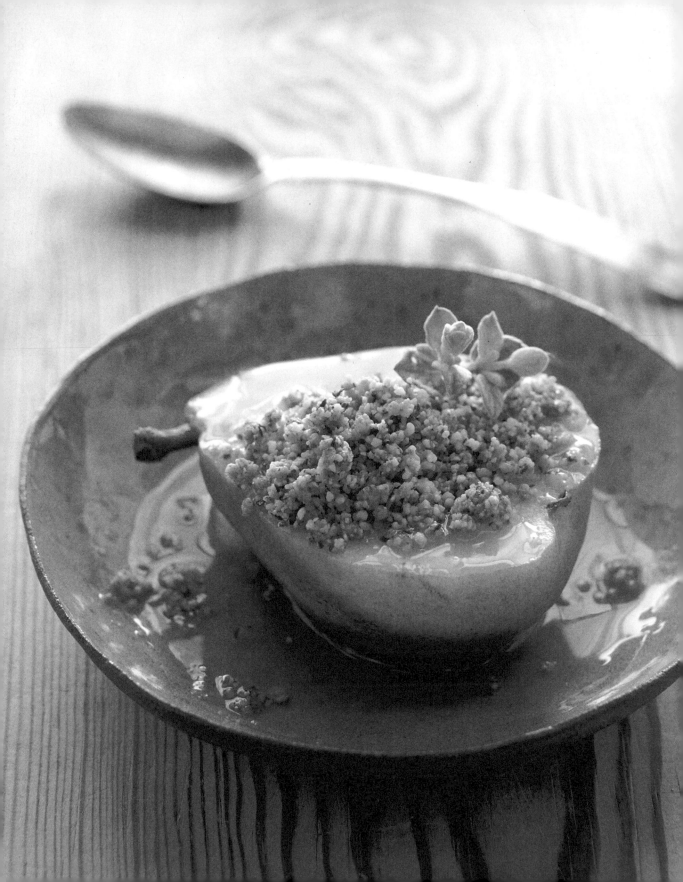

Candied Ginger Pears

I love this recipe with the maple syrup drizzled on top at the end, but the dessert itself is so sweet that you may not need it. Find out for yourself!

SERVES 4 TO 6

1 cup ground almonds

2 tablespoons brown rice syrup

3 large or 4 small pears, halved and core scooped out

1½ cups pear or apple juice

1 teaspoon ginger juice (grate 1" fresh ginger and use your fingers to squeeze out the juice)

Pinch of fine sea salt

1 tablespoon kuzu mixed with 1 tablespoon cold pear juice

1 tablespoon fresh lemon juice

1 teaspoon lemon zest

4 teaspoons maple syrup (optional)

Heat a dry skillet over medium heat. Add the almonds, and toast for 3 to 5 minutes, stirring constantly, until fragrant and golden brown. Transfer to a small bowl to cool. When cool, buzz the almonds in a food processor or blender until very finely ground. Heat the rice syrup in a small saucepan. Add the ground almonds, and stir over medium-low heat until the mixture thickens. Set aside.

Arrange the pears in a deep skillet, cut sides up. Add the pear or apple juice to the pan along with the ginger juice and salt. Cover the pan, bring to a boil, then reduce the heat to medium, and simmer for 7 to 10 minutes, or until the pear halves are soft. Using a slotted spoon, transfer the pears to a serving platter, reserving the cooking liquid. Fill the hollow of each pear with some of the ground almond mixture.

Stir the diluted kuzu into the reserved cooking liquid, and heat for 3 to 5 minutes, stirring constantly, until the sauce thickens. Remove from the heat, and stir in the lemon juice and zest. Pour the sauce over the pears, and serve. For extra sweetness and some color, drizzle each pear with 1 teaspoon maple syrup.

Plum Soup

Back in the day, I was served a fruit soup for dessert at a fancy French restaurant. I'd never heard of fruit soup, so I found it exciting, elegant, and really delicious.

This recipe is easy; it will take only a few minutes to make. You could have a cup of this every day and not gain an ounce—*and* stay really healthy. If you can't get plums, substitute about 2 cups of any seasonal fruit or berries, peeled and cut into large chunks.

SERVES 2 OR 3

1 cup apple juice

1 cinnamon stick

1 tablespoon currants

Pinch of fine sea salt

8–10 small plums, peeled, pitted, and halved

1½ tablespoons brown rice syrup

1 tablespoon kuzu mixed with 1 tablespoon water

Combine the apple juice, cinnamon stick, currants, and salt in a medium saucepan. Bring to a boil over medium heat, then reduce the heat to low and simmer for 10 minutes. Add the plums, return to a boil, then simmer for 20 minutes over low heat. Add the syrup and kuzu. Cook for another minute, stirring constantly, until thickened. Pour into a bowl and allow to cool before serving.

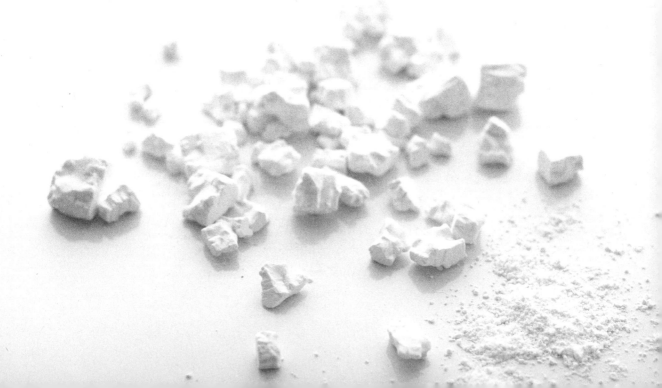

Strawberry Kanten

Kantens contain a sea vegetable called agar agar, which makes liquids set like Jell-o. This works well with any kind of berry, or use a combination of berries if you like. Superheroes can have kanten 3 or 4 times a week, and it will last about 4 days in the fridge.

SERVES 4 TO 6

1 pint fresh or 1 cup frozen and thawed strawberries (or any berry of your choosing)

4 cups apple juice

1 tablespoon fresh orange juice

Pinch of fine sea salt

3 generous tablespoons agar agar

A few drops ginger juice (grate 1" piece of ginger and use your fingers to squeeze out the juice)

Slice the berries thinly, and arrange them in an 8" × 8" heatproof glass dish or baking dish.

Combine the apple juice and orange juice in a saucepan over medium heat. Add the salt and agar agar. Bring to a boil, and let simmer for 10 to 15 minutes, stirring often to make sure the agar agar doesn't stick to the bottom of the pot. Simmer until all the agar agar has dissolved. (If it doesn't dissolve completely, it will make little lumps in your kanten.) Stir in the ginger juice and pour over the berries.

Allow the kanten to cool to room temperature, and then refrigerate, uncovered, until chilled and set, about 2 hours. The kanten is now ready to serve or may be covered and kept in the fridge for up to 4 days.

Variations:

You can make this with any kind of juice you like, including peach, apricot, or pear. A combination I especially like is peach juice with fresh apricots and blueberries. Because apricots are only around 1 month of the year, I try to use them in all sorts of dishes. They are my favorite!

To make a lovely fruit pudding, increase the agar agar to 4 tablespoons, let the kanten set completely, and then whiz it all in a blender with 1 tablespoon tahini. Serve in a wine glass!

BREAKFAST AND SPECIAL DRINKS

My idea of a great breakfast is one that is nourishing, satisfying, and makes me feel great for the rest of the day. Generally, that means a grain porridge, a cup of miso soup, and some steamed leafy greens with some yummy seeds. For more ideas on greens, see page 63.

Of course, there are times I like a fun breakfast with cereal, tempeh bacon, or waffles, but that's for when friends are over or I'm having a lazy weekend with my husband.

Quick breakfast ideas:

- If you want something super quick, try puffed kamut or puffed rice crisps with some nondairy milk. There are some really good cereals out there with clean ingredients and no white sugar.
- Lightly steam a piece of sourdough bread for a few seconds until it's soft. Spread some tahini and all-fruit jam on it . . . sounds weird, but it's totally yummy.
- Sometimes I just eat leftovers. I pull out any grain or vegetables from the day before, pour on some dressing or some seeds, and I'm good to go.

In this section I'm also including a few of my favorite drink recipes. I make these only as needed to treat cold and menstrual symptoms, hangovers, and other assorted minor ailments. Any of the teas below are fine to drink whenever you like.

Roasted barley tea: I love barley tea; I drink it hot when it's cold out and cold when it's hot out—it just tastes that great. Barley is great for the skin and has an overall cooling effect on the body. I buy big barley tea bags and just keep refilling my cup with water throughout the day.

Kukicha tea: Bancha and kukicha come from the same tea plant, but the bancha is made from leaves and the kukicha from the twigs. Bancha—which is a type of green tea—has a noticeable amount of caffeine in it, whereas kukicha has only trace amounts of caffeine. Kukicha also contains some calcium and is naturally alkalizing, which is why it's used in my Cure-All Tea on page 290.

Bancha tea: Green tea is fine to drink every once in a while, but you might find it has too much caffeine. All that said, if you're a big coffee drinker, make the transition with green tea.

Scrambled Tofu

Scrambled tofu is an easy way to clean out your fridge and end up with a great, simple meal. In fact, it's good for lunch or dinner as well, so for those of you who don't want too much protein in the morning, consider this as an anytime dish.

SERVES 2 TO 4

2 tablespoons sesame oil

2 cups chopped mixed vegetables (such as leeks, broccoli, zucchini, sugar snap peas, corn, mushrooms, red onion, sliced burdock, lotus root, and/or shredded cabbage)

1–2 tablespoons shoyu

1 tablespoon mirin (optional)

1 teaspoon umeboshi vinegar (optional)

Fine sea salt to taste

1 (14-ounce) package firm tofu, mashed or crumbled

¼ cup toasted seeds (such as sunflower, sesame, or pumpkin)

Chopped fresh scallions, cilantro, or parsley for garnish

Heat the oil in a skillet and, when hot, add the vegetables. Sauté until the vegetables are tender, about 5 to 8 minutes, depending on which vegetables you are using. If the vegetables start to stick or scorch, add a bit of water to the pan. Season the vegetables with shoyu, mirin (if using), ume vinegar (if using), and salt. Add the tofu, and cook, stirring constantly, until heated through, about 2 to 3 minutes. Add more seasoning to taste, if necessary. Serve sprinkled with the seeds, scallions, cilantro, or parsley.

Alicia's Soft Rice Porridge

In the morning, you are basically waking up from a night-long fast, hence the word *breakfast*. Because your body is empty and needs some gentle waking up, try grains that have been cooked soft to make them more digestible. I feel really good when I start the day with warm porridge.

SERVES 1

1 cup leftover rice

4 dried apricots (or any dried fruit you like), chopped

Toasted sunflower seeds

⅓ umeboshi plum, pit removed and cut into little pieces

Chopped fresh parsley

Place the rice, 2 cups of water, and the apricots into a saucepan. Bring to a boil, cover, and simmer (on a flame deflector if you have one) for 15 minutes. Remove from the heat and pour into a bowl. Top with the seeds, plum, and parsley. Good morning!

Variation:

Skip the apricots, and add ½ diced onion and 1 small carrot also diced. Simmer as usual and add 1 teaspoon diluted miso during the last 3 minutes of cooking. Garnish with scallions, torn nori, and the toasted seeds. A savory, hearty start to the day.

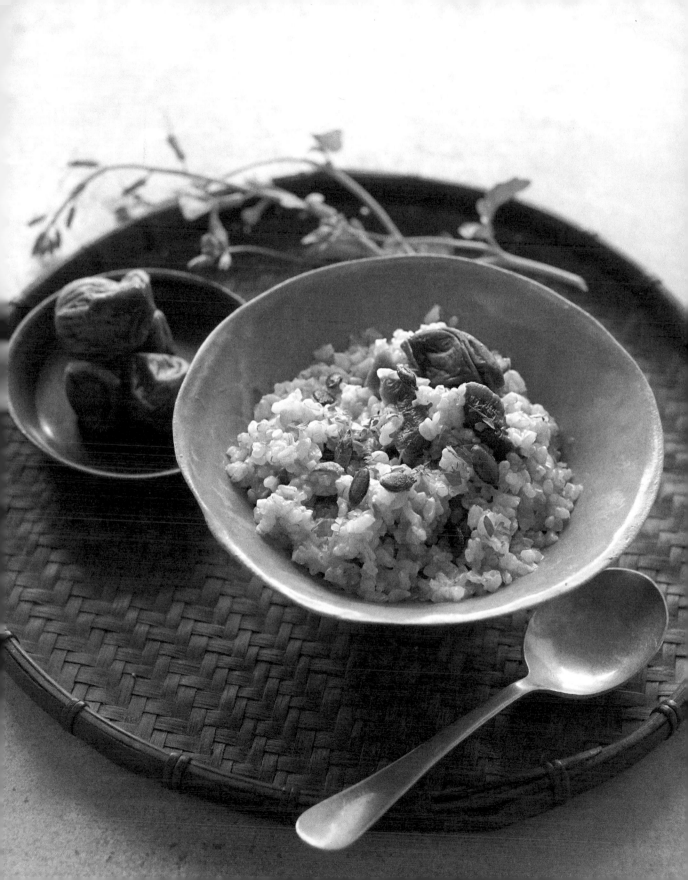

Mochi Waffles Drizzled with Lemon–Walnut–Rice Syrup

These are delicious. Mochi waffles are fun and easy for everyday eating, but they're also great to offer guests. Serve with a bowl of steamed collards and some tempeh bacon or Smart Bacon, and you have a quick, fantastic brunch.

MAKES 4 OR 5 WAFFLES

1 cup walnuts

1–1½ packages plain mochi
 (Grainaissance brand is good)

½ cup brown rice syrup

Juice of ½ lemon

Toast the walnuts in a dry skillet over medium heat until just starting to turn golden and fragrant, about 5 minutes, stirring often. Transfer to a bowl to cool, and chop coarsely. Set aside.

Preheat a waffle iron. Cut a package of mochi into 3 large pieces, widthwise. Slice each piece into long fingerlike pieces, about ¼"-wide. Using 6 to 8 strips for each waffle, place the mochi strips on the hot, ungreased waffle iron and close the top. Cook until puffed and slightly crispy but not too hard and dry, about 3 minutes, or until your waffle iron signals that it's done. Remove the waffle and place on a plate. Do not stack the waffles because they will stick together. Serve and eat waffles as soon as possible—they are best hot and crispy.

While the waffles cook, combine the rice syrup with 3 tablespoons of water, lemon juice, and toasted walnuts in a saucepan. Stir together over medium heat just until warmed. Pour over the waffles, and serve.

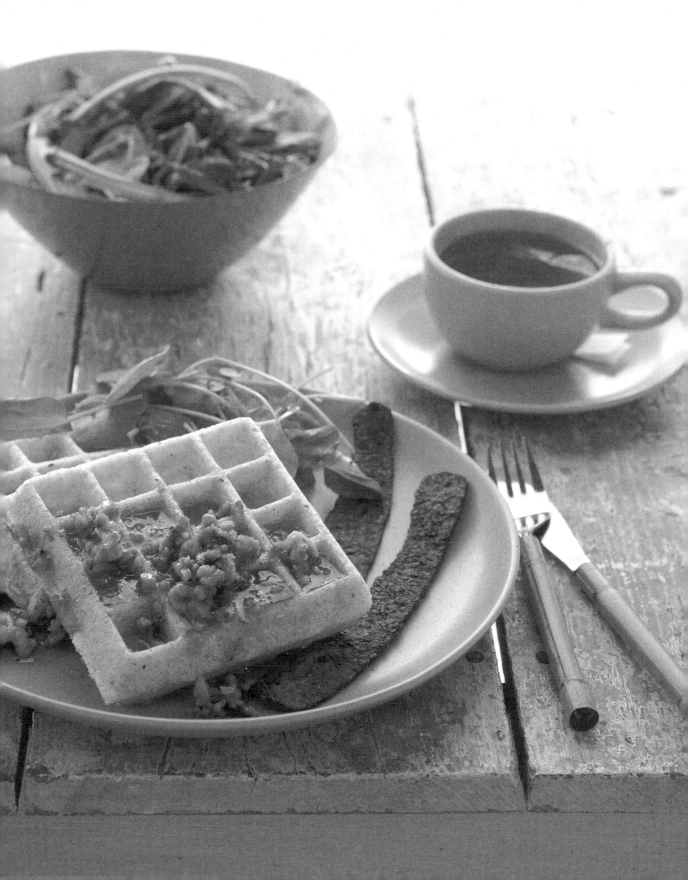

Millet and Sweet Vegetable Porridge

Millet is an underappreciated grain, but this porridge should change all that—it's really great. Naturally alkalizing and rich in B vitamins, millet is soothing to the stomach, spleen, and pancreas. It makes me feel settled and deeply nourished.

SERVES 6 TO 8

1" piece kombu

1 yellow onion, finely diced

2 stalks celery, finely diced

1 cup finely diced kabocha or butternut squash

½ cup yellow millet

2–3 teaspoons white miso

2–3 scallions, white and green parts, thinly sliced on the diagonal

Layer the kombu, onion, celery, squash, and millet in a soup pot. Gently add 5 cups of water to the pot, cover, and bring to a boil. Reduce the heat to low and simmer until the vegetables are tender and the millet is creamy, about 35 minutes.

Place the miso in a small bowl. Stir in a few tablespoons of the cooking liquid to dissolve it, and stir the miso back into the porridge.

Simmer gently, uncovered, for 3 to 4 minutes to avoid destroying the miso's enzymes. Serve sprinkled with the scallions.

Barley with Sweet Rice and Corn

According to Oriental medicine, barley is a tonic for the liver and gallbladder and helps to cool the body in spring and summer. It's also great for the skin. Sweet rice is a sticky form of brown rice that is used to make mochi and amasake. It's one of my favorite grains.

SERVES 2

⅔ cup sweet rice

⅓ cup barley

Pinch of fine sea salt

½ cup fresh or frozen and thawed corn kernels

Gomashio (page 232, optional)

Chopped fresh parsley, cilantro, or scallions (optional)

Place the rice and barley in a fine sieve, and rinse under running water. Transfer the grains to a saucepan, add 2 cups of water and the salt, and bring to a boil over medium-high heat. Reduce the heat to low, cover the pan, and cook for 50 minutes. Add the corn, cover again, and cook 5 minutes longer. Serve topped with gomashio and a bit of parsley, cilantro, or scallions, if you like.

Hot Polenta, Millet, and Corn Cereal

Another great way to serve millet.

SERVES 2

½ cup polenta

1 tablespoon millet

⅓ cup fresh or frozen and thawed corn kernels

Pinch of fine sea salt

2 teaspoons roasted and ground pumpkin seeds (see Note)

Stir together the polenta and millet in a small saucepan. Add 2 cups of water, and soak for 6 to 8 hours or overnight.

The next day, add the corn and salt to the saucepan, cover, and bring to a boil. Reduce the heat to a very low simmer, and cook for 25 minutes. Serve topped with the seeds.

Note: If you have a suribachi, you can use it to grind your pumpkin seeds; otherwise, whir them briefly in a small food processor or blender just until finely ground. Don't overprocess or it will get too oily and butterlike.

Cure-All Tea

Because it restores minerals to the blood, this tea is great:

- For hangovers
- When you've eaten white sugar
- To soothe digestion and release trapped gas
- To reduce heartburn
- For nausea
- If you're just feeling weak and spacey

SERVES 1

1 kukicha tea bag (if you're using loose-leaf tea, follow the package instructions)

¼–½ umeboshi plum, pit removed and chopped very fine

3–5 drops shoyu

Steep the tea in 1 cup of boiling water. While the tea steeps, place the umeboshi plum into a teacup with the shoyu. Pour the hot tea over the umeboshi plum in the teacup, and stir well. Drink hot. The umeboshi pit is also good to suck on, if you want.

Menstrual Cramp Tea (Daikon Drink)

Make this drink if you're feeling crampy; it will magically make you feel better. Daikon helps to relax the liver, and, in Chinese medicine, the liver is the organ that governs female reproduction. So when the liver relaxes, our female discomforts quiet down. This drink will also help to reduce swelling in the ankles.

SERVES 1

½ cup grated (into a pulp) daikon

½ cup spring water

1–2 drops shoyu

Combine the daikon and water in a small saucepan and bring to a boil over medium heat. Add the shoyu, reduce the heat to low, and simmer for 2 or 3 minutes. Drink hot, warm, or at room temperature.

P.S. It's important to eat lighter, fresher dishes right before your period. Skip bread and go easy on the salt. Eat more veggies, especially lightly cooked green ones. It's not unusual to crave sugar or chocolate before menstruating, so let yourself have some good-quality sweets. You might even want an organic beer or sake to help you relax. If you don't drink alcohol, try a glass of warm apple juice or even warm carrot juice. Sounds weird, but tastes great.

Phlegm-Fixer Tea (Lotus Root Tea)

I drink this when I have a cough or any kind of congestion in my chest. It's also good for asthma symptoms, allergies, and sinus conditions because lotus root dries up excess fluid and helps you to breathe easy. This drink is thick and creamy. Drink it as soon as it's made, while it's still hot.

SERVES 1

1 medium lotus root

Fine sea salt

Few drops of ginger juice (grate 1" fresh ginger root and use your fingers to squeeze out the juice, optional)

Using the finest grater you have, grate about ½ cup of lotus root onto a plate to catch any excess lotus root juice. Gather the grated shreds and squeeze the juice into a measuring cup. Discard the squeezed pulp. Add an equal amount of water to the juice in the measuring cup. Add the salt, and pour the lotus juice mixture into a saucepan. Bring to a boil, reduce the heat, and simmer for 2 to 3 minutes. Flavor the drink with a few drops of grated ginger juice during the last minute of cooking, if you like.

Variation: Lotus root is in season between September and February (cold season!). If you need this tea at other times of the year or can't find fresh lotus root (often found in better health food stores or Oriental markets), Lotus Root Tea Powder also exists and can be ordered through Goldmine Natural Foods and the Kushi Institute Store.

Appendix: Further Reading

The China Study by T. Colin Campbell. Perfect for the scientifically minded people in your life.

The Food Revolution by John Robbins

Any book by Dr. Neal Barnard: They include *Food for Life, Foods That Fight Pain*, and *Eat Right, Live Longer.*

My Beautiful Life by Mina Dobic. Inspiration for anyone fighting illness.

Mad Cowboy by Howard Lyman. Lyman was a rancher and carnivore himself who got a firsthand look at the meat industry.

The Hip Chick's Guide to Macrobiotics by Jessica Porter. A friendly, funny macro primer with recipes.

The Real Food Daily Cookbook by Ann Gentry and Anthony Head. Try the nachos!

Babycakes by Erin McKenna. Try the cinnamon buns and the cookie sandwich!

Vegan Cupcakes Take Over the World by Isa Chandra Moskowitz, Terry Hope Romero, and Sara Quin.

The Eco Chick Guide to Life: How to Be Fabulously Green by Starre Vartan

Conscious Style Home by Danny Seo. A beautiful book about decorating your home in environmentally friendly ways.

Thanking the Monkey: Rethinking the Way We Treat Animals by Karen Dawn. A groovy, hip book for anyone who loves animals and wants to help them.

Don't Sweat the Small Stuff—and It's All Small Stuff by Richard Carlson. A lovely collection of thoughts on what's truly important. It would be bathroom reading, but on the Kind Diet, you don't need bathroom reading.

The Joy Diet: 10 Daily Practices for a Happier Life and *Finding Your Own North Star* by Martha Beck

Organizing from the Inside Out: The Foolproof System for Organizing Your Home, Your Office, and Your Life by Julie Morgenstern

Endnotes

CHAPTER 2

1. Dr. Leslie Van Romer, "But Won't Eating Chicken and Fish Lower My Cholesterol?," EzineArticles.com, http://ezinearticles.com/?But-Wont-Eating-Chicken-and-Fish-Lower-My-Cholesterol?&id=179070.

2. ActionPA, "Dioxin Homepage," managed by ActionPA.org, http://www.ejnet.org/dioxin.

3. Arnold Schecter and others, "Intake Of Dioxins and Related Compounds from Food in the U.S. Population," *Journal of Toxicology and Environmental Health, Part A,* 63:1-18, 2001, http://www.ejnet.org/dioxin/dioxininfood.pdf.

4. Nutrition Scientists with The Cancer Project, Media Report, August 24, 2005, "New Report Names Five Worst Foods to Grill: Chicken Tops the List with the Most Cancer-Causing Chemicals," The Cancer Project, http://www.cancerproject.org/media/news/release_grill.php.

5. Neal Barnard, MD, *Foods That Fight Pain* (New York: Three Rivers Press, 1998), 16.

6. Laurie Barclay, MD, *"Diet May Influence Relapse in Ulcerative Colitis,"* citing a University of Newcastle (UK) study, Medscape Medical News, http://www.medscape.com/viewarticle/489613.

7. Debra Wood, RN, "Diverticulitis," Aurora Health Care, http://www.aurorahealthcare.org/yourhealth/healthgate/getcontent.asp?URLhealthgate=%2211898.html%22.

8. American Cancer Society News Center, "Eating Lots of Red Meat Linked to Colon Cancer," American Cancer Society, http://www.cancer.org/docroot/NWS/content/NWS_1_1x_Eating_Lots_of_Red_Meat_Linked_to_Colon_Cancer.asp.

9. Hyon K. Choi, M.D., Dr.P.H. and others, "Purine-Rich Foods and the Risk of Gout in Men," *New England Journal of Medicine,* http://content.nejm.org/cgi/content/short/350/11/1093.

10. From Medscape Medical News, December 12, 2004, "Too much red meat linked to increased risk of RA," citing a University of Manchester (UK) report, Medscape, http://www.medscape.com/viewarticle/538046.

11. W. G. Robertson, M. Peacock, P. J. Heyburn, et al. "Should recurrent calcium oxalate stone formers become vegetarians?" *British Journal of Urology* 51 (1979): 427–31.

12. Julie Vorman, "Raw ground beef often tainted with E. coli, " Organic Consumers Association, March 1, 2000, http://www.organicconsumers.org/Irrad/patties.cfm.

13. Division of Foodborne, Bacterial, and Mycotic Diseases, "Campylobacter," Centers for Disease Control and Prevention, http://www.cdc.gov/nczved/dfbmd/disease_listing/campylobacter_gi.html#2.

14. John Robbins, *The Food Revolution* (Berkeley, CA: Conari Press, 2001), 128.

15. Mitchell Satchell and Stephen J. Hedges, "The next bad beef scandal? Cattle feed now contains things like chicken manure and dead cats," *US News & World Report,* September 1, 1997.

16. www.ncbi.nlm.nih.gov/pubmed/4037499

17. Environmental Working Group, www.ewg.org/reports/farmedPCBs

18. Ashley Glacel (contact), "Senators welcome endorsements from PHRMA, ADVAMED, ASTRAZENECA, and MERCK of Physician Payments Sunshine Act," United States Senate Special Committee on Aging, http://aging.senate.gov/record.cfm?id=298258.

19. E. Haavi Morreim, "Prescribing Under the Influence," The Markkula Center for Applied Ethics, http://www.scu.edu/ethics/publications/submitted/morreim/prescribing.html.

20. American Dietetic Association, "How much did your doctor learn about nutrition in medical school?," http://www.eatright.org/cps/rde/xchg/ada/hs.xsl/nutrition_8555_ENU_HTML.htm.

21. www.reuters.com/article/marketsNews/idUSBNG12204220090109

22. www.nytimes.com/2009/03/03/business/03medschool.html?pagewanted=1&_r=1

23. Natasha Singer, "Lawmakers Seek to Curb Drug Commercials," *New York Times*, July 26, 2009, http://www.nytimes.com/2009/07/27/business/media/27drugads.html?scp=5&sq=spending%20on%20prescription%20drugs&st=cse.

24. Adapted from Environmental Protection Agency documents, "Climate Change," August 14, 2002, Almanac of Policy Issues, http://www.policyalmanac.org/environment/archive/climate_change.shtml.

25. Opinion, "Killer cow emissions," *Los Angeles Times*, October 15, 2007, http://articles.latimes.com/2007/oct/15/opinion/ed-methane15.

26. Opinion, "Killer cow emissions," *Los Angeles Times*, October 15, 2007, http://articles.latimes.com/2007/oct/15/opinion/ed-methane15.

27. Juliette Jowit, environment editor, "UN says eat less meat to curb global warming," *The Observer*, Sunday 7 September 2008, http://www.guardian.co.uk/environment/2008/sep/07/food.foodanddrink.

28. Jeff Tietz, "Boss Hog," Rolling Stone, http://www.rollingstone.com/politics/story/12840743/porks_dirty_secret_the_nations_top_hog_producer_is_also_one_of_americas_worst_polluters.

29. Joel Achenbach, "A 'Dead Zone' in The Gulf of Mexico," *Washington Post,* July 31, 2008, p. A02, http://www.washingtonpost.com/wp-dyn/content/story/2008/07/31/ST2008073100349.html.

30. John Robbins, *The Food Revolution* (Berkeley, CA: Conari Press, 2001), p. 245.

31. Earth Trends Country Profiles, "Water Resources and Freshwater Ecosystems—United States," Earth Trends, http://earthtrends.wri.org/pdf_library/country_profiles/wat_cou_840.pdf.

32. John Robbins, *The Food Revolution* (Berkeley, CA: Conari Press, 2001).

33. National Corn Growers Association, "Livestock," National Corn Growers Association, http://www.ncga.com/livestock.

34. National Corn Growers Association, "U.S. Corn Growers: Producing Food &Fuel," National Corn Growers Association, http://74.125.47.132/search?q=cache:ba7xFU5lUtcJ:www.ncga.com/files/pdf/FoodandFuelPaper10-08.pdf+%25+u.s.+corn+to+human&cd=4&hl=en&ct=clnk&gl=us&client=firefox-a, p. 4.

35. DairyBusiness, "USDA forecast: 2009 corn acreage down; soybeans, dry hay acreage up," March 31, 2009, DairyBusiness Communications, http://dairywebmall.com/dbcpress/?p=2187.

36. Rural Migration News, "US Fruits and Vegetables," *Rural Migration News,* July 2007 Volume 13 Number 3, http://migration.ucdavis.edu/rmn/comments.php?id=1231_0_5_0.

37. David Pimentel and Marcia Pimentel, "Sustainability of meat-based and plant-based diets and the environment," American Society for Clinical Nutrition, *American Journal of Clinical Nutrition,* Vol. 78, No. 3, 660S-663S, September 2003, www.ajcn.org/cgi/content/full/78/3/660S.

38. Tom Gorey (contact), "Fact Sheet on the BLM's Management of Livestock Grazing," Updated March 2009, U.S. Department of the Interior, Bureau of Land Management (BLM), www.blm.gov/wo/st/en/prog/grazing.html.

39. Howard F. Lyman, *Mad Cowboy* (Scribner, 1998).

40. Newsroom, "Farmed vs. Fresh Fish," National Cooperative Grocers Association, www.ncga.coop/newsroom/fish.

41. April McKettrick and others, "Rainforest Destruction," Cal Poly Pomona, www.csupomona.edu/~admckettrick/projects/ag101_project/html/destruction.html.

42. CuringOxygen.com, "What's Happening to our Oxygen?," CuringHerbs.com, http://curingoxygen.com/oxygen_problem.htm.

43. Steve Boyan, PhD, "How Our Food Choices Can Help Save the Environment," EarthSave International, www.earthsave.org/environment/foodchoices.htm.

44. The Nature Conservancy, "Facts about Rainforests," The Nature Conservancy, www.nature.org/rainforests/explore/facts.html.

45. www.nature.org/rainforests/explore/facts.html

46. Editorial, "What Humans Owe to Animals," *The Economist,* August 19, 1995.

47. Compassion Over Killing, "Eggs-Aggerated Claims," Compassion Over Killing, www.cok.net/camp/egg_labeling/

CHAPTER 3

1. http://www.adweek.com/aw/content_display/news/agency/e3i1751753614c1db77d493e602f21b59ff?pn=2

2. Neal D. Barnard, MD, *Breaking the Food Seduction* (New York: St. Martin's Griffin, 2004).

3. Roberta Larson Duyff, *American Dietetic Association Complete Food and Nutrition Guide* (Hoboken, NJ: John Wiley and Sons, 2006), 524.

4. Michael Pollan, *In Defense of Food: An Eater's Manifesto* (New York: Penguin Books, 2009), 102.

5. William J. Cromie, "Growth Hormone Raises Cancer Risk," *The Harvard University Gazette,* April, 1999, President and Fellows of Harvard College, http://www.news.harvard.edu/gazette/1999/04.22/igf1.story.html.

6. T. Colin Campbell, *The China Study* (Dallas: BenBella Books, Inc., 2006).

7. Andrew Weil, M.D., "Does Milk Cause Cancer?," citing a Study by Ganmaa Davaasambuu, M.D., Ph.D., Weil Lifestyle, LLC, http://www.drweil.com/drw/u/id/QAA400175.

8. National Cancer Institute, "Breast Cancer," U.S. National Institutes of Health, http://www.cancer.gov/cancertopics/types/breast.

9. N. Seppa, "Cows' milk, diabetes connection bolstered," in Science News Online, *Science News,* Vol. 155, No. 26, June 26, 1999, p. 404, Science Service, http://www.sciencenews.org/sn_arc99/6_26_99/fob2.htm.

10. National Institute of Diabetes and Digestive and Kidney Diseases, "National Diabetes Statistics, 2007 fact sheet," Bethesda, MD: U.S. Department of Health and Human Services, National Institutes of Health, 2008, http://diabetes.niddk.nih.gov/DM/PUBS/statistics/#deaths.

11. S. Renaud and M. de Lorgeril, "Dietary Lipids and Their Relation to Ischaemic Heart Disease: From Epidemoiology to Prevention," citing the Seven Countries Study and recent statistics from WHO and the OECD, *Journal of Internal Medicine* (suppl.), 225, No. 731 (1989), 39-46, Abstract Web site: http://www.ncbi.nlm.nih.gov/pubmed/2650697.

12. M. J. Brouk and others, "Drinking water requirements for lactating dairy cows", RBST-Facts.com, http://www.rbstfacts.org/rbst-facts/rbst-and-farm-economics/drinking-water-requirements-for-lactating-dairy-cows.html.

CHAPTER 4

1. Cathleen Genova, "Missing link between fructose, insulin resistance found," biowww.net, http://biowww.net/bioblog/html/17/n-717.html.

2. National Center for Biotechnology Information, "Insulin and cancer," Integr Cancer Ther. 2003 Dec;2(4):315-29, U.S. National Library of Medicine and the National Institutes of Health [PubMed—indexed for MEDLINE], http://www.ncbi.nlm.nih.gov/pubmed/14713323.

3. Holistic Healing Web Page, "Sucralose Toxicity Information Center," Holistic Medicine Resource Center, http://www.holisticmed.com/index.shtml.

4. http://www.webmd.com/diet/news/20041228/more-americans-getting-caffeine-buzz

CHAPTER 5

1. Dan Buettner, "The Secrets of Long Life," National Geographic Society, November 2005, http://ngm.nationalgeographic.com/ngm/0511/feature1/.

2. Joel Fuhrman, MD, *Eat to Live: The Revolutionary Formula for Fast and Sustained Weight Loss* (New York: Little, Brown and Company, 2003), xi.

3. John Robbins, *The Food Revolution* (Berkeley, CA: Conari Press, 2001), p. 63.

4. Brit Amos, "Death of the Bees: GMO Crops and the Decline of Bee Colonies in North America," Global Research.ca, March 25, 2008, http://www.globalresearch.ca/index.php?context=va&aid=8436.

5. John Robbins, *The Food Revolution* (Berkeley, CA: Conari Press, 2001), p. 370.

6. Simone Gabbay, RNCP, "Whole vs. Processed Foods," Source: *alive* #248, June 2003, Alive Publishing Group, http://www.alive.com/1377a4a2.php?subject_bread_cramb=491.

CHAPTER 6

1. *Journal of the National Cancer Institute* (2009, February 26). "Million Women Study Shows Even Moderate Alcohol Consumption Associated With Increased Cancer Risk." in *ScienceDaily*, http://www.sciencedaily.com/releases/2009/02/090224163555.htm.

2. Joel Fuhrman, *Eat to Live: The Revolutionary Formula for Fast and Sustained Weight Loss,* from the Foreword by Mehmet Oz, (New York: Little, Brown and and Company, 2003).

CHAPTER 7

1. http://www.epa.gov/waterscience/fish/advice/factsheet.html

Acknowledgments

My heartfelt thanks for contributions large and small go to:

Sampson, my dearest love, for sharing your life with me and being my inspiration and teacher. You were so funny and sweet. I love you forever and miss you so much.

All the animals, for making me smile and opening my heart.

My husband, Christopher Jarecki, for being nice to me and showing me love like no one ever has before. You have supported my growth, been the best friend anyone could imagine, and completely changed my life.

Mother Nature, for the ocean, sand, gentle breezes, sun, rain, and all of your beauty. And for love in this amazing life.

All undercover activists who document the cruelty to animals—God bless you. And to the not-so-undercover activists and volunteers dedicated to ending suffering.

Mina Dobic, for your heart, spirit, and dedication, and for making me feel so cared for.

My grandfather, Sydney Silver. For being cute and for loving me truly and easily with no agenda or mess. I miss you.

Dad, for taking us on trips to see the world when I was little, and for taking me to the theater.

My collaborator, Jessica Porter. The dream to write this book has been alive in me for well over 8 years, and I was so lucky to find you to help me realize it with your sass, wisdom, kindness, and fun. Thank you, rice and universe, for introducing us!

My editor, Pam Krauss, for your enthusiasm, kindness, brains, and hard work. Thanks also to Zach Greenwald; Yelena Gitlin; Hope Clarke; Christina Gaugler; Wayne Wolf of Blue Cup Studio; Ruthanne Secunda; Elizabeth Much; Peter Steinberg; Johnny Stuntz, hair stylist; Kerry Malouf, makeup; Dr. Neal Barnard; Paul McCartney; Stella McCartney; John Robbins; Andrea Beaman; Joy Pierson; and Bart Potenza for your talent, energy, and support.

Photographer Victoria Pearson and the crew that made the photography in this book so insanely beautiful: Michelle Reiner; food stylist Rori Trovato; prop stylist Ann Johnstad; digital technician Luke Sommers; retoucher Gus Dering; I am forever grateful to you all.

Megan Lipshultz, for supporting me every day and taking care of a million details for this book and my life. You make everything better.

Lisa Addy, for changing my life.

Ida Kendall, for being an amazing, wise goddess who supports my independence and intuition with love.

Ana Avelar, for your cute laugh and sweet self and hard work with love.

Renée Loux, for your passion for the planet and for feeding me insane food.

Mrs. Phoner, my fourth-grade teacher, for telling me to get organized. I did it.

Colin Russell, my first ballet teacher, for putting so much love into this world.

And to all the starving children in the world—I'm sorry we steal your food.

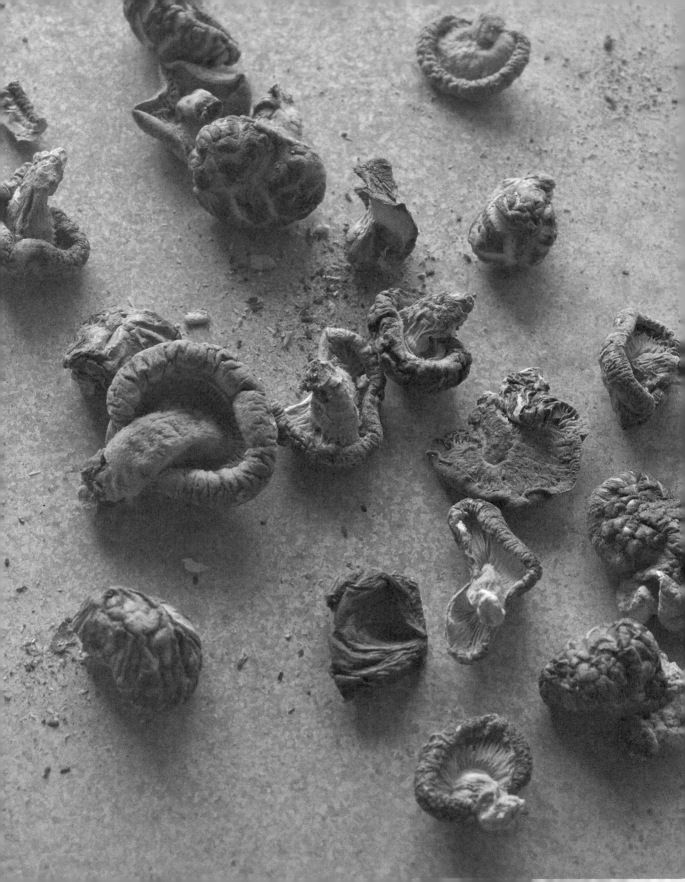

Index

Underscored page references indicate boxed text and tables. **Boldface** references indicate photographs.